Farm Toxicology

William J. Meggs • Ricky L. Langley
Editors

Farm Toxicology

A Primer for Rural Healthcare Practitioners

Springer

Editors
William J. Meggs
Brody School of Medicine
East Carolina University
Greenville, NC, USA

Ricky L. Langley
Department of Biological Sciences
North Carolina State University
Raleigh, NC, USA

ISBN 978-3-031-80443-4 ISBN 978-3-031-80441-0 (eBook)
https://doi.org/10.1007/978-3-031-80441-0

This Springer imprint is published by the registered company Springer Nature Switzerland AG
The registered company address is: Gewerbestrasse 11, 6330 Cham, Switzerland

I would like to dedicate this book to my wife Sandra, my children Patrick, Nicholas, and Megan, my grandchildren Jacob, Ella, and Lucas, and the agricultural community that produces our food.

—Ricky L. Langley MD, MPH, FACP, FACOEM

To my wife Susan Martin Meggs for your unswerving support while tolerating the difficulties of being the spouse of a practicing physician.

To the medical students, residents, physician colleagues, and patients who have challenged and educated me over decades of practice.

—William Joel Meggs, MD, PhD, FACMT, FACEP

Foreword

Preserving the health of farmers, farm workers, and their families is vital to creating a healthy and sustainable food supply. I grew up on a small farm in Eastern North Carolina and had my share of adventures and misadventures on the farm. I carried these experiences with me to pursue medical training and became a family physician who returned to the rural county where I was raised. When in practice, I discovered health problems that farmers and farm workers brought to me, which had not been part of my medical training. There was not a textbook to help me address these questions from my rural patients. For example, my training did not prepare me for cases of pesticide poisonings, fire ant stings, or snake bites. At the medical center, patients did not ask me about working outdoors in hot weather or whether it was safe for their animals to drink water from ponds with algal blooms. While my medical training was valuable, it did not address more common rural concerns, presenting each day to the clinician caring for these workers. Now this book *Farm Toxicology: A Primer for Rural Healthcare Practitioners* is the reference I longed to have. It is a great resource for the variety of problems unique to the agricultural community and any healthcare provider practicing in rural areas should have a copy in their personal medical library. Drs. Meggs and Langley have assembled an outstanding group of farm toxicology experts to guide us as we care for this important community.

Department of Family Medicine
University of Washington
Seattle, WA, USA

Paul James

Preface

Farm Toxicology: A Primer for Rural Healthcare Practitioners was conceived and written to address the needs of healthcare providers practicing in rural area as a resource to address the numerous hazards that occur in farm environments. Farmers, farm workers, and farm families have daily exposures to a complex environment that contains a host of toxicants and toxins. Practitioners in rural areas, including physicians, nurses, nurse practitioners, physician assistants, and paramedics, often find themselves ill-equipped to recognize, diagnose, and treat farm-related illnesses and injuries. A comprehensive source of information on potential farm-related exposures with clinical presentations and management of the exposed patient is needed. The present publication is designed to fill the gap as no such comprehensive text exists.

We also recognize there are many professionals who are involved in training, education, evaluation, and amelioration of various hazards that occur on the farm and can benefit from much of the information provided in this book. These professionals include medical toxicologists, veterinary toxicologists, occupational and environmental physicians, public health and preventive medicine physicians, agricultural health and safety professionals, environmental health specialists, cooperative extension agents, pesticide trainers and applicators, and veterinarians, to name a few.

This book opens with a chapter on the approach to the acutely ill farm worker, which involves considerations of a broad differential diagnosis that goes beyond chemical exposures. This is followed by a chapter on first aid and pre-hospital management that will be invaluable to first responders. Personal protective equipment is covered in depth due to the overwhelming need for practitioners (as well as farmers and farm workers) to protect themselves from hazards and to care for the exposed.

Since information is needed about explicit exposures, a chapter follows on sources of information. The internet revolution and search engines have put safety data sheets for commercial products within a mouse-click reach of practitioners. State and Federal regulations require medical information on chemical labels that can be invaluable when product containers are available. Proper interpretation of labels and safety data sheets is essential and information is provided on what to look for when evaluating these materials. Poison centers are a toll-free phone call away and have medical toxicologists—licensed physicians who have completed 2-year fellowships after primary specialty training—who can assist with management of exposed patients.

Chemical exposures found on the farm are presented by classes, as pesticides of specific classes have similar toxicities and treatments. In addition to pesticides, chapters are presented on algal toxins, toxic gases, endotoxins and mycotoxins, welding hazards, and a chapter on miscellaneous toxins/exposures which the rural practitioner needs to be able to recognize and respond to. Arthropod bites and stings and snake bites/envenomations are discussed as well as a chapter on plant and mushroom poisoning. This book ends with discussions on chronic disabilities and diseases associated with chemical exposures on the farm and an overview of the epidemiology of farm hazards.

Greenville, NC, USA William J. Meggs
Raleigh, NC, USA Ricky L. Langley

Disclaimer

Medicine is a constantly changing science. Standard safety precautions must be followed, but as new research and clinical experience increase our knowledge, changes in treatment and drug therapy may become necessary or appropriate. This book is for informational purposes only and is not intended to diagnose, treat, cure, or prevent any condition or disease. The authors and the publisher of this work have checked with sources believed to be reliable in their efforts to provide information that is complete and generally in accord with the standards accepted at the time of publication. However, in view of the possibility of human error or changes in medical sciences, neither the authors nor the publisher nor any other party that has been involved in the preparation or publication of this work warrants that the information contained herein is in every respect accurate or complete, and they disclaim all responsibility and liability to persons or property for any errors or omissions or for the results obtained from use of the information contained in this work. Readers are encouraged to confirm the information contained herein with other sources. In particular, readers are advised to check the product information sheet included in the package of each drug they plan to administer to be certain that the information contained in this work is accurate and that changes have not been made in the recommended dose or in the contraindications for administration. In cases of suspected poisoning, readers are encouraged to consult with a medical toxicologist or call the Poison Control Center in your country (800-222-1222 in the USA) for advice.

Contents

Contributors

Dalia Alwasiyah North Carolina's Poison Center, Charlotte, NC, USA

Chad Andicochea Department of Emergency Medicine – Division of EMS, East Carolina University, Greenville, NC, USA

Jo Anne G. Balanay Environmental Health Sciences Program, Department of Health Education and Promotion, College of Health and Human Performance, East Carolina University, Greenville, NC, USA

Wayne Buhler Department of Horticultural Science, North Carolina State University, Raleigh, NC, USA

Tim Cookson Department of Emergency Medicine – Division of EMS, East Carolina University, Greenville, NC, USA

Jason Dietz Division of Medical Toxicology, Ronald O. Perelman Department of Emergency Medicine, NYU Grossman School of Medicine, New York, NY, USA

Beth Dittman North Carolina Department of Agriculture and Consumer Services, Structural Pest Control and Pesticides Division, Raleigh, NC, USA

Benjamin German Emergency Medicine, WakeMed Health and Hospitals, Raleigh, NC, USA

Jason B. Hack Department of Emergency Medicine, Brody School of Medicine, East Carolina University, Greenville, NC, USA

Gregory D. Kearney Department of Public Health, Brody School of Medicine, East Carolina University, Greenville, NC, USA

Ricky L. Langley Department of Biological Sciences, North Carolina State University, Raleigh, NC, USA

David Lipton North Carolina Department of Health and Human Services, Occupational and Environmental Epidemiology Branch, Raleigh, NC, USA

William J. Meggs Brody School of Medicine, East Carolina University, Greenville, NC, USA

Jennifer Parker-Cote Division of Medical Toxicology, Department of Emergency Medicine, East Carolina University-Brody School of Medicine, Greenville, NC, USA

Roberto Portela Department of Emergency Medicine – Division of EMS, East Carolina University, Greenville, NC, USA

Stephanie L. Richards Environmental Health Sciences Program, Department of Health Education and Promotion, College of Health and Human Performance, East Carolina University, Greenville, NC, USA

Mina W. Shehee Biology Department, Indian River State College, Fort Pierce, FL, USA

H. Thomas Cusick III Duke University, Durham, NC, USA
Concentra Urgent Care, Durham, NC, USA

Avian White Environmental Health Sciences Program, Department of Health Education and Promotion, College of Health and Human Performance, East Carolina University, Greenville, NC, USA

1 Approach to the Acutely Ill Farmworker

William J. Meggs

Approach to Ill Patient: History and Physical Examination

When a farmworker becomes acutely ill while working on a farm, an ambulance may be summoned. Farm fields may be remote and difficult to locate by emergency medicine personnel. In rural settings, distances and travel times may be prolonged, leading to delays in assessment and definitive treatment. Sometimes the ill farmworker is loaded into the back of a pickup truck and driven to a rural primary care office or hospital by individuals with little or no knowledge of first aid. Healthcare providers, including paramedics, triage nurses, physician assistants, nurse practitioners, and physicians, must be prepared to rapidly assess the ill farmworker, formulate a differential diagnosis, and initiate treatment.

The approach, as always, begins with obtaining a history. Since many farmworkers are migrants who do not speak English, facilities must be prepared to obtain a history in Spanish (or other non-English languages). Acutely ill farmworkers often cannot give a history, so coworkers, a foreman, or farm owners may be called upon to give information about the event.

In addition to the standard medical history, practitioners need to ask about the occupation/environment and activity the person was doing when he/she became ill. Elements of an environmental and occupational history (Papali & Hines 2015) are given in Table 1.1.

Where did the onset of illness take place? If the person became ill while working in a field, what were the weather conditions? What tasks were being performed? When did symptoms first begin? The crop being cultivated or harvested can be important. Were any pesticides being used or applied? Were there any other exposures? If chemicals were involved, did the patient wear personal protective equipment? What medications was the person taking? Did other workers experience any symptoms?

Travel history should be obtained because some farmworkers have recently crossed borders.

Table 1.1 Elements of an environmental and occupational history

- Occupation
- Location
- Weather conditions
- Tasks performed (what crop?)
- Exposures
- Personal protective equipment
- Home environment
- Travel
- Hobbies and recreational activities
- Family members
- Nearby facilities

W. J. Meggs (✉)
Brody School of Medicine, East Carolina University, Greenville, NC, USA
e-mail: meggsw@ecu.edu

W. J. Meggs, R. L. Langley (eds.), *Farm Toxicology*, https://doi.org/10.1007/978-3-031-80441-0_1

Recent travelers have possibly been exposed to infectious agents, such as the fungus causing coccidioides (also known as San Joaquin Valley fever), if they traveled through the American Southwest. They may present with an acute illness such as seizures, which in a migrant may suggest neurocysticercosis. Ask about hobbies and recreational activities since these can involve harmful exposures. Alcohol and illicit drug use should be a part of any occupational and exposure history. Concurrent illnesses among coworkers or family members can be a clue to diagnosis. The onset of illness among contacts at the same time favors a chemical exposure, while staggering onset favors an infectious cause. It is important to ask about nearby activities and facilities. Though no pesticides may have been used in the field where the patient was working, pesticide drift from a neighboring field may cause illness in workers in nearby fields.

History of exposure to agricultural chemicals is important. Route of exposure is an essential aspect of history. Dermal exposures can cause contact dermatitis and other skin problems; however, many agricultural chemicals are absorbed through the skin and can result in systemic toxicity. Inhalational exposures to pesticides are most likely to result in irritant effects on the airway but seldom cause systemic toxicity. Ingestions are potentially the most lethal route of exposure due to the higher doses. Ingestions in adults and adolescents are generally from suicide attempts, while unintentional ingestions occur in small children.

Physical examination can give clues to the diagnosis. Vital signs are important. Elevated core temperature suggests heat-related illness or infection or amphetamine/methamphetamine/cocaine overdose. Hypertension can result from organochlorine insecticide exposures. Organophosphate insecticide exposures can cause bradycardia or tachycardia. Attention should be given to neurological, respiratory, and dermal examinations. Muscle weakness and pinpoint pupils can occur with organophosphate and carbamate insecticide exposures but pinpoint pupils may also suggest opioid overdose. Organochlorines can cause rigidity and hyperreflexia. Many agricultural products affect the respiratory system and can cause airway inflammation and/or hypoxia such as anhydrous ammonia, nitrogen dioxide, hydrogen sulfide, and carbon monoxide.

A differential diagnosis of the illness should be formulated. In addition to a potential work-related toxic exposure, healthcare providers should consider weather-related illnesses, stings and bites, and toxicity from contact with crops or other plants.

Chemical Exposures

The class of a chemical to which a person was exposed can offer clues to the diagnosis. For example, the toxicity of insecticides can be dramatically different from herbicides or rodenticides (Roberts & Reigart 2013). Subclasses can also vary in toxicity. For example, the toxicity of the dipyridyl herbicides paraquat and diquat is very different from glyphosate herbicides. Table 1.2 gives the classes of insecticides with findings that can direct healthcare providers to the exposure class (United States Environmental Protection Agency, 2021; EPA). Detailed specifics about the different classes will be discussed in subsequent chapters.

Severe illness and fatalities have occurred in farmworkers from exposure to toxic gases. Anhydrous ammonia is a water-soluble irritant that can cause massive edema of the upper air-

Table 1.2 Classes of insecticides with acute toxic effects

Class	Examples	Toxic effects
Organochlorines	DDT and aldrin	Neurological and excitatory
Organophosphates	Chlorpyrifos and malathion	Cholinergic and paralysis
Carbamates	Aldicarb and carbaryl	Cholinergic and paralysis
Pyrethroid	Pyrethrums	Irritant, allergic, and neuropathy
Nicotine and neonicotinoids	Dinotefuran and nitenpyram	Autonomic stimulation

ways, leading to airway obstruction, freezing skin burns, and severe eye damage. Carbon monoxide from fossil fuel exhaust can cause multisystem illnesses including myocardial infarction, coma, and death. Hydrogen sulfide from decay of organic matter including manure has a noxious odor and is a respiratory irritant, neurotoxin, and the cause of many on-the-farm deaths from chemical hypoxia.

Healthcare workers, from paramedics in the field to nurses and physicians at a healthcare facility, should protect themselves from secondary exposures. Medical personnel should use personnel protective equipment that is appropriate for the chemical. Information about what personnel protective equipment should be used can be found on product labels and safety data sheets (see Chap. 2 for details). For example, latex gloves do not protect the hands from some pesticides, so butyl rubber or other gloves should be used. A patient's skin, hair, and clothing can be contaminated. The body must be completely decontaminated with copious amounts of water. Special care should be given to areas such as the axilla, groin, and under the nails that are easily missed. Clothing should be removed and treated as contaminated waste. Emergency departments should have a decontamination room where the water is captured as contaminated waste.

Practitioners evaluating farm-related illnesses should be aware that workers' compensation insurance claims can result. Hence, the documentation including exposure history should be detailed. If there is exposure to a farm chemical for which the container is available, photographs of the label should be made and preserved. The standard for causation in a workers' compensation claim is a reasonable degree of medical certainty, which means more likely than not, or more than a 50% chance, that the agent caused the problem.

Weather-Related Exposures

Weather-related illnesses and injuries occur in farmworkers. Field workers can be caught in severe thunderstorms that appear suddenly with high winds, blowing debris, toppled trees, and downed power lines. Lightning strikes cause serious injury and death. Tornados can cause devastating traumatic injury and death. They can form with little warning in isolated rural areas, giving little chance for field workers to seek shelter.

Extremes of temperature (both heat and cold) can cause acute illness. Heat-related illnesses include heat syncope, heat cramps, heat exhaustion, and heatstroke (CA; CA 2006; Centers for Disease Control (CDC) 2020). In addition to environmental exposure, other causes of hyperthermia should be considered in the differential diagnosis (Table 1.3).

Heatstroke can be fatal (Centers for Disease Control (CDC) 2008; Bonauto et al. 2007). The risk of heat-related illness increases with temperature and relative humidity and is more common when the heat index is greater than 100° Fahrenheit. The human body's defenses against environmental heat exposures include increased blood flow to the skin and evaporative cooling through sweating. When these defenses are overwhelmed, body temperature can rapidly rise to 104° Fahrenheit (40° Celsius) or higher. In heatstroke, dizziness, confusion, and delirium can progress to seizure, coma, and death (California State (CA) 2006; National Institute of Occupational Safety and Health (NIOSH) 2020). The mainstay of treatment is to reduce body temperature as rapidly as possible while rehydrating the worker. Cold water baths and ice packs are options. Evaporative cooling is the technique of blowing a fan over wet skin.

Medication history is important because many medicines can inhibit the body's ability to regu-

Table 1.3 Differential diagnosis of hyperthermia

• Environmental exposures
• Overdose of sympathomimetic drugs
– Cocaine
– Amphetamines
• Overdoses of anticholinergic medications
• Ingestion or smoking anticholinergic plants (e.g., Jimson weed and belladonna)
• Neuroleptic malignant syndrome
• Serotonin syndrome
• Malignant hyperthermia

Table 1.4 Medications that alter thermoregulation and increase the risk of heatstroke

- Diuretics
  - HCTZ, furosemide
- Psychiatric medications
  - Antipsychotics
  - Antidepressants
- Antihistamines
  - Benztropine
- Anticholinergic
  - Atropine
  - Scopolamine

Table 1.5 Physiological adaptation to heat stress

- Increased sweating efficiency
- Stabilization of the circulation
- The ability to perform work with lower core temperature and heart rate
- Increased skin blood flow at a given core temperature

late temperature (Table 1.4) and increase the risk of heatstroke. These include diuretics such as hydrochlorothiazide (HCTZ) and furosemide, antipsychotic and antidepressant medications, antihistamines, and anticholinergic such as atropine and scopolamine (Levine et al. 2012).

Farmworkers new to heat exposure are at greater risk of heat-related illnesses. A strategy of limiting the hours in the field for the first few days of employment has been shown to reduce the risk of heatstroke. This is known as acclimation. Acclimation (NIOSH 2018; OSHA) to heat exposure occurs from several mechanisms (Table 1.5).

One recommendation to reduce the risk of heat-associated illness in new workers is to limit heat exposure for new workers to 20% on day 1 of fieldwork with increases to no more than 20% on subsequent days. For experienced workers, no more than 50% on day 1, 60% on day 2, 80% on day 3, and 100% on day 4 is recommended (CDC 2018).

Heat-related skin conditions can also occur such as heat rash (miliaria) and sunburn from ultraviolet (UV) (sunlight) exposure (Campbell et al 2017). Miliaria rubra, also known as heat rash, sweat rash, or prickly heat, is common among farmworkers and is caused by eccrine

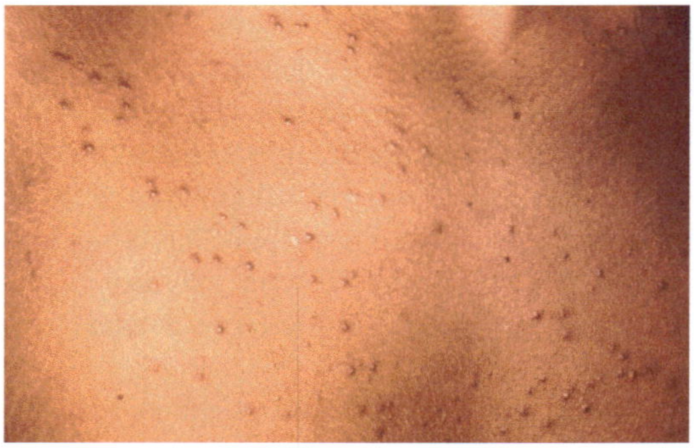

Fig. 1.1 Erythematous, papular rash on a patient's torso, illustrating a case of heat rash, a skin irritation caused by excessive sweating during hot, humid weather. (Source: CDC Public Health Image Library)

sweat duct blockage (Fig. 1.1). It is associated with the hot, humid environments on farms during the growing season. Potentiating factors include strenuous activity, fever, poor unairconditioned housing in hot humid seasons, and skin occlusion. Skin manifestations are variable, from 4 mm red papules to diffuse erythema, vesicles, and bulla. Removal from hot humid environments is ideal but not always practical. Loose-fitting clothing and topical corticosteroids can be considered. Secondary infections can occur and require antibiotic therapy.

Hypothermia and frostbite can also occur among farmworkers exposed to cold weather. Winter activities on farms include fruit tree pruning, repairing fences and barns, and attending to winter crops such as kale. Diagnosis of hypothermia is made by a history of a worker becoming ill on a cold day while working outside and measurement showing a decrease in core body temperature. Clinical manifestations include confusion, hypotension, and bradycardia. Severe cases can lead to coma and cardiac arrest. An Osborn wave (J wave) may be noted on an electrocardiogram (ECG). The treatment is to warm the patient. Warming blankets can shunt blood to the skin and worsen hypotension, so internal warming is preferred. Nebulization treatments with heated saline, gastric lavage with warm water, and bladder irrigation with warm water can raise the core body temperature. A patient with severe hypothermia in cardiac arrest should not have resuscitative efforts terminated until warming to normal body temperature because clinical experience has shown remarkable recoveries from severe hypothermia with coma and cardiac arrest. As with hypothermia, a number of drugs including opioids can cause temperature dysregulation and be synergistic with cold environmental exposures in producing hypothermia.

Crops and Toxic/Irritating Plants

Skin conditions are common complaints among farmworkers. Exposure to crops and toxic and irritating plants can cause systemic illness and/or dermal irritation and sensitization. The most notable illness from crops is green tobacco syndrome, where nicotine from tobacco plants (Fig. 1.2) is absorbed through the skin (NIOSH 2014). Illness is most likely to occur in tobacco workers in wet fields with exposed skin. Symptoms can include nausea, emesis, headaches, and dizziness. Dehydration can occur. Since nicotine is rapidly metabolized, most cases resolve with supportive care. During the tobacco season, workers handling tobacco can be chronically ill with headaches and nausea.

Contact dermatitis can occur from exposure to plants with the oily resin urushiol. The major sources are poison ivy, poison oak, and poison sumac. Corticosteroids (topical and systemic) and calamine topically are useful in the management of symptoms.

Phytophotodermatitis (Ellis and Elston 2021) is skin inflammation caused by a combination of the ultraviolet A in sunlight and furocoumarins found in plants, including psoralen. Exposure can occur through direct skin contact or secondary to ingestion. Plants containing furocoumarins include celery, carrots, lemons, limes, hogweed, and some herbs. Acutely, the lesions can resemble sunburn with erythema and bulla. Persistent hyperpigmentation can result. The sap of hogweed can cause skin blistering and scarring, with eye contact being particularly hazardous. Cases of temporary and permanent blindness have been

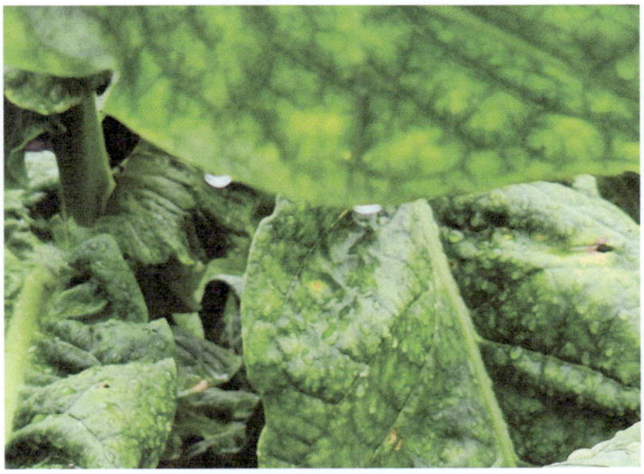

Fig. 1.2 Water on tobacco leaves contains nicotine that can be absorbed through the skin and cause nicotine poisoning, known as green tobacco sickness

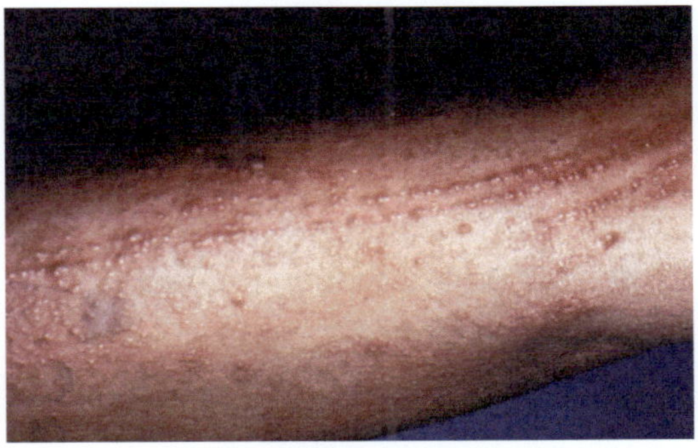

Fig. 1.3 Linear pattern of blistering rash from a linear swipe of an arm against poison oak leaves, with contact with the oily resin urushiol being a potent cause of contact dermatitis. The rash appears within 12–48 h of exposure. (Source: CDC Public Health Image Library)

reported from hogweed sap (Fig. 1.3) (Ohio State University Extension 2024).

Plants can cause mechanical injury to farmworkers from briars, thorns, and burrs (Fig. 1.4). Hands are particularly susceptible to injury such as when picking blackberries or other crops with infestations of unwanted plants with sharp protrusions. Sharp edges of leaves can cause cutting injuries. The risk of infection and retained plant materials can complicate these injuries. Wounds should be antiseptically cleaned. Foreign material should be removed with forceps if possible. For small plant parts, tape can be an effective method of removal. Instructions should be given to return for care for any signs of infection such

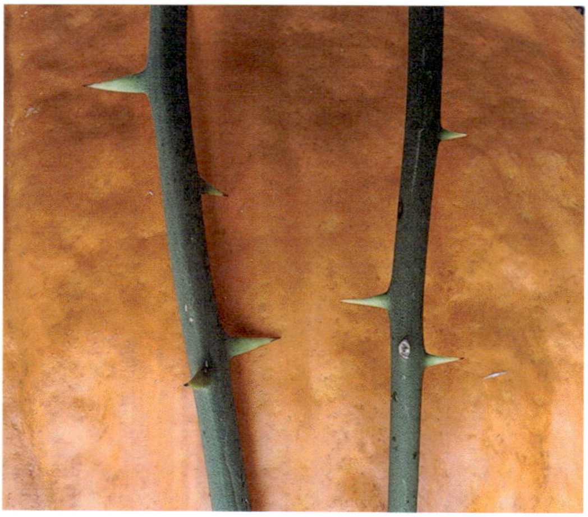

Fig. 1.4 Thorns can cause mechanical injury to farmers, such as these in a pumpkin patch

as redness, swelling, purulent drainage, and red streaks consistent with lymphangitis.

Stinging Insects and Snake Bites

Stinging insects include bees, wasps, hornets, and yellow jackets. Farmworkers are at risk for stings while working with flowering trees and crops. Acute illnesses related to stings are allergic reactions and toxic effects from multiple stings. Allergic reactions are variable and can include wheezing, urticaria, airway edema, and shock. Diagnosis is made by a history of the sting and manifestations of allergic reactions including anaphylaxis. The mainstay of treatment is to administer an initial dose of 0.3–0.5 mg epinephrine (1:1000) by intramuscular injection in adults and 0.01 mg/kg in children. The dose should be repeated as needed for persistent hypotension or hypoxia. Studies have shown that the onset of action of epinephrine from intramuscular injections is twice as fast as subcutaneous injections. Intravenous injections of epinephrine are reserved for cardiac arrest. Corticosteroids are indicated to prevent late-phase reactions. After resuscitation, referral to an allergist for possible desensitization and prescriptions for epinephrine autoinjectors are the standards of care. See Chap. 18 for further details of treatment.

Hymenoptera venom has systemic toxicity that is different from allergic reactions, though the dose received from a single sting is unlikely to result in systemic toxicity. Multiple stings such as those of Africanized honeybees can have serious toxic manifestations. A severe envenomation syndrome has been described (Ferreira Jr et al. 2012) that can result in multiple organ system failure mediated by a surge in cytokines including tumor necrosis factor. Diagnosis is made by a history of attack by a swarm of bees and multiple sting sites on the skin. Clinical manifestations of hypotension, respiratory failure, hemolysis, and kidney failure can occur. See Chap. 18 for details.

Poisonous snake bites occur in farm settings and are a major cause of death and disability among agricultural workers in some countries. Though uncommon in the United States, they do occur from both pit vipers and coral snakes. Diagnosis is made by a history of a bite, though sometimes patients did not see what bit them. Pit viper bites are characterized by severe local pain and swelling that progresses up the extremity. Two fang marks at the site of the bite are usually seen with pit viper envenomation. Systemic toxicity including coagulopathy can occur. Definitive treatment is with antivenom, with two products available in the United States. Coral snakes have neurotoxic venom that causes muscle paralysis and respiratory failure. At the current time, there is no Food and Drug Administration antivenom being marketed in the United States for coral snake bites though limited supplies of expired horse serum antivenom are available. Respiratory support with endotracheal intubation and mechanical ventilation is the treatment though ventilation must be maintained until recovery occurs, which can take days. See Chap. 14 for details.

References

Bonauto D, Anderson R, Rauser E, Burke B. Occupational heat illness in Washington State, 1995–2005. Am J Ind Med. 2007;50:940–50.

CA. https://www.dir.ca.gov/dosh/etools/08-006/whatis.htm. Accessed 25 Apr 2023.

CA 2006. Investigations of heat related illnesses. 2006. https://www.dir.ca.gov/dosh/heatillnessinvestigations-2005.pdf.

California State, Department of Industrial Relations, Division of Occupational Safety and Health. Cal/OSHA investigations of heat related illnesses. 2006. https://www.dir.ca.gov/dosh/heatillnessinvestigations-2005.pdf. Accessed 15 Apr 2021.

Campbell K, Baker B, Tovar A, Economos E, Williams B, McCauley L. The association between skin rashes and work environment, personal protective equipment, and hygiene practices among female farmworkers. Workplace Health Saf. 2017;65:313–21.

CDC. Heat-related deaths among crop workers—U.S., 1992–2006. MMWR Morb Mortal Wkly Rep. 2008;57:649–53.

CDC 2018. Acclimatization. 2018. https://www.cdc.gov/niosh/topics/heatstress/acclima.html.

CDC. 2020. https://www.cdc.gov/niosh/topics/heatstress/default.html.

DHHS. Key principles of toxicology and exposure. US Department of Health & Human Services; 2021. https://chemm.nlm.nih.gov/toxprinciples.htm

Ellis CR, Elston DM. Psoralen-induced phytophotodermatitis. Dermatitis. 2021;32:140–3.

EPA. Agricultural Worker Protection Standard (WPS), Pesticide Worker Safety. 2021. https://www.epa.gov/pesticide-worker-safety/agricultural-worker-protection-standard-wps. Accessed 15 Apr 2021.

EPA. Exposure assessment tools by chemical classes—pesticides. https://www.epa.gov/expobox/exposure-assessment-tools-chemical-classes-pesticides. Accessed 18 May 2021.

Ferreira RS Jr, Almeida RA, Barraviera SR, Barraviera B. Historical perspective and human consequences of Africanized bee stings in the Americas. J Toxicol Environ Health B Crit Rev. 2012;5:97–108.

Levine M, LoVecchio F, Ruha AM, Chu G, Roque P. Influence of drug use on morbidity and mortality in heatstroke. J Med Toxicol Off J Am Coll Med Toxicol. 2012;8(3):252–7.

NIOSH. Green tobacco sickness. 2014. https://www.cdc.gov/niosh/topics/greentobaccosickness/. Accessed 15 Apr 2021.

NIOSH. Acclimatization. 2018. https://www.cdc.gov/niosh/topics/heatstress/acclima.html. Accessed 15 Apr 2021.

NIOSH. Heat stress. 2020. https://www.cdc.gov/niosh/topics/heatstress/default.html. Accessed 15 Apr 2021.

Ohio State University Extension. Giant Hogweed. 2024. https://www.ohioline.osu.edu/factsheet/anr-35#. (Accessed December 20, 2024).

OSHA. Heat safety tool. https://www.osha.gov/heat/heat-app. Accessed 15 Apr 2021.

Papali A, Hines SE. Evaluation of the patient with an exposure-related disease: the occupational and environmental history. Curr Opin Pulm Med. 2015;21(2):155–62.

Roberts JR, Reigart JR. Recognition and management of pesticide poisonings. 6th ed. Office of Pesticide Programs, U.S. Environmental Protection Agency; 2013.

First Aid and Prehospital Management in Rural Areas

2

Tim Cookson, Chad Andicochea, and Roberto Portela

Introduction

Farming is the largest occupation worldwide with 1.3 billion workers. The International Labor Organization (ILO) estimates that worldwide 170,000 persons die each year working in agriculture, with 11,000 deaths from pesticide poisoning. Millions of others are injured in various agricultural activities, and the ILO estimates that 44% of farmers are poisoned by farm chemicals each year (International Labor Organization 2023). In the United States, the National Institute for Occupational Safety and Health (NIOSH) reported 453 agricultural deaths in 2021 with a rate of 19.5 deaths/100,000 (National Institute for Occupational Safety and Health 2023).

Farming holds countless dangers for its workers and a potential risk to rescuers. The amount of chemicals and machinery involved in modern-day farming, together with the usual remote location of farms, makes prehospital care challenging. The yearly fatality rate among farmworkers in the United States is among the highest of all occupations, with the number one cause being traumatic in nature, specifically with the use of tractors (Puvvula et al. 2022). In Iowa, one-fifth of all severe occupational injuries entered in the trauma registry are farm-related. Farmers were less likely to reach definite care in a given time compared to non-farmers (Swanton et al. 2020).

Aside from traumatic injuries, farmworkers can be exposed to various chemicals such as pesticides. About 75% of pesticides used in the United States are used in agriculture (Calvert et al. 2008). Improper handling or inadequate protective equipment can result in acute intoxication (Maroni et al. 1999; Woodruff et al. 1994). Healthcare professionals involved in prehospital care of patients with farming exposures must consider the possible hazards, the location, and the distance to care. Knowledge of the chemicals involved in farming is necessary to provide optimal care to the patient while maintaining the safety of the rescuers.

When activating the local emergency medical services (EMS) system, it is important to be as clear as possible with the 911 emergency dispatcher (i.e., exposure to what chemical). The rural location of most farming incidents makes finding victims and responding in a timely manner challenging. It is common for rural EMS units to cover large response areas. Distance to EMS incidents is typically greater in rural areas compared to urban areas (Jarman et al. 2016). One study showed that the 90th percentile response time in rural areas was 26 min compared to 12 min in urban areas. Around 10% of EMS responses took 30 min from 911 call to

T. Cookson · C. Andicochea · R. Portela (✉)
Department of Emergency Medicine – Division of EMS, East Carolina University, Greenville, NC, USA
e-mail: cooksont23@ecu.edu; andicocheac22@ecu.edu; portelar@ecu.edu

W. J. Meggs, R. L. Langley (eds.), *Farm Toxicology*, https://doi.org/10.1007/978-3-031-80441-0_2

arrival in rural areas (Mell et al. 2017). Longer response times make total EMS call time in rural areas longer than in suburban and urban areas, making it harder for that rural EMS unit to be back in service and available for the next call. Although air ambulances can provide faster transport to definite care over longer distances, they are not always available in rural areas and are easily impacted by weather.

It is important that first responders and health care professionals relay accurate location information to EMS dispatch centers. Healthcare professionals and rescuers should obtain as much information about the circumstances as possible. In exposure cases, information such as time of onset, type of substance involved, quantity, and route of exposure are crucial elements to elicit. Look for chemical placards, warning labels, or containers. If possible, take pictures of labels and/or containers to help hospital personnel. When doing a physical exam, the health care professional should look for possible toxidromes that would point to a certain kind of poison. Smells could point to a particular chemical or gas exposure (Murphy 2021). Look for injuries or bite marks on the skin. When dealing with animal bites and stings, it is valuable but not necessary to try to identify the culprit. Treatment at the scene will depend on the offending agent or type of injury. Maintaining the patient's airway and ensuring adequate ventilation should be a priority. The lungs should be auscultated, listening for crackles or wheezing. Pulse oximetry should be established to guide oxygen administration. Rescuers should be mindful of inaccurate readings in the setting of carbon monoxide poisoning. Elevated carboxyhemoglobin falsely elevates oxygen saturation measurements by the pulse oximeter, thereby overestimating arterial oxygenation (Hampson 1998). Intravenous access should be established and complete vital signs taken. EMS agencies will often have specific protocols for common toxic exposures like organophosphates, cyanide, and carbon monoxide. Local healthcare providers that interact with EMS agencies must understand their scope of practice and limitations. EMS personnel operate under written standing orders (protocols) authorized by the agency's medical director and are unable to practice outside their scope of practice, regardless of what healthcare profesional is on the scene. EMS stock some common antidotes like naloxone, atropine, pralidoxime, and cyanide antidote kits. Regardless of the setting, healthcare professionals should not forget about common medical problems that could occur around a farm like acute myocardial infarctions, seizures, hypoglycemia, and arrhythmias.

The safety of the on-scene healthcare personnel is essential when dealing with toxic exposures. There might be the need to use personal protective equipment (PPE) such as respirators and self-contained breathing apparatus (SCBA) in the case of gaseous toxins such as carbon monoxide, cyanide, nitrogen dioxide, or hydrogen sulfide gas. Protection against vapors might also be required if dealing with substantial amounts of organophosphates. PPE provides various levels of protection, classified from A to D. Level A provides the highest level of protection. It includes a fully encapsulated suit that provides eye, skin, and airway protection with its own source of breathing air. It is indicated when the rescuer needs protection from vapors and/or exposure to mucosal membranes. Examples could be large spills of liquid organophosphate pesticides or corrosive gases. Level B provides lower skin protection but the same level of respiratory protection as level A. This level of PPE should be used when there is no risk of skin contamination but there is considerable risk of toxic gas or low oxygen concentration in the atmosphere. Examples are nitrogen dioxide gas inside grain silos and carbon monoxide. Level C has a lower level of both skin and respiratory protection. It relies on a respirator to filter the ambient air from particles, spores, chemicals, solvents, and toxic gases. To use a respirator, there should be normal oxygen content in the atmosphere. To protect the rescuer from chemicals, the right cartridge must be used with the respirator. Respirators can protect you from chemicals like chlorine gas, ammonia, and sulfur dioxide. Level D offers the lowest level of protection to the rescuer and consists of standard work clothes. It is used when there is no danger of chemical exposure and no need for respiratory protection (Blackwell et al. 2021; Respiratory protection for the farm and ranch 2012).

Additional safety concerns in some toxic exposures may delay transport to definite care. There might be the need for decontamination of the victim as in the case of cutaneous exposure to organophosphates or other chemicals. Contamination can occur by direct exposure to vapors, spray, or air particles (aerosols); liquid spills on an individual; or by contacting a wet surface. These toxic substances adhere to clothes, surfaces, and equipment. Healthcare professionals should take care not to get contaminated while taking care of the victim. Every effort should be taken to minimize the risk of transporting a contaminated victim, thereby moving the hazardous condition to the emergency department and exposing other healthcare personnel. Although a complete guide to proper decontamination of victims is beyond the scope of this chapter, general guidelines apply. Ensure proper PPE when caring for the victim. Remove contaminated clothes and put them in a sealed plastic bag, if possible, to minimize off-gassing. Wash any chemicals off the skin with large amounts of water; use soap if possible. If the eyes were exposed, irrigate with water or saline solution continuously for 10–15 min. More detailed information regarding decontamination for mass exposures can be found on the Office of the Assistant Secretary of Preparedness and Response website (ASPR 2023).

There are several clinical resources at the disposal of the prehospital healthcare professionals. The poison control center is an excellent, easily accessible resource in the United States. Calling 1-800-222-1222 will get you 24/7 access for consultation in any suspected poisoning. Field guides like the "Emergency Response Handbook" (U.S. Department of Transportation 2023) will give you information on how to identify chemicals as well as what safety precautions and dangers to consider. The U.S. Environmental Protection Agency (EPA) publishes the manual "Recognition and Management of Pesticide Poisonings," which gives healthcare providers a quick reference for toxicology and treatment of patients with pesticide exposures (US EPA 2013).

Insect Bites and Stings

The prehospital literature on insect envenomation is limited; however, management has remained relatively unchanged with priority on early recognition of anaphylaxis, supportive treatment, and early transport to an appropriate facility, regardless of the envenomation type. Prehospital protocols or education should exist especially when certain 3s are known to be endemic to the area; however, protocols rarely exist for specific insect envenomation. While identification of the insect is extremely valuable information for clinicians and toxicologists, it is not required. Safety is of utmost concern. EMS crew members should avoid unnecessary risks when trying to identify an insect to prevent exposing themselves, the patient, or other bystanders. Capturing insects is not encouraged, especially if they are still alive. In this case, it may be reasonable to obtain a photograph for the clinicians, if able.

There are numerous insects around the world that have the capability to induce toxic envenomation resulting in varying degrees of physiological responses, both systemically and locally. However, most reactions are not unique to the insects themselves. It is important to recognize that while insect bites or stings may seem commonplace, there is not ample literature on prehospital management. Thus, the purpose of this chapter is to focus on the identification of the insects that are commonly found in a rural setting in the United States.

Lepidoptera are also known as butterflies, moths, and their larvae form, caterpillars. The primary Lepidoptera native to the United States and involved in envenomation include: puss caterpillar, flannel moth caterpillar, Io moth, and saddleback caterpillar. Of the available data from 2000 to 2016 in Texas poison centers, 3484 stings were reported from southern flannel moth, with roughly 89% being managed without healthcare facility management (Seldeslachts et al. 2020). Unlike most insect envenomation, their toxic effects are mediated via direct contact with the venom on their spines or hairs. Systemic symptoms include nausea, vomiting, or, less commonly, seizures in extreme cases such as ingestion. Their cutaneous effect can include severe pain, edema, erythema, and even skin ulceration with necrosis. Broadly speaking, Lepidoptera venom is not well-studied. However, it is thought that their hairs release toxins with proteolytic enzymes and other pro-inflammatory proteins including histamine (Villas-Boas et al. 2018). The prehospital management is supportive with antihistamines and analgesia. Other measures include washing the site with soap/water and air drying, isopropyl alcohol cooling for topical comfort, and using strong adhesive tape to remove spines/hairs.

The most common rural scorpion endemic to the American Southwest region is the *Centruroides sculpturatus* or "bark scorpion." They can be identified via UV light bioluminescence and are often found in dark crevices, loose-fitting clothes, linen, or boots. It is important to identify and treat due to its potentially severe systemic effects. According to the 2019 Annual Report of the American Association of Poison Control Centers' National Poison Data System, there were 9756 reported single-exposure scorpion stings, with 542 cases with moderate systemic symptoms and 28 with major symptoms for potentially life-threatening effects but no reported deaths (Burns 2021). The bark scorpion injects its toxin through the sting of the tail. Its venom is a neurotoxin that activates catecholamine and acetylcholine release. Signs and symptoms include diaphoresis, muscle fasciculations with cramping, tachycardia, and respiratory depression. Prehospital management is supportive with emphasis on opioid analgesia, benzodiazepines for neurotoxic effects, and early aggressive airway management, if needed (Skolnik and Ewald 2013). Icepacks may be considered for topical relief.

The Hymenoptera that are relevant in the rural setting and have toxin-mediated effects include three families: Apidae, Vespidae, and Formicidae. Hymenoptera venom is more commonly known for its allergic reaction and high anaphylactic potential. The venom for Apidae, Vespidae, and Formicidae are similar in that they consist of a blend of low-molecular-weight proteolytic enzymes and high-molecular-weight allergens. The low-molecular-weight components are responsible for local inflammatory reactions, whereas the high-molecular-weight proteins are more involved in systemic findings (Arif and Williams 2023). In 2019, there were 2537 single-incident exposure to Apidae and Vespidae as well as 592 total Formicidae exposures reported to American poison control centers (Gummin et al. 2020). Despite how common Hymenoptera envenomation and allergic reactions may seem, it is a grossly underestimated condition since many cases go unreported or managed without medical intervention. Apidae or honeybees and bumblebees do release a toxic venom that is potentiated when they are swarming. *Apis mellifera scutellata*, also known as "killer bees," are aggressive honeybees. They become more lethal due to their swarming nature, thus increasing the risk of severe reactions (Lovecchio et al. 2007). Vespidae are more commonly known as yellow jackets, hornets, and wasps. In contrast to the Apidae, they are more solitary and aggressive and do not have a barbed stinger, making them capable of stinging multiple times. Formicidae or fire ants are named for their severe burning pain, swelling, and pustule formation that has the potential for skin necrosis. Formicidae use a stinger located on the tip of the abdomen that can penetrate the skin. There will usually be multiple stings, with about a 6% chance of developing anaphylaxis (Desforges et al. 1990). Compared to other insects, Hymenoptera account for most of the severe allergic reactions. They do not require previous exposure or sting to develop a severe reaction (Klotz et al. 2009), and it is thought that if you are allergic to one type, it is likely that you are allergic to other types (Graft 2006). Prehospital management is aimed at early identification of airway compromise and recognition of anaphylaxis, with the mainstay treatment being epinephrine and antihistamines. Epinephrine can be administered to adults via an auto-injector EpiPen® or by epinephrine 1:1000 solution 0.3–0.5 mg intramuscularly. For pediatric patients, the dose is 0.01 mg/kg intramuscularly. The rest of prehospital treatment is supportive with an emphasis on early transport, especially when anaphylaxis is identified. The use of steroids is thought to aid with reduction of inflammation. In the prehospital setting, it may have a role when considering the time of onset of steroid therapeutic effects and delay in reaching definitive care.

There are two clinically relevant species of spiders in the rural setting of North America: *Lactrodectus* and *Loxosceles reclusa*. *Lactrodectus* or black widow spider is easily recognized by its red hourglass marking on the abdomen. It is responsible for more than 2600 exposures each year according to the National Poison Data System (Williams et al. 2023). There are over 30 distinct types of black widow spiders, several of which are endemic to different regions of North America. They prefer warmer climates and are commonly found in firewood, sheds, equipment, barns, etc. The primary toxin found in its venom is the latrotoxin, which binds irreversibly to protein receptors on presynaptic neurons that results in a large release of neurotransmitters that include acetylcholine, dopamine, norepinephrine, epinephrine, and glutamate (Williams et al. 2023). The release of various neurotransmitters is responsible for the syndrome of pain, rigidity, vomiting, diaphoresis, tachycardia, tachypnea, and hypertension. The bite produces extreme, localized pain before systemic symptoms develop and sometimes an associated fang mark. Prehospital management is supportive with analgesia for pain control and benzodiazepines for dampening the amplified excitatory neurotransmission. Benzodiazepines may also aid in the reduction of elevated blood pressure, tachycardia, and muscle spasms. Early transport to a hospital should be made, especially with preference for a facility that possesses antivenin if possible.

Loxosceles reclusa or brown recluse spiders are found primarily in the Southwest, Southeast, and Mississippi River Valley. They have similar hiding places as the bark scorpion, with emphasis on dark areas around rocks, wood, farms, attics, or anything with crevices. The venom is considered cytotoxic, with many enzymes that can also cause hemolysis and other proteins that participate in indiscriminate cellular destruction, resulting in coagulative necrosis. The findings are mostly cutaneous; however, systemic findings such as nausea, headache, and weakness can occur. The bite may go unnoticed for several hours until the pain develops. Bite marks are identified by two small puncture wounds with surrounding erythema. Days later, the wound will evolve from a blister into a necrotic ulcer with a dark eschar (Anoka et al. 2023). Prehospital management includes simple first aid with elevation of affected extremity and analgesia. The activity of one of the enzymes in the cytotoxin is heat-activated; therefore, icepacks can be helpful. This may not only aid in pain control but also reduce cellular breakdown (Anoka et al. 2023). Corticosteroids are thought to aid in the abatement of hemolytic anemia, but their prehospital role has not been demonstrated in the literature. Hemolytic anemia, rhabdomyolysis, disseminated intravascular coagulation (DIC), renal failure, and death are features of "systemic loxoscelism" (Saucier 2004) that usually develop several days after the bite. This is more common in the pediatric and geriatric populations.

Snake Bites

Snake envenomation presents a significant health concern worldwide with over 2.5 million people bitten annually, resulting in up to 125,000 deaths according to the World Health Organization (Cruz et al. 2009). In the United States, the annual incidence of snake bites ranges from 5000 to 10,000 (Greene et al. 2020; Ruha et al. 2017). Death in the United States from snake bites is rare. Cases from the National Poison Data System from 1989 to 2018 identified only 101 fatal snake bites (Greene et al. 2020). In the United States, 20% of snake bites are considered "dry bites" with no venom injected into the wound. Blood vessel envenomation tends to lead to the rapid onset of severe systemic symptoms and have higher lethality rates compared to muscle or subcutaneous delivery.

Snake venom is comprised of peptides and proteins stored in the snake's venom gland and delivered through the fangs during a strike, or bite, of their victim (Osipov and Utkin 2023).

Venom type is commonly divided into neurotoxic and hemotoxic (Osipov and Utkin 2023), with a few snake species in the United States expressing a mixed venom type such as the Mojave rattlesnake, or *Crotalus scutulatus*. Neurotoxic venom, found in the coral snake, targets and inhibits neuromuscular transmission while hemotoxic venom impairs blood coagulation (Osipov and Utkin 2023). Bites are delivered into the subcutaneous tissue, muscle, vein, or artery (Parker-Cote and Meggs 2018). Muscle and subcutaneous deliveries utilize the lymphatic system to bring venom to the central circulation (Parker-Cote and Meggs 2018).

In the United States, a majority of snake bite envenomation are by snakes with hemotoxic venom such as rattlesnakes and copperheads, which are of the family Viperidae, subfamily crotaline (Nazim et al. 2008). The initial signs and symptoms usually include puncture marks at the wound, redness, swelling, pain at the site, and development of systemic signs such as tachycardia, nausea, vomiting, and low blood pressure. Neurotoxic snake venom such as from the coral snake tends to have similar initial symptoms as hemotoxic snake venom but progresses to neuromuscular depression with symptoms such as muscle paralysis, diplopia, respiratory distress, and respiratory failure.

Center for Disease Control and Prevention's List of Snake Bite Symptoms:

- Puncture marks at the wound
- Redness, swelling, bruising, bleeding, or blistering around the bite
- Severe pain and tenderness at the site of the bite
- Nausea, vomiting, or diarrhea
- Labored breathing (in extreme cases, breathing may stop altogether)
- Rapid heart rate, weak pulse, and low blood pressure
- Disturbed vision
- Metallic, mint, or rubber taste in the mouth
- Increased salivation and sweating
- Numbness or tingling around face and/or limbs
- Muscle twitching

In the prehospital setting, healthcare professionals should start by ensuring a safe scene and wearing appropriate PPE. Although transportation to a facility that stocks and administers antivenin is of high priority, initial medical intervention should utilize the same primary survey recommended for most medical emergencies, namely hemorrhage control and ensuring patent airway and adequate breathing and circulation. Experts do recommend noting the physical traits of the snake and/or obtaining a photograph, if safe and feasible. Capturing and/or killing the snake to bring to a treatment facility should be avoided as even a decapitated snake can envenomate. To reduce systemic toxicity, the patient should be placed in a supine position and limit the mobility of the affected limb. Splinting the limb can be considered to reduce the lymphatic return to central circulation (Parker-Cote and Meggs 2018). Keep the limb below the level of the heart when snake venom is known to induce severe systemic toxicity and at the level of the heart when the snake venom is known to have severe local tissue damage (Parker-Cote and Meggs 2018). Loosening or removing clothing from the affected extremity may reduce complications like compartment syndrome if edema were to develop. Remove wrist watches, bracelets, rings or other jewelry if the distal arms are involved before edema develops. Apply standard wound dressing to prevent unnecessary bleeding and contamination of the wound. Do not apply ice to the bite site. If it is not known which medical facilities have access to antivenin, calling the poison control center can be a simple first step to help with destination decisions. Supportive care may be necessary for patients who start demonstrating advanced signs of system-toxic symptoms such as shock and/or respiratory muscle paralysis with intravenous fluids and assisted ventilation.

There has been interest in devices such as tourniquets, venom extractors, pressure immobilization bandages, and herbal medicines to name a few (Parker-Cote and Meggs 2018). Overall, many of these techniques have not yet shown benefits for reducing lethality and, in fact, tend to increase harm of the affected limb including cellulitis, tissue necrosis, and osteomyelitis. The

American Heart Association's 2010 and 2015 guidelines do offer recommendations for a pressure immobilization bandage, arguing for the potential of decreased lymphatic spread. This technique, however, may require training and skill maintenance to achieve the recommended 40–70 mmHg and 55–70 mmHg in the upper and lower extremities, respectively, while refraining from a tourniquet-like compression. This may be an option in regions where prolonged field care is required with significant delays in medical transport. Unfortunately, a bite that penetrates to the level of a blood vessel may make this technique obsolete.

Toxic Gases

Agriculture and farmworkers also have high rates of respiratory diseases owing to dust, particles, and toxic gases with long-term health consequences such as asthma, silo-filler's disease, farmer's lung, chronic bronchitis, pneumonitis, and pulmonary edema, to name a few (Puvvula et al. 2022). As a result, protective measures have been recommended such as filter masks and self-contained breathing apparatuses. In a report, however, only 50% of agriculture workers reported using recommended protective equipment half of the time, which is likely an important cause of the lifetime prevalence of any respiratory condition of 18% (Puvvula et al. 2022). The purpose of this section is not to discuss long-term health consequences; however, the known issues of health hazards from toxic gases and the limited use of the necessary protective equipment increase the risk of acute toxic exposure and medical emergencies that may be encountered.

Toxic farm gas exposures can occur in confined or open spaces. Confined spaces include grain silos, manure pits, grain bins, and controlled atmospheric storages. Many of these are regulated by the Occupational and Safety Health Administration (OSHA) and require adequate ventilation to prevent injury to workers by the accumulation of toxic gases (Occupational Safety and Health Administration 2009). Silos produce nitrogen dioxide (NO_2), and workers should not enter within 10 days of filling to avoid exposure to dangerous levels of the gas (Donham and Thelin 2016). Open spaces include open manure pits which produce hydrogen sulfide (H_2S), ammonia (NH_3), methane (CH_4), and carbon dioxide (CO_2), as well as concentrated animal feeding operations (CAFOs), which produce ammonia (NH_3), hydrogen, sulfide (H_2S), and carbon dioxide (CO_2). Other sources are open agricultural fields and animal storage areas due to the increased production of dust, microbes, animal dander, proteins, insects, and pesticides (Puvvula et al. 2022).

Many exposure cases start with mucous membrane irritation and burning. However, many of these gases can be odorless and undetectable until elevated levels are reached, causing severe medical symptoms. For example, CO_2 is odorless and colorless and may produce slight symptoms such as headaches, before causing suffocation leading to cardiopulmonary failure. Hydrogen sulfide (H_2S) is also colorless but may have the distinct smell of rotten eggs. At elevated levels, the gas may also be odorless to the victim (olfactory fatigue) and can lead to initial headaches, nausea, and dizziness, before causing loss of consciousness and respiratory failure (Reiffenstein et al. 1992). Ammonia (NH_3) initially causes milder symptoms with eye irritation and/or ulceration, before causing severe irritation to the respiratory tract leading to respiratory distress (Doss and Tilma 2009). Odorless methane (CH_4) works as an asphyxiant, leading to respiratory distress and failure. NO_2 typically has a sweet odor with a reddish-brown color when in high enough concentrations to be visible. NO_2, when inhaled, reacts with water and produces nitrous acid, which produces tissue damage, leading to initial symptoms such as dyspnea, productive cough, chest pain, light-headedness, shortness of breath, and choking and could lead to pulmonary edema and resulting respiratory collapse (Schultz 2016).

In most cases of concern for toxic gas exposure causing an acute medical emergency, the healthcare professional should assume that levels of exposure are extreme. As such, most recommended PPE for rescue personnel includes the use of a positive-pressure, self-contained breathing apparatus (SCBA) and a safety line for rapid exit (Occupational Safety and Health Administration 2023).

After ensuring an appropriate level of PPE for all responders, the victim should be moved out of the exposure area. A standard approach to the critical patient in the prehospital setting should be done, including assessment and intervention following airway evaluation, breathing, and circulation. Given the likelihood of a victim collapsing due to the effects of the toxic gas, trauma considerations should include cervical spinal protection and head injuries. Most acute toxic gas exposures cause respiratory failure due to simple asphyxiation from CO_2 or CH_4 inhalation, and supplemental oxygen, with or without assisted ventilation, is the most important first line of treatment. Concerns for pneumonitis and/or pulmonary edema in the cases of possible NO_2 exposure also require, as initial treatment steps in the prehospital setting, supplemental oxygenation and assisted ventilation. If the patient is demonstrating spontaneous breathing and has the capability to respond to noninvasive ventilation (NIV) or continuous positive airway pressure (CPAP), this may ensure restoration of alveolar recruitment and improve ventilation and oxygenation (Bello et al. 2018). Those without adequate spontaneous breathing may need to be considered for endotracheal intubation for positive pressure ventilation (Bello et al. 2018).

References

Anoka IA, Robb EL, Baker MB. Brown recluse spider toxicity. In: StatPearls [Internet]. Treasure Island: StatPearls Publishing; 2023. [cited 2023 Dec 8].

Arif F, Williams M. Hymenoptera stings. In: StatPearls [Internet]. Treasure Island: StatPearls Publishing; 2023. [cited 2023 Dec 8].

ASPR. Homepage [Internet]. 2023. [cited 2023 Dec 11]. Available from: https://aspr.hhs.gov:443/Pages/Home.aspx.

Bello G, De Santis P, Antonelli M. Non-invasive ventilation in cardiogenic pulmonary edema. Ann Transl Med. 2018;6(18):355.

Blackwell TH, DeAtley C, Yee A. Medical support for hazardous materials response. In: Cone DC, Brice JH, Delbridge TR, Brent Myers J, editors. Emergency medical services: clinical practice and systems oversight. 3rd ed. John Wiley & Sons, Ltd; 2021. p. 337–51. https://doi.org/10.1002/9781119756279.ch103. [cited 2023 Dec 11].

Burns D Insect bites: background, pathophysiology, epidemiology. 2021. Oct 13 [cited 2023 Dec 8]; Available from: https://emedicine.medscape.com/article/769067-overview?form=fpf.

Calvert GM, Karnik J, Mehler L, Beckman J, Morrissey B, Sievert J, et al. Acute pesticide poisoning among agricultural workers in the United States, 1998–2005. Am J Ind Med. 2008;51(12):883–98.

Cruz LS, Vargas R, Lopes AA. Snakebite envenomation and death in the developing world. Ethn Dis. 2009;19(1 Suppl 1):S1-42–6.

Desforges JF, deShazo RD, Butcher BT, Banks WA. Reactions to the stings of the imported fire ant. N Engl J Med. 1990;323(7):462–6.

Donham KJ, Thelin A. Agricultural respiratory diseases. In: Agricultural medicine: rural occupational and environmental health, safety, and prevention. 2nd ed. Wiley; 2016. [cited 2023 Dec 19]. p. 95–154. https://doi.org/10.1002/9781118647356.ch3.

Doss HJ, Tilma C. NASD—confined space hazards a threat to farmers [Internet]. 2009. [cited 2023 Dec 13]. Available from: http://nasdonline.org.

Graft DF. Insect sting allergy. Med Clin North Am. 2006;90(1):211–32.

Greene S, Folt J, Wyatt K, Brandehoff N. Epidemiology of fatal snakebites in the United States 1989–2018. Am J Emerg Med. 2020;45:309–16. https://doi.org/10.1016/j.ajem.2020.08.083.

Gummin DD, Mowry JB, Beuhler MC, Spyker DA, Brooks DE, Dibert KW, et al. 2019 Annual report of the American Association of Poison Control Centers' National Poison Data System (NPDS): 37th annual report. Clin Toxicol Phila Pa. 2020;58(12):1360–541.

Hampson NB. Pulse oximetry in severe carbon monoxide poisoning. Chest. 1998;114(4):1036–41.

International Labour Organization. Chemicals in agriculture [Internet]. 2023. [cited 2023 Dec 19]. Available from: http://www.ilo.org/global/topics/safety-and-health-at-work/areasofwork/chemical-safety-and-the-environment/WCMS_871784/lang%2D%2Den/index.htm.

Jarman MP, Castillo RC, Carlini AR, Kodadek LM, Haider AH. Rural risk: geographic disparities in trauma mortality. Surgery. 2016;160(6):1551–9.

Klotz JH, Klotz SA, Pinnas JL. Animal bites and stings with anaphylactic potential. J Emerg Med. 2009;36(2):148–56.

Lovecchio F, Cannon RD, Algier J, Ruha A-M, Curry SC, Wallace KL, et al. Bee swarmings in children. Am J Emerg Med. 2007;25(8):931–3.

Maroni M, Fait A, Colosio C. Risk assessment and management of occupational exposure to pesticides. Toxicol Lett. 1999;107(1–3):145–53.

Mell HK, Mumma SN, Hiestand B, Carr BG, Holland T, Stopyra J. Emergency medical services response times in rural, suburban, and urban areas. JAMA Surg. 2017;152(10):983–4.

Murphy CM. Principles of toxicology. In: Cone DC, Brice JH, Delbridge TR, Myers JB, editors. Emergency medical services: clinical practice and systems oversight. 3rd ed. John Wiley & Sons, Ltd; 2021. [cited 2023 Dec 11]. p. 371–82.

Nazim MH, Gupta S, Hashmi S, Zuberi J, Wilson A, Roberts L, et al. Retrospective review of snake bite victims. W V Med J. 2008;104(5):30–4.

NIOSH | CDC. 2023. National farm safety and health week: no one can take your place [Internet]. [cited 2023 Dec 19]. Available from: https://www.cdc.gov/niosh/newsroom/feature/national-farm-safety-and-health.html.

Occupational Safety and Health Administration. 2009. 1926.55—Gases, vapors, fumes, dusts, and mists [Internet]. [cited 2023c Dec 12]. Available from: https://www.osha.gov/laws-regs/regulations/standardnumber/1926/1926.55.

Occupational Safety and Health Administration 2023 Hydrogen sulfide—evaluating and controlling exposure [Internet]. [cited 2023 Dec 12]. Available from: https://www.osha.gov/hydrogen-sulfide/evaluating-controlling-exposure.

Osipov A, Utkin Y. What are the neurotoxins in hemotoxic snake venoms? Int J Mol Sci. 2023;24(3):2919.

Parker-Cote J, Meggs WJ. First aid and pre-hospital management of venomous snakebites. Trop Med Infect Dis. 2018;3(2):45.

Puvvula J, Baccaglini L, Johnson A, Du Y, Bell JE, Rautiainen RH. Prevalence and risk factors for pulmonary conditions among farmers and ranchers in the Central United States. J Agromedicine. 2022;27(4):378–90.

Reiffenstein RJ, Hulbert WC, Roth SH. Toxicology of hydrogen sulfide. Annu Rev Pharmacol Toxicol. 1992;32:109–34.

Respiratory Protection for the Farm and Ranch 2012 Respiratory protection on the farm and ranch—ag safety and health [Internet]. [cited 2023 Dec 11]. Available from: https://ag-safety.extension.org/respiratory-protection-on-the-farm-and-ranch/.

Ruha A-M, Kleinschmidt KC, Greene S, Spyres MB, Brent J, Wax P, et al. The epidemiology, clinical course, and management of snakebites in the North American Snakebite Registry. J Med Toxicol Off J Am Coll Med Toxicol. 2017;13(4):309–20.

Saucier JR. Arachnid envenomation. Emerg Med Clin North Am. 2004;22(2):405–22, ix

Schultz C. Comparing silo filler disease with farmer's lung disease. Gen Intern Med Clin Innov. 2016;1 https://doi.org/10.15761/GIMCI.1000123.

Seldeslachts A, Peigneur S, Tytgat J. Caterpillar Venom: A Health Hazard of the 21st Century. Biomedicines. 2020;8(6):143.

Skolnik AB, Ewald MB. Pediatric scorpion envenomation in the United States: morbidity, mortality, and therapeutic innovations. Pediatr Emerg Care. 2013;29(1):98–103; quiz 104–5.

Swanton A, Peek-Asa C, Torner J. Time to definitive care among severely injured farmers compared to other work-related injuries in a Midwestern state. Inj Epidemiol. 2020;7:33.

U.S. Department of Transportation. Emergency Response Guidebook (ERG). PHMSA [Internet]; 2023. [cited 2023 Dec 19]. Available from: https://www.phmsa.dot.gov/training/hazmat/erg/emergency-response-guidebook-erg

US EPA. Recognition and management of pesticide poisonings [Internet]. 2013. [cited 2023 Nov 16]. Available from: https://www.epa.gov/pesticide-worker-safety/recognition-and-management-pesticide-poisonings.

Villas-Boas IM, Bonfá G, Tambourgi DV. Venomous caterpillars: from inoculation apparatus to venom composition and envenomation. Toxicon. 2018;153:39–52.

Williams M, Sehgal N, Nappe TM. Black widow spider toxicity. In: StatPearls [Internet]. Treasure Island: StatPearls Publishing; 2023. [cited 2023 Dec 8].

Woodruff TJ, Kyle AD, Bois FY. Evaluating health risks from occupational exposure to pesticides and the regulatory response. Environ Health Perspect. 1994;102(12):1088–96.

3 Sources of Information

William J. Meggs

Introduction

A healthcare provider evaluating an ill farmworker after a potential exposure may have limited information. Sometimes only the class of chemical—insecticide, herbicide, rodenticide, etc.—is known. Even that information may be incorrect. An example is the insecticide Aldicarb used off-label as rat poison in a watermelon patch (D'Haenens et al. 2013). In an ideal situation, the precise exposure is known. Knowing the brand name of a product or its active ingredients opens the door to a wealth of information about the product.

Regional Poison Centers

Information about poisons can be obtained 24 hours a day from a regional poison center. In the United States, the number is +1-800-222-1222. Poison centers are staffed by specialists in poison information (SPIs). Most are pharmacists or nurses. A certification examination for SPIs under the auspices of America's Poison Centers (formerly known as the American Association of Poison Control Centers) can be taken. SPIs have access to databases of products and are trained to quickly provide information in response to calls from both the public and healthcare professionals. For critically ill patients, a medical toxicologist is available to assist in management.

Poison centers can help with triage. SPIs can give advice about when an asymptomatic subject can be observed at work or home and what signs and symptoms motivate a higher level of care.

Medical Toxicology Consultation

Medical toxicology is a subspecialty that diagnoses and treats acute and chronic poisonings, from drug overdoses to environmental exposures and envenomation. Becoming a medical toxicologist requires training in a primary residency—usually emergency medicine, pediatrics, or environmental and occupational medicine—followed by a two-year fellowship with supervised practice. In-person consultations are available at many tertiary care hospitals. Telephone consultations and management of severe poisonings are available through poison centers. Board certification and lifelong learning assessment are administrated as sub-boards of the American Board of Emergency Medicine. Information about the specialty is available at the American College of Medical Toxicology (ACMT n.d.) website.

W. J. Meggs (✉)
Brody School of Medicine, East Carolina University, Greenville, NC, USA
e-mail: meggsw@ecu.edu

W. J. Meggs, R. L. Langley (eds.), *Farm Toxicology*, https://doi.org/10.1007/978-3-031-80441-0_3

Product Labels

Often, the container of a product of concern accompanies an acutely ill farmworker to a healthcare setting. Product labels can be a valuable source of information about potential illnesses associated with exposure to the product. These labels are legally enforceable and contain the statement: "It is a violation of Federal law to use this product in a manner inconsistent with its labeling."

The following information is required on pesticide labels:

- Ingredients: What is in the product?
- Signal word: The three signal words are *Caution*, *Warning*, and *Danger*. *Caution* labels a product as slightly toxic if ingested, absorbed dermally, or inhaled or can cause mild skin and eye irritation. *Warning* labels a product as being moderately toxic, while *Danger* indicates that the product is highly toxic by one or more exposure routes. A dangerous product may be corrosive and cause irreversible damage to the skin or eyes or be extremely poisonous by ingestion, inhalation, or dermal absorption. Products labeled as dangerous must have the word *POISON* on the front panel of the container in bold red letters.
- Precautionary statements: These tell the dangers of the product.
- First aid information: What should be done immediately if the product gets on the skin or in the eyes or is inhaled or ingested?
- Environmental hazards: Damage of a pesticide to the environment and danger to wildlife must be spelled out on the label.
- Personal protective equipment (PPE): PPE can range from simple to complex. The label tells what type of gloves should be worn, what type of respiratory protection is necessary, and if whole-body protection is necessary.
- Directions for use: These directions dictate where and when the product can be used and can include amounts.
- Storage and disposal: Legal restrictions on how the product can be stored and how to dispose of unused products are spelled out on the label.
- Manufacturer's contact information: Labels contain the name and address of the manufacturer.
- Phone number: Usually, the number is a toll-free number that can be used to obtain a variety of information about the product, including what to do in an emergency and safe handling.
- EPA (Environmental Protection Agency 2023a) registration number: By law, pesticide products marketed in the United States must be registered with the federal EPA. Pesticides are given a unique registration number.

Safety Data Sheets

A safety data sheet (SDS) for a product was formerly known as a material safety data sheet (MSDS). Both terms are still used. Manufacturers and importers of chemical products, including pesticides and other chemicals used on the farm, are required by law to provide safety data sheets for the product, with contents prescribed by law. Further, employers are required to provide employees with safety data sheets for any product that the employee could be exposed to. The contents of SDSs are like the information on the label but more detailed. The sections of an SDS are listed below (Occupational Safety and Health Administration (OSHA)). Sections 4 (First aid measures) and section 11 (toxicological information) are of particular interest to healthcare providers.

Section 1: Identification includes product identifier; manufacturer's or distributor's name, address, and phone number; emergency phone number; recommended use; and restrictions on use.

Section 2: Hazard(s) identification includes all hazards regarding the chemical and required label elements.

Section 3: Composition/information on ingredients includes information on chemical ingredients and trade secret

claims.

Section 4: First aid measures include important symptoms/effects, acute and delayed, and required treatment.

Section 5: Fire-fighting measures list suitable extinguishing techniques, equipment; and chemical hazards from fire.

Section 6: Accidental release measures list emergency procedures, protective equipment, and proper methods of containment and cleanup.

Section 7: Handling and storage list precautions for safe handling and storage, including incompatibilities.

Section 8: Exposure controls/personal protection lists OSHA's permissible exposure limits (PELs); American Conference of Governmental Industrial Hygienists (ACGIH) Threshold Limit Values (TLVs); and any other exposure limit used or recommended by the chemical

manufacturer, importer, or employer preparing the SDS, where available, as well as appropriate engineering controls and personal protective equipment (PPE).

Section 9: Physical and chemical properties list the chemical's characteristics.

Section 10: Stability and reactivity information lists chemical stability and the possibility of hazardous reactions.

Section 11: Toxicological information includes routes of exposure, related symptoms and acute and chronic effects, and numerical measures of toxicity.

Section 12: Ecological information*.

Section 13: Disposal considerations*.

Section 14: Transport information*.

Section 15: Regulatory information*.

Section 16: Other information includes the date of preparation or last revision.

*Note: Agencies other than OSHA regulate this information, so

OSHA does not enforce Sections 12 through 15 (29 CFR 1910.1200(g)(2)).

Federal, State, and Local Health Departments

Health departments can be helpful in cases of farm poisonings and send trained investigators to the scene though they may not be immediately available. They are of particular benefit in cases of mass poisonings or disease outbreaks. Agencies that can assist state and local health agencies with toxic investigations include:

EPA Regional Response teams.

Agency for Toxic Substances and Diseases Registry (ATSDR).

There are 13 EPA Regional Response Teams that provide a forum for federal-agency field offices and state agencies to exchange information about their abilities to respond to on-scene coordinator's (OSC's) requests for assistance. RRT members do not respond directly to releases or spills but may be called upon to provide technical advice, equipment, or manpower to assist with a response (EPA 2023b).

ATSDR is an operational division of the U.S. Department of Health and Human Services and reports to the same director as the National Center for Environmental Health of the Centers for Disease Control and Prevention (CDC). Since the local, state, and federal agencies work closely together, a call to one generally activates the resources of all levels.

Requirements for reporting poisonings vary in different states. Some states require that all poisoning episodes be reported, while some only require that pesticide poisonings be reported. A call to a poison center can be a source of local information and often satisfies the requirement.

Reference Books

A reference book that is highly recommended for rapid access to vital information in the clinical setting is *Poisoning & Drug Overdose* (Olsen), a relatively inexpensive paperback reference produced by the faculty and staff associated with the California Poison Control System. The publisher is the Lange division of McGraw Hill. Poisons and drug classes are listed alphabetically and organized for rapid retrieval of essential information, with sections on mechanism, clinical presentation, diagnosis, and treatment. Specific antidotes and decontamination are given when applicable. An online version of this book is available through Access Medicine, an electronic resource to which many medical libraries have subscriptions.

For an in-depth analysis, *Goldfrank's Toxicological Emergencies*, also published by McGraw Hill, is a comprehensive reference. While *Poisoning & Drug Overdose* tells a clinician what to do in a concise format, *Goldfrank's Toxicological Emergencies* also discusses why certain treatments are effective in comprehensive detail.

Online Resources and Use of Online Search Engines

Since the information revolution, a tremendous amount of information is available online. The advent of rapid search engines that access large databases has greatly facilitated access to critical information in a timely manner. Google searches are recommended as a search engine platform noted for accuracy, speed and comprehensiveness. Beam and Yahoo are also available. If a product name or ingredients are known, searching for the safety data sheet for the product is generally an almost instantaneous way to gain information. Information about the toxicity of the product and treatment of poisoning by the product can be essential.

Government websites for agencies like the Environmental Protection Agency, Occupational Health and Safety Administration, and Centers for Disease Control and Prevention have information on poisons that undergo extensive internal reviews and verifications and are reliable. National Institute for Occupational Safety and Health (NIOSH) is a division of the CDC that provides research on numerous chemicals used in the workplace. The Agency for Toxic Substances and Diseases Registry has online toxicological profiles for a number of hazardous substances. These can be downloaded without charge. The National Pesticide Information Center (NPIC), formed as a cooperative agreement between Oregon State University and the U.S. Environmental Protection Agency, has information on pesticides. The National Toxicology Program (NTP) of the National Institutes of Health has evaluated more than 2800 environmental substances for potential human health effects. The World Health Organization also provides toxicologic information on numerous chemicals including pesticides and investigates carcinogenic potential of chemicals through its International Agency for Research on Cancer (IARC) program.

In addition to governmental agencies, there are nongovernmental agencies in many countries that research and make recommendations on levels of exposure to workers. For example, in the United States, the American Conference of Governmental Industrial Hygienists (ACGIH) develops Threshold Limit Values (TLVs) and Biological Exposure Indices (BEIs) for numerous chemicals to which workers may be exposed.

References

ACMT. https://www.acmt.net/.

D'Haenens JP, McDonald KW, Langley RL, et al. Aldicarb: a case series of watermelon-borne carbamate toxicity. J Agromedicine. 2013;18:174–7.

EPA. 2023a. https://www.epa.gov/pesticide-labels/pesticide-label-review-training.

EPA. 2023b. https://www.epa.gov/emergency-response/regional-response-teams.

Goldfrank L, et al. editors. Goldfrank's toxicologic emergencies. McGraw Hill. Frequent Revisions.

Olsen K, editor. Poisoning & drug overdose. Lange Division of McGraw Hill. Frequent Revisions.

OSHA. n.d. https://www.osha.gov/sites/default/files/publications/OSHA3493QuickCardSafetyDataSheet.pdf. Accessed 21 Jan 2024.

Personal Protective Equipment 4

Wayne Buhler, Beth Dittman, and Ricky L. Langley

Introduction

Hazards exist in every workplace in a variety of forms including sharp edges, falling objects, flying sparks, chemicals, heat/cold, noise, dust particles, and gases/vapors. The Occupational Safety and Health Administration (OSHA) within the U.S. Department of Labor (USDOL) requires that employers protect their employees from workplace hazards that can cause injury (OSHA 1970). A "Hierarchy of Controls" (Fig. 4.1) has been recommended to lower worker exposures and reduce the risk of illness or injury (NIOSH (b) 2023). There are five levels of actions in the preferred order of general effectiveness:

1. Elimination
2. Substitution
3. Engineering controls
4. Administrative controls
5. Personal protective equipment (PPE)

The hierarchy of controls is a way of determining which actions will best control or mitigate exposures. Depending on the hazard or workplace conditions, OSHA recommends the use of engineering or work practice controls to manage or eliminate hazards to the greatest extent possible. When engineering, work practice, and administrative controls are not feasible or do not provide sufficient protection, employers must provide personal protective equipment (PPE) to their employees and provide training on its use. PPE refers to clothing and devices worn to protect the wearer from contact with chemicals or other hazards. Coveralls or protective suits, footwear, gloves, aprons, respirators, eyewear, and headgear are examples of PPE (OSHA 2023).

Wearing personal protective equipment (PPE) can greatly reduce the potential for exposure to hazards but does not necessarily eliminate it. PPE offers various levels of protection, depending on the type of material the equipment is made from. When working with chemicals such as pesticides, PPE protects only if the chemical remains on the outside of the protective clothing. If the chemical gets inside the PPE being worn next to the skin, the protective clothing works against the user by holding the chemical in contact with the skin. This increases the likelihood of local contact or

W. Buhler (✉)
Department of Horticultural Science,
North Carolina State University, Raleigh, NC, USA
e-mail: wayne_buhler@ncsu.edu

B. Dittman
North Carolina Department of Agriculture and Consumer Services, Structural Pest Control and Pesticides Division, Raleigh, NC, USA
e-mail: Beth.Dittman@ncagr.gov

R. L. Langley
Department of Biological Sciences,
North Carolina State University,
Raleigh, NC, USA
e-mail: rllangley@ncsu.edu

W. J. Meggs, R. L. Langley (eds.), *Farm Toxicology*, https://doi.org/10.1007/978-3-031-80441-0_4

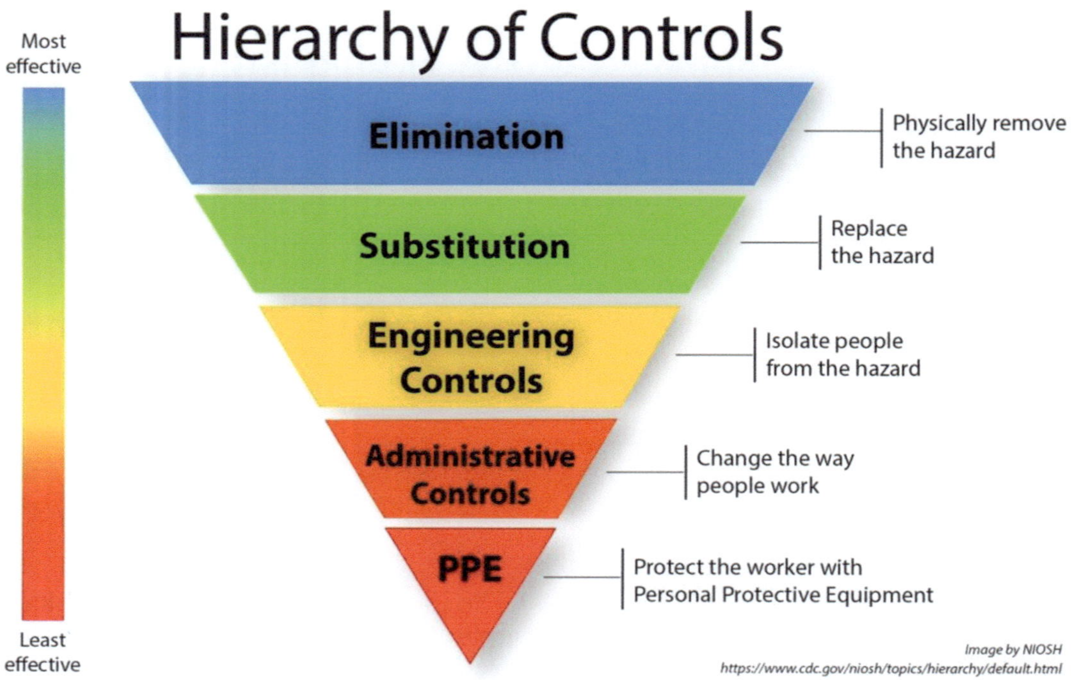

Fig. 4.1 Hierarchy of controls of workplace hazards

systemic injury. The likelihood of adverse effects from any hazardous exposure depends on several factors, including the inherent toxicity of the hazard, the length and frequency of exposure, the concentration of the chemical, and underlying health issues. When exposure does occur, it is important to address the hazard immediately to reduce the length of exposure.

All pesticide handlers and early-entry agricultural workers are legally required to follow all PPE instructions that appear on the product label. Sometimes a label has different PPE requirements for pesticide handlers and early-entry workers. A pesticide label lists the minimum PPE that a person must wear. If the label does not require PPE or requires only one or two pieces of PPE, a pesticide handler can always add extra PPE for increased safety. Consult labels and Safety Data Sheets (SDS) for instructions about protective equipment and clothing, and remember that protective equipment has limitations. A person is never completely protected and must still use caution and common sense to prevent chemicals from contacting the body.

Dermal Protection

The skin is the largest organ of the human body and accounts for more than 10% of the body's mass. It enables the body to readily interact with the environment and also serves as a defense barrier. Skin poses as a significant exposure pathway for many chemicals because of the potential for contact on a large surface area [1.5–2.5 squared meters (m^2)] (USEPA 2011). Dermal exposures to chemicals can result in either temporary or permanent adverse health impacts (NIOSH 2017). These adverse impacts may occur at the point of contact with the chemical, or the chemical may be taken into the body through non-intact skin (such as an open wound or a puncture) or by permeating the skin. Temporary or permanent damage may occur to body organs or systems as a result of chemical absorption across the skin.

Temporary health impacts may include dry, red, and cracked skin (irritation) from contact with water, soaps, gasoline, and certain types of solvents. These disorders usually heal quickly when skin contact with the chemical has abated, but they can increase the chance of infection when breaks in the skin are present. Permanent impacts may result if the skin is exposed to certain chemicals. For example, a chemical burn may leave a permanent scar while exposure to some chemicals can result in permanent loss of skin color or hyperpigmentation.

The major types of adverse dermal effects are (NIOSH 2017):

1. Direct: Exposure to chemicals can cause effects at the point of contact which may include defatting/drying, irritation, corrosion, changes in pigmentation, chloracne, and skin cancer.
   (a) Defatting/drying: The most frequent causes of defatted or dry skin are exposures to soaps, solvents, and moisture. This effect is temporary if the exposure ceases.
   (b) Irritation: Irritation is most frequently caused by fiberglass, food products, oils and lubricants, and solvents. If caught in time, no permanent effects occur.
   (c) Corrosion: A chemical burn can result from a brief exposure to a corrosive substance. Corrosive substances include strong alkali (basic) materials and acids. Scarring is a common outcome. Effects resulting from exposure to corrosives are often permanent.
   (d) Pigmentation changes: A permanent change in skin color may result from exposure to certain chemicals, such as tar and asphalt products and some disinfectants.
   (e) Chloracne: Chloracne is a type of acne caused by certain halogenated aromatic chemicals. It can occur after exposure to polychlorinated hydrocarbons (PCBs) and certain pesticides.
   (f) Skin cancer: Several chemicals found in the workplace contain cancer-producing substances (carcinogens). When these contact the skin, a tumor (benign or malignant) may form at the site of contact. Exposure to coal tar, PCBs, and arsenic are examples. Exposure to ultraviolet (UV) radiation, especially from sunlight-exposed skin, is a major cause of skin cancer in agricultural workers.
2. Systemic: Chemicals that are absorbed across the skin can enter the bloodstream and be distributed throughout the body. They may then cause or contribute to health problems in other tissues or organs in the body. Exposure to organophosphate pesticides, which can enter the body through the skin (intact or broken skin), may cause damage to the nervous system. Liver and kidney damage may occur from exposure to solvents such as toluene and xylene, trichloroethylene, and tetrachloroethylene.
3. Sensitization: Chemicals may cause a sensitization effect, in which an individual becomes unusually susceptible to a chemical or group of chemicals. From then on, exposure to even very small amounts of the substance can cause an allergic reaction. Sensitization effects include allergic contact dermatitis and airway sensitization. Allergic contact dermatitis is an allergic response (immunological response) of the skin because of exposure to a chemical. Examples of chemicals causing allergic contact dermatitis include epoxy resins, chromates, rubber chemicals, amine hardeners, and phenol-formaldehyde resins. An allergic reaction of the mucous membranes or airways may result when the skin is exposed to certain chemicals. Skin exposure, as well as inhalation of isocyanates (contained in many paints, glues, and other building materials, like spray-on insulation and roofing materials), can result in airway sensitization.
4. Combined: Chemical exposure to the skin may cause multiple health effects. For example, contact with cement may result in irritation at the point of contact from the alkaline nature of the cement. In addition, workers may also become sensitized to cement due to the chrome salts present in the material.

To reduce the risk of adverse health effects from chemical exposures to the skin, the exposure must be either prevented or controlled. The use of PPE as described below can help prevent adverse exposures to hazards on the farm. Anytime a person handles chemicals or works around chemical (pesticide) residues, they should wear at least a long-sleeved shirt (fasten the shirt collar completely to protect the lower part of the neck), long pants, socks, and shoes and use eye protection. The product label must be checked to see if it requires wearing chemical-resistant clothing, a coverall (a second layer of clothing), or a chemical-resistant apron over work clothes. If working around physical hazards such as sharp objects or hot materials (such as welding), then appropriate clothing, including heat-resistant/cut-resistant materials should be worn.

Chemical-Resistant Clothing

Different materials are resistant to different substances.

- Water-resistant refers to PPE that keeps a small amount of fine spray particles or small liquid splashes from penetrating the clothing and reaching the skin.
- Waterproof (liquid-proof) material keeps water-soluble materials out, but it may not keep out oil solvent–based products. Waterproof materials include items made of plastic or rubber.
- Chemical-resistant means that no measurable movement of the chemical through the material occurs during a specified period of use.

There are differences among materials in how long they provide protection from a particular chemical. Thin materials, such as disposable plastic gloves, shoe covers, or aprons may provide the necessary protection for only a few minutes. Longer jobs usually require heavier materials. Chemical resistance is often stated in exposure time. For example, neoprene is resistant to acetone for 30 min or less and diesel fuel for more than 4 h. The type of PPE recommended or required is based largely on the type of solvent used in the chemical (in agricultural operations, usually a pesticide) formulation. Workers should always read the chemical labeling to see if it tells which materials are resistant to the chemical product and check the PPE manufacturer's information on the allowable length of exposure to specific chemicals. Cotton, leather, canvas, and other absorbent materials are NOT chemically resistant—even to dry formulations. Powders and dust may move through cotton and other woven materials, and they may remain in the fibers even after several washings. For pesticides that require chemical-resistant PPE, workers should not use a hat that has a cloth or leather sweatband and cloth or cloth-lined gloves, footwear, or aprons. All these materials are difficult or impossible to clean after they have contacted a pesticide. Gloves, boots, aprons, and hoods come in a variety of chemical-resistant materials.

Generally, the best choices of materials are:

- Plastics, such as polyvinyl chloride (PVC)
- Rubber, such as butyl, nitrile, neoprene, or viton rubber Nonwoven fabrics coated with plastic or another barrier material such as Tyvek®

Workers should watch for signs that the material is not chemically resistant to the chemical product being used. Sometimes it is easy to see when plastic or rubber is not resistant to a pesticide or other chemical. The material may change color, become soft or spongy, swell or bubble up, dissolve, turn to a jelly consistency, crack or develop holes, or become stiff or brittle. If any of these changes occur, the item should be discarded and another type of resistant material should be chosen. Another factor to consider is the exposure situation. Chemical-resistant materials do not protect when they become damaged during the chemical-handling task. For tasks that involve handling sharp or pointed objects or walking through rough terrain, workers should select a heavy-duty or sturdy material.

Workers should be aware that the use of chemical-resistant clothing during hot weather can increase the risk of heat stress. Signs to look for include heavy sweating; cold, pale, and clammy skin; fast but weak pulse; nausea or vomiting; muscle cramps; tiredness or weakness; dizziness; headache; and thirst. If these symptoms develop, the worker should leave the area where the chemical is being applied, move to a cool area, remove the chemical-resistant clothing, place cool wet clean cloths on the body or take a cool shower, if possible, rest, and sip water. If symptoms do not resolve, then the worker should call 911 for emergency assistance (CDC 2017).

Coveralls

Coveralls must be loose-fitting, one- or two-piece garments that cover the entire body except the head, eyes, hands, and feet. A coverall can be made of woven (like cotton or twill) or nonwoven fabrics. It should be either easy to clean and sturdy enough for laundering and repeated use or disposable. Wearing a disposable coverall reduces decontamination time and lowers the risk of contaminating the wearer, the application equipment, and the vehicle. Disposable coveralls differ in their level of protection. Most importantly, wearing coveralls lessens the chance that pesticides will be taken home. Workers should handle disposable coveralls carefully so as not to contaminate other people or equipment.

Very few pesticides require a chemical-resistant coverall. If one is required, this usually indicates that the pesticide is very hazardous and extra care is needed to prevent the pesticide from getting on the person using it. When wearing a two-piece outfit, workers should not tuck the shirt or coat in at the waist but should have the shirt extend below the waist of the pants and fit loosely around the hips.

Chemical-Resistant Apron

Workers may consider wearing an apron whenever handling pesticide concentrates. The product label may require the use of a chemical-resistant apron when mixing or loading a pesticide or cleaning application equipment. The apron should extend from the neck to at least the knees. However, an apron can pose a safety hazard when working around equipment with moving parts. If an apron can get caught in machinery or get in the way, workers should wear a chemical-resistant suit instead.

Gloves and Footwear

Pesticide handlers get the most exposure from pesticides on their hands and forearms. Wearing chemical-resistant gloves can reduce exposure of the hands by 99 percent. Most product labels require the use of waterproof or chemical-resistant gloves during handling and mixing activities. Gloves come in many materials. Workers must read the product label to find the right gloves for the product. Pesticide handlers often get pesticides on their feet. Sturdy shoes and socks are sufficient to protect the feet during handling activities that do not require chemical-resistant PPE. When handling pesticide concentrates or making applications or when residues pose a high hazard to your feet, workers should wear waterproof or chemical-resistant footwear. Some product labels require waterproof or chemical-resistant footwear, which could mean shoe covers or boots. If a pesticide is likely to get on the lower legs or feet, chemical-resistant boots that extend past the ankle and at least halfway up to the knee should be worn. Workers should put pant legs outside boots to avoid pesticides running down pants legs and into their boots. Wearing waterproof boots is especially important if entering or walking through treated areas before the spray has dried, such as pesticide applications made to lawns. Use of steel-toed shoes may be appropriate if working with material or equipment that could injure the foot from physical trauma.

Fumigants require especially careful handling due to their high toxicity and chemical behavior in the environment. Like other pesticides, fumigant labels specify the appropriate PPE required to protect the applicator from exposure. In certain fumigants' cases, it may be advisable to not wear gloves or footwear when handling as the gloves and footwear can trap the fumigant gas near the skin and cause burns. Rings, watches, and other tight-fitting jewelry should also be removed.

Other fumigants specify that gloves made of cotton or similar material be worn when handling the product.

Care must be taken to avoid contamination, which often occurs when applicators remove their gloves during an application to adjust the equipment or their PPE, open a pesticide container, or wipe their faces, and then replace the gloves over their contaminated hands. If gloves must be removed during a handling activity, workers should wash the gloves thoroughly before taking them off, wash hands thoroughly and dry them before touching anything, and then put the gloves on again upon returning to work. Another common mistake is putting on footwear with contaminated hands, thereby transferring pesticides from their hands to the feet and socks. To avoid chemicals from running down sleeves and into gloves while performing tasks in which the arms are mostly lowered, workers should place sleeves outside the gloves that go up over the wrist and at least halfway to the elbow. For jobs in which the arms are mostly raised, workers should leave the gloves outside the sleeves and fold the cuff of the gloves up 1 or 2 inches toward the fingers to catch the pesticide before it runs down the arm. For many jobs, the person will be working some of the time with the arms raised and some of the time with them lowered. In these cases, close the glove cuff tightly outside the sleeve and put heavy-duty tape or an elastic band around the end of the glove where it meets the sleeve. Some gloves have a built-in method of tightening the cuff like a strap or string so the pesticide cannot run down the sleeve into the glove.

Hats

For overhead exposure or exposure to a lot of airborne particles, wearing a wide-brimmed hat or chemical-resistant hood can help protect the worker. Plastic safari hats with plastic sweatbands are a good choice because they are relatively cool in hot weather. More flexible hats and hoods are also available in chemical-resistant materials. Hats must not contain absorbent material such as cotton, leather, or straw. Many chemical-resistant jackets or coveralls can be purchased with a protective hood attached. Also, the use of hard hats should be considered if work involves construction activities.

Eye Protection

Eye injuries from dust and particles, chemicals, and exposure to welding light are not uncommon on the farm. Often these injuries occur because workers are not wearing eye protection or using the wrong eye protection. Although some eye injuries are minor, even a simple scratch from wood, cement, or drywall dust can cause significant pain from a damaged cornea. Metal slivers from a grinding wheel or rebounding nails from routine hammering and carpentry can puncture the eye and lead to significant vision impairment, which may be permanent. Welding light can cause "welders' flash" that damages the corneas and surrounding soft tissue. Nearby workers and bystanders are also at risk. Work-related eye injuries can have life-long consequences (NIOSH 2022).

The eyes are very sensitive to chemicals contained in some pesticide formulations, especially concentrates. As a result, some product labels require a handler to wear protective eyewear. Goggles, a face shield, or safety glasses with shields at both the brow and sides are examples of protective eyewear. Some labels specify that a particular type of eye protection must be worn. People who wear contact lenses should consult their ophthalmologist or optometrist before using pesticides to see what the proper eye protection to use is. Shielded safety glasses and full-face shields are good choices in many handling situations because they are comfortable, do not cause fogging or sweating, and give good eye protection. Face shields that are cupped inward toward the throat give better protection from splashes than straight face shields. Goggles should fit tightly against the face if the worker is in an open cab during an air-blast application; applying mists, fogs, or aerosols indoors; or in any other situation in which the person will be exposed to a spray, mist, or dust.

Select goggles made of polycarbonate and that have protected air baffles to avoid fogging. Either goggles or shielded safety glasses can be worn with a half-face respirator. Full-face respirators are supplied with their own face shields, so additional eye protection is not required. Under the revised U.S. EPA Agricultural Worker Protection Standard of 2015 (US EPA 2024), if the label requires goggles for eye protection, then the handler must have immediate access to an eyewash dispenser at all times. Eyewashes can be portable or set in a fixed location such as an eyewash station in a greenhouse. Any user who handles pesticide products that require goggles should have an eyewash readily available. If a pesticide gets past the goggle's protection, any delay in flushing the eye increases the risk of eye damage. Carrying an eyewash dispenser on the worker is recommended because some corrosive and irritant products can cause injury within a few seconds.

NIOSH recommends the following ways to prevent eye injuries (NIOSH 2022):

- Identify eye hazards before starting work.
- Always wear the correct eye protection for those hazards.
- Wear safety glasses marked with "Z87+" on the frame or lenses as an indicator of impact protection (ANSI 2020).
- Use vented goggles for dust, such as cement dust, and non-vented goggles for chemicals.
- Use face shields with safety glasses or goggles for protection from flying objects or chemical splashes.
- When welding, use a welding helmet or goggles with the correct lens shade for the job (shades 10–14 are for arc welding, 4–8 for gas welding, and 3–6 for torch brazing). Helpers and bystanders also need UV protection.
- Take care of the eye protection equipment and replace it when damaged.
- Do not rub the eyes if injured by small particles such as wood, cement or drywall dust, or chemicals. Use the eyewash station. Rinse with clean water for at least 15–20 min and seek medical evaluation if symptoms do not resolve.
- Get medical help for cuts, punctures, and objects in the eyes such as metal slivers, rebounding nails, or wood shavings. Do not wash out the eyes or try to remove objects yourself.

OSHA provides information on selecting eye and face protection depending on the work exposure anticipated (Fig. 4.2).

Notes to Eye and Face Protection Selection Chart

(1) Care should be taken to recognize the possibility of multiple and simultaneous exposure to a variety of hazards. Adequate protection against the highest level of each of the hazards should be provided. Protective devices do not provide unlimited protection.

(2) Operations involving heat may also involve light radiation. As required by the standard, protection from both hazards must be provided.

(3) Face shields should only be worn over primary eye protection (spectacles or goggles).

(4) As required by the standard, filter lenses must meet the requirements for shade designations in § 1915.153(a)(4). Tinted and shaded lenses are not filter lenses unless they are marked or identified as such.

(5) As required by the standard, persons whose vision requires the use of prescription (Rx) lenses must wear either protective devices fitted with prescription (Rx) lenses or designed to be worn over regular prescription (Rx) eyewear.

(6) Wearers of contact lenses must also wear appropriate eye and face protection devices in a hazardous environment. It should be recognized that dusty and/or chemical environments may represent an additional hazard to contact-lens wearers.

(7) Caution should be exercised in the use of metal frame protective devices in electrical hazard areas.

(8) Atmospheric conditions and the restricted ventilation of the protector can cause lenses

EYE AND FACE PROTECTION SELECTION CHART

Source	Assessment of hazard	Protection
Impact:		
Chipping, grinding machining, masonry work, woodworking, sawing, drilling, chiseling, powered fastening, riveting, and sanding	Flying fragments, objects, large chips, particles, sand, dirt, etc	Spectacles with side protection, goggles, face shields. See notes (1), (3), (5), (6), (10). For severe exposure, use face shield.
Heat:		
Furnace operations, pouring, casting, hot dipping, and welding	Hot sparks	Face shields, goggles, spectacles with side protection. For severe exposure use face shield. See notes (1), (2), (3).
	Splash from molten metals	Face shields worn over goggles. See notes (1), (2), (3).
	High temperature exposure	Screen face shields, reflective face shields. See notes (1), (2), (3).
Chemicals:		
Acid and chemicals handling, degreasing, plating	Splash	Goggles, eyecup and cover types. For severe exposure, use face shield. See notes (3), (11).
	Irritating mists	Special-purpose goggles.
Dust:		
Woodworking, buffing, general dusty conditions	Nuisance dust	Goggles, eyecup and cover types. See note (8).
Light and/or Radiation:		
Welding: Electric arc	Optical radiation	Welding helmets or welding shields. Typical shades: 10-14. See notes (9), (12).
Welding: Gas	Optical radiation	Welding goggles or welding face shield. Typical shades: gas welding 4-8, cutting 3-6, brazing 3-4. See note (9).
Cutting, Torch brazing, Torch soldering	Optical radiation	Spectacles or welding face-shield. Typical shades, 1.5-3. See notes (3), (9).
Glare	Poor vision	Spectacles with shaded or special-purpose lenses, as suitable. See notes (9), (10).

Fig. 4.2 OSHA eye and face protection selection chart. (Source: OSHA (USDOL) 2002)

to fog. Frequent cleansing may be necessary.

(9) Welding helmets or face shields should be used only over primary eye protection (spectacles or goggles).

(10) Non-side shield spectacles are available for frontal protection only but are not acceptable eye protection for the sources and operations listed for "impact."

(11) Ventilation should be adequate but well protected from splash entry. Eye and face protection should be designed and used so that it provides both adequate ventilation and protects the wearer from splash entry.

(12) Protection from light radiation is directly related to filter lens density. See note (d). Select the darkest shade that allows task performance.

Figure 4.3 shows examples of safety glasses and goggles frequently used by workers.

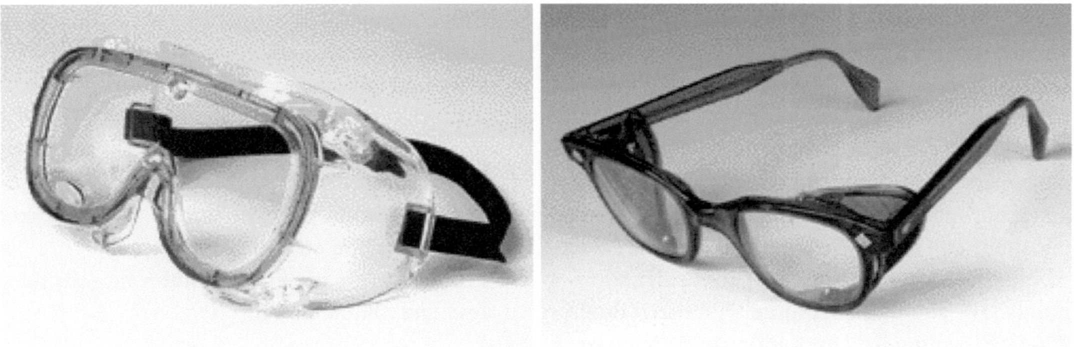

Fig. 4.3 Examples of safety goggles and glasses

Respiratory Protection

Air contaminants can exist in several forms that are dependent on their identity, how the exposure is generated, and their physical form or state of matter. These include particulates, fumes, mists, gases, and vapors (Geddie 2015).

Particulates include dusts, fibers, mists, and fumes. Dusts are generated during the handling, crushing, grinding, detonation, impact, and decrepitation (breaking apart by heat) of solid materials and have a general range of particle sizes ranging from 0.1 to 25 microns (1/25,400 inch) in diameter. The health consequences of dust exposure by inhalation depend on the dust particle size and the toxicity of the material from which the dust is generated. Examples of dusts that are known to produce hazardous health effects include organic dust from grains and raw cotton, inorganic dusts such as crystalline silica and asbestos, and metals such as inorganic lead, nickel, cadmium, and chromium. A fiber is a particle that has a length-to-diameter ratio of 3 to 1 or greater. In the workplace, exposure to fibers can arise from asbestos-containing materials and man-made mineral fibers (MMMF, also referred to as synthetic vitreous fibers (SVF)) such as refractory ceramic fibers, fiberglass (glass wool and glass filament), and mineral wool (Rockwool and slag wool). The concentration of particulates in air is expressed in terms of milligrams per cubic meter (mg/m^3). However, the measured concentration of airborne fibers, especially asbestos fibers, is expressed in fibers per cubic centimeter (f/cc) (Geddie 2015).

A fume is formed when volatilized particles condense in the air during operations such as welding, brazing, and torch cutting. Fume particulates generally have a particle diameter that is less than 1 micron. In most cases, the hot vapor reacts with oxygen in the air to form oxides such as iron oxide fume, zinc oxide fume, and chromium (VI) oxide fume. Mists are suspended liquid droplets generated by the condensation of liquids from vapor back to liquid or breaking up liquid into a dispersed state, for example, by atomization or splashing. Mists may occur in electroplating and pickling operations.

The size of the particulate determines what part of the respiratory system will be affected. Particles that are 10 microns or greater in diameter will be deposited in the upper airways and will not usually impact the alveolar (gas exchange) region of the lungs. These are referred to as non-respirable particles. Particles that are less than 10 microns in diameter (especially 1–5 microns) are small enough to reach the alveolar sacs of the lungs in great quantities and referred to as respirable particles.

Vapors are normally in a non-gaseous state (liquid) at normal temperature and pressure. Vapors can be returned to the liquid state either by lowering the temperature or by increasing the pressure. At room temperature and normal pressure, a gas expands to assume the shape and size of the container it occupies. Unlike vapors, gases can be compressed. Additionally, they can be returned to a liquid state by lowering the temperature and increasing the pressure. The water solubility of gases and vapors influences where in the respiratory tract the effects of exposure occur. Highly water-soluble gases such as ammonia, hydrogen chloride, and hydrogen fluoride will most often cause adverse effects in the upper nasopharynx and mucus membranes, whereas insoluble gases such as nitrogen dioxide and phosgene can readily reach the alveoli. Chlorine, of intermediate solubility, can cause irritation at points all along the respiratory tract (Proctor 2004). Sampling for gases and vapors in the work environment is often performed to determine oxygen content and the presence and concentrations of toxic gases and identify whether explosive levels of gases exist. Gases and vapors are measured in units of parts per million (ppm).

In general, the nose, throat, and lungs are much more absorbent than the skin. Even if a chemical label does not require it, workers should consider wearing a respirator if handling any product for which the label states "do not breathe vapors or spray mist" or "harmful or fatal if inhaled." In addition, advise workers to wear a respirator if exposed to any pesticide that can potentially be inhaled. Some fumigants and a few other pesticide formulations contain a chemical warning additive that alerts the worker when he/she begins to inhale the pesticide. Such warning agents are often used when the pesticide-active ingredient is highly toxic but is not easily detected by smell.

Respirators

Respirators protect the worker from breathing contaminated air. If the job requires the use of a respirator to provide proper protection of the worker, the federal Occupational Safety and Health Administration (OSHA)–developed regulations for a respiratory protection program must be followed. The regulations require these elements (OSHA 2019):

- Written procedures to select the proper respirator for your work site or job
- Medical evaluation to determine the ability to use a respirator
- Fit testing for tight-fitting respirators
- Procedures for the proper use of respirators in routine work and emergency situations
- Care and maintenance of respirators
- Procedures to ensure adequate air quality, quantity, and flow of breathing air for supplied-air respirators
- Training on hazard recognition, dangers, and proper use and care of respirators
- Program evaluation on respirator fit, selection, use, and maintenance

The National Institute for Occupational Safety and Health (NIOSH), a part of the Centers for Disease Control and Prevention (CDC) in the U.S. Department of Health and Human Services (DHHS), is the federal agency responsible for testing and certifying respirators used with pesticides (and other non-mining respiratory protection needs). Approval numbers beginning with the letters TC (Tested and Certified) are assigned to all respirators reviewed by the agency and must be on the box containing the facepiece. Pesticide product labels often specify the type of respirator required by listing its TC number. In addition, filters are classified based on filter efficiency and how well they resist oil. There are three classification levels for oil degradation: N, not oil-resistant; R, oil-resistant; and P, oil-proof. The filter efficiency for each classification level may be 95, 99, or 100 percent. For example, R-95 refers to a filter that is oil-resistant (R) and 95% efficient in removing particles from the air you breathe.

Workers must always follow the manufacturer's instructions when operating any respirator. Two major groups of respirators, air-supplying and air-purifying, are used when dealing with pesticides:

- Air-supplying respirators: Air-supplying respirators provide clean, uncontaminated air from an outside source. They are used in low-oxygen environments and are generally more expensive. There are two types of air-supplying respirators:
  - Supplied-air respirators pump clean air through a hose. This limits the distance the applicator can go from the air source.
  - Self-contained breathing apparatus (SCBA) supplies clean air from cylinders carried by

the applicator. These allow more movement but are often heavy and contain a limited air supply and require additional training for use.

- Air-purifying respirators: Air-purifying respirators use physical and chemical filters (cartridges) to trap and remove contaminants as they pass through the respirator (Fig. 4.4). Filters and cartridges are chemical-specific or dust/mist-specific. A combination of chemical and dust/mist cartridges is also available. When handling some pesticides, an organic vapor (OV) cartridge is required. Pesticide labels provide guidance on which type of filters or cartridges to use. Adequate oxygen must be present in the air because this type of respirator filters the surrounding air. Air-purifying devices may be powered or non-powered:
  - Powered air-purifying respirators (PAPR) use a blower to move the contaminated air through a purifying filter and can be used with either a tight-fitting facepiece or a loose-fitting hood.
  - Non-powered devices can be either half-mask or full-face devices that place a filtration unit between the breathing passage and the contaminated air source.

Proper Respirator Use

When a pesticide label requires a respirator, workers must wear a NIOSH-approved respirator for use with that specific pesticide. Different pesticides or different formulations may require different types of respirators. A single type of respirator does not adequately protect from every pesticide or formulation that may be used.

To work properly and provide the necessary protection, a respirator must fit tightly. The fit test is a method used to select the right-size respirator for the user. OSHA's Respiratory Protection Standard requires a fit test prior to initial use of a respirator, whenever a different respirator facepiece is used, and at least annually thereafter. An additional fit test is required whenever there are changes in the user's physical condition that could affect respirator fit (for example, facial scarring, dental changes, cosmetic surgery, or an obvious change in body weight). A full-facemask respirator may be necessary if glasses interfere with the fit of a half facemask. Special glasses can be purchased that fit inside a full facemask. All employees using either a negative or positive pressure, tight-fitting, facepiece respirator must pass an appropriate fit test.

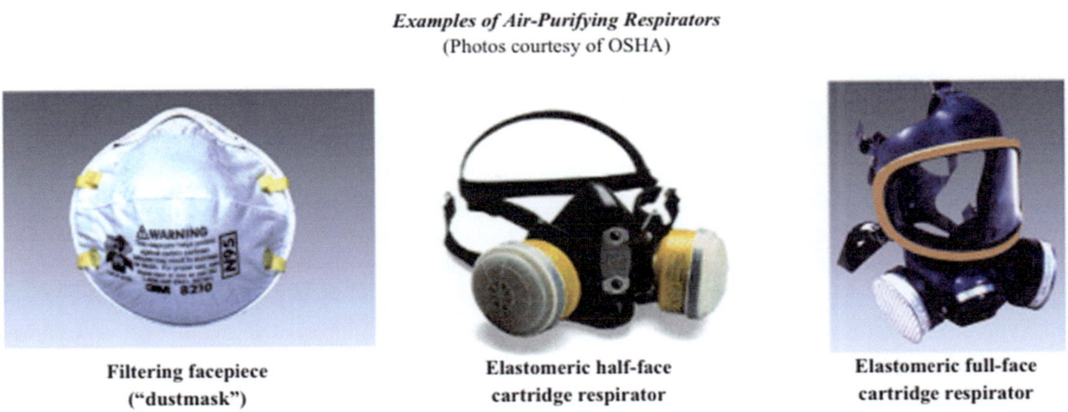

Fig. 4.4 Examples of air-purifying respirators. (Source: OSHA (USDOL))

Medical Clearance for Respirator Use

Medical clearance is required by the U.S. EPA prior to completing a respirator fit test for individuals subject to Risk Mitigation Measures for Soil Fumigants and the Worker Protection Standard and the Occupational Safety and Health Administration when respirators are required by agricultural operations having more than 10 full-time employees. Although medical clearance is not required for other respirator uses in agriculture, it is highly recommended (NCAI 2024). A physician or other licensed healthcare professional (PLHCP) must perform the medical evaluation using OSHA's respirator medical evaluation questionnaire or an initial medical exam that obtains the same information as the OSHA questionnaire. This questionnaire can be found on the OSHA website: https://www.osha.gov/sites/default/files/publications/OSHA3790.pdf. An example of the questionnaire is included in Fig. 4.5.

As noted by OSHA, the purpose of a medical evaluation program is to determine if employees can tolerate the physiological burden associated with respirator use, including the burden imposed by the respirator itself (e.g., its weight and breathing resistance during both normal operation and under conditions of filter, canister, or cartridge overload); musculoskeletal stress (e.g., when the respirator to be worn is an SCBA); limitations on auditory, visual, and olfactory sensations; and isolation from the workplace environment. Because certain jobs and workplace conditions in which a respirator is used can also impose a physiological burden on the user, the employer must provide the following information to the PLHCP before or at the time of evaluation:

- Type of respirator used
- Frequency of use
- Duration of use
- Physical demands while wearing a respirator
- Environmental conditions (e.g., heat)
- Other protective equipment worn

While most persons are able to wear a respirator, there are physiologic consequences to the use of respirators that the healthcare provider should be aware of including:

- Pulmonary effects:
  - Increased breathing resistance
  - Increased work on breathing
  - Decreased endurance
  - Decrease in exercise performance
- Cardiac effects:
  - Increased cardiac work
  - Increased heart rate
  - Increased blood pressure

In addition, there are medical conditions that may increase the risks from wearing respirators that should be considered when evaluating a person (ATS 1996; NCAI 2024; OSHA 1999). Examples of medical conditions that may warrant clearance with restrictions, follow-up medical exam, or denial of clearance include but are not limited to:

- Cardiovascular: hypertension, myocardial infarction, angina, cerebrovascular accident, and dysrhythmia
- Respiratory: chronic obstructive pulmonary disease (chronic bronchitis and emphysema), decreased pulmonary function, asthma, tuberculosis, lung cancer, asbestosis, and silicosis
- Neurological: tinnitus, impaired sense of smell/taste, and seizure disorder
- Psychological: claustrophobia, and severe anxiety
- Musculoskeletal: arthritis, lack of dexterity in hands, upper extremity amputation, and chronic back pain
- Other: facial deformities, poorly controlled diabetes mellitus, and perforated eardrum

A follow-up physical evaluation is required for anyone who gives a positive response to any of questions 1–8 of the mandatory OSHA questionnaire and can be given at the PLHCP's discretion. The respirator standard requires the employer to medically reevaluate an employee under certain circumstances. This is required when the employee reports medical signs or symptoms that are related to the employee's abil-

OSHA INFOSHEET

Respirator Medical Evaluation Questionnaire

Respirators must be used in workplaces in which employees are exposed to hazardous airborne contaminants. When respiratory protection is required employers must have a respirator protection program as specified in OSHA's Respiratory Protection standard (29 CFR 1910.134). Before wearing a respirator, workers must first be medically evaluated using the mandatory medical questionnaire or an equivalent method. To facilitate these medical evaluations, this INFOSHEET includes the mandatory medical questionnaire to be used for these evaluations.

Medical Evaluation and Questionnaire Requirements

The requirements of the medical evaluation and for using the questionnaire are provided below:

- The employer must identify a physician or other licensed health care professional (PLHCP) to perform all medical evaluations using the medical questionnaire in Appendix C of the Respiratory Protection standard or a medical examination that obtains the same information. (See Paragraph (e)(2)(i).)
- The medical evaluation must obtain the information requested in Sections 1 and 2, Part A of Appendix C. The questions in Part B of Appendix C may be added at the discretion of the health care professional. (See Paragraph (e)(2)(ii).)
- The employer must ensure that a follow-up medical examination is provided for any employee who gives a positive response to any question among questions 1 through 8 in Part A Section 2, of Appendix C, or whose initial medical examination demonstrates the need for a follow-up medical examination. The employer must provide the employee with an opportunity to discuss the questionnaire and examination results with the PLHCP. (See Paragraph (e)(3)(i).)
- The medical questionnaire and examinations must be administered confidentially during the employee's normal working hours or at a time and place convenient to the employee and in a manner that ensures that he or she understands its content. The employer must not review the employee's responses, and the questionnaire must be provided directly to the PLHCP. (See Paragraph (e)(4)(i).)

Excerpt from Appendix C of 29 CFR 1910.134:
OSHA Respirator Medical Evaluation Questionnaire

To the employer: Answers to questions in Section 1, and to question 9 in Section 2 of Part A, do not require a medical examination.

To the employee: Your employer must allow you to answer this questionnaire during normal working hours, or at a time and place that is convenient to you. To maintain your confidentiality, your employer or supervisor must not look at or review your answers, and your employer must tell you how to deliver or send this questionnaire to the health care professional who will review it.

Once filled out, this form must be given to the PLHCP. This form should **not** be submitted to OSHA.

1

Fig. 4.5 OSHA's respirator medical evaluation questionnaire from https://www.osha.gov/sites/default/files/publications/OSHA3790.pdf

Part A Section 1. (Mandatory) The following information must be provided by every employee who has been selected to use any type of respirator (please print).

1. Today's date:
2. Your name:
3. Your age (to nearest year):
4. Sex (circle one): Male/Female
5. Your height: ft. in.
6. Your weight: lbs.
7. Your job title:
8. A phone number where you can be reached by the health care professional who reviews this questionnaire (include the Area Code):
9. The best time to phone you at this number:
10. Has your employer told you how to contact the health care professional who will review this questionnaire (circle one): Yes/No
11. Check the type of respirator you will use (you can check more than one category):

    a. ___ N, R, or P disposable respirator (filter-mask, non-cartridge type only).

    b. ___ Other type (for example, half- or full-facepiece type, powered-air purifying, supplied-air, self-contained breathing apparatus).

12. Have you worn a respirator (circle one): Yes/No If "yes," what type(s):

Part A. Section 2. (Mandatory) Questions 1 through 9 below must be answered by every employee who has been selected to use any type of respirator (please circle "yes" or "no").

	YES	NO
1. Do you *currently* smoke tobacco, or have you smoked tobacco in the last month?	☐	☐
2. Have you *ever had* any of the following conditions?	☐	☐
a. Seizures	☐	☐
b. Diabetes (sugar disease)	☐	☐
c. Allergic reactions that interfere with your breathing	☐	☐
d. Claustrophobia (fear of closed-in places)	☐	☐
e. Trouble smelling odors	☐	☐
3. Have you *ever had* any of the following pulmonary or lung problems?	☐	☐
a. Asbestosis	☐	☐
b. Asthma	☐	☐

2

Fig 4.5 (continued)

	YES	NO
c. Chronic bronchitis	☐	☐
d. Emphysema	☐	☐
e. Pneumonia	☐	☐
f. Tuberculosis	☐	☐
g. Silicosis	☐	☐
h. Pneumothorax (collapsed lung)	☐	☐
i. Lung cancer	☐	☐
j. Broken ribs	☐	☐
k. Any chest injuries or surgeries	☐	☐
l. Any other lung problem that you've been told about	☐	☐
4. Do you *currently* have any of the following symptoms of pulmonary or lung illness?	☐	☐
a. Shortness of breath	☐	☐
b. Shortness of breath when walking fast on level ground or walking up a slight hill or incline	☐	☐
c. Shortness of breath when walking with other people at an ordinary pace on level ground	☐	☐
d. Have to stop for breath when walking at your own pace on level ground	☐	☐
e. Shortness of breath when washing or dressing yourself	☐	☐
f. Shortness of breath that interferes with your job	☐	☐
g. Coughing that produces phlegm (thick sputum)	☐	☐
h. Coughing that wakes you early in the morning	☐	☐
i. Coughing that occurs mostly when you are lying down	☐	☐
j. Coughing up blood in the last month	☐	☐
k. Wheezing	☐	☐
l. Wheezing that interferes with your job	☐	☐
m. Chest pain when you breathe deeply	☐	☐
n. Any other symptoms that you think may be related to lung problems	☐	☐
5. Have you *ever had* any of the following cardiovascular or heart problems?		
a. Heart attack	☐	☐
b. Stroke	☐	☐
c. Angina	☐	☐
d. Heart failure	☐	☐

3

Fig 4.5 (continued)

		YES	NO
	e. Swelling in your legs or feet (not caused by walking)	☐	☐
	f. Heart arrhythmia (heart beating irregularly)	☐	☐
	g. High blood pressure	☐	☐
	h. Any other heart problem that you've been told about	☐	☐
6.	Have you *ever had* any of the following cardiovascular or heart symptoms?	☐	☐
	a. Frequent pain or tightness in your chest	☐	☐
	b. Pain or tightness in your chest during physical activity	☐	☐
	c. Pain or tightness in your chest that interferes with your job	☐	☐
	d. In the past two years, have you noticed your heart skipping or missing a beat	☐	☐
	e. Heartburn or indigestion that is not related to eating	☐	☐
	f. Any other symptoms that you think may be related to heart or circulation problems	☐	☐
7.	Do you *currently* take medication for any of the following problems?	☐	☐
	a. Breathing or lung problems	☐	☐
	b. Heart trouble	☐	☐
	c. Blood pressure	☐	☐
	d. Seizures	☐	☐
8.	If you've used a respirator, have you *ever had* any of the following problems? (If you've never used a respirator, check the following space and go to question 9.) ☐	☐	☐
	a. Eye irritation	☐	☐
	b. Skin allergies or rashes	☐	☐
	c. Anxiety	☐	☐
	d. General weakness or fatigue	☐	☐
	e. Any other problem that interferes with your use of a respirator	☐	☐
9.	Would you like to talk to the health care professional who will review this questionnaire about your answers to this questionnaire?	☐	☐

Questions 10 to 15 below must be answered by every employee who has been selected to use either a full-facepiece respirator or a self-contained breathing apparatus (SCBA). For employees who have been selected to use other types of respirators, answering these questions is voluntary.

		YES	NO
10.	Have you *ever* lost vision in either eye (temporarily or permanently)?	☐	☐
11.	Do you *currently* have any of the following vision problems?	☐	☐
	a. Wear contact lenses	☐	☐
	b. Wear glasses	☐	☐
	c. Color blind	☐	☐
	d. Any other eye or vision problem	☐	☐

4

Fig 4.5 (continued)

	YES	NO
12. Have you *ever had* an injury to your ears, including a broken eardrum?	☐	☐
13. Do you *currently* have any of the following hearing problems?	☐	☐
a. Difficulty hearing	☐	☐
b. Wear a hearing aid	☐	☐
c. Any other hearing or ear problem	☐	☐
14. Have you *ever had* a back injury?	☐	☐
15. Do you *currently* have any of the following musculoskeletal problems?	☐	☐
a. Weakness in any of your arms, hands, legs, or feet	☐	☐
b. Back pain	☐	☐
c. Difficulty fully moving your arms and legs	☐	☐
d. Pain and stiffness when you lean forward or backward at the waist	☐	☐
e. Difficulty fully moving your head up or down	☐	☐
f. Difficulty fully moving your head side to side	☐	☐
g. Difficulty bending at your knees	☐	☐
h. Difficulty squatting to the ground	☐	☐
i. Climbing a flight of stairs or a ladder carrying more than 25 lbs.	☐	☐
j. Any other muscle or skeletal problem that interferes with using a respirator	☐	☐

This infosheet does not include the questions in Part B because they are not mandatory; rather, they may be added to the questionnaire at the discretion of the health care professional who will review the questionnaire.

OSHA Educational Materials

OSHA has an extensive publications program. For a listing of free items, visit OSHA's web site at www.osha.gov/publications or contact the OSHA Publications Office, U.S. Department of Labor, 200 Constitution Avenue, N.W., N-3101, Washington, DC 20210. Telephone (202) 693-1888 or fax to (202) 693-2498.

Contacting OSHA

To report an emergency, file a complaint or seek OSHA advice, assistance or products, call (800) 321-OSHA (6742) or contact your nearest OSHA regional, area, or State Plan office; TTY: 1-877-889-5627.

This InfoSheet is not a standard or regulation, and it creates no new legal obligations. It contains recommendations as well as descriptions of mandatory safety and health standards. The recommendations are advisory in nature, informational in content, and are intended to assist employers in providing a safe and healthful workplace. The *Occupational Safety and Health Act* requires employers to comply with safety and health standards and regulations promulgated by OSHA or by a state with an OSHA-approved state plan. In addition, the Act's General Duty Clause, Section 5(a)(1), requires employers to provide their employees with a workplace free from recognized hazards likely to cause death or serious physical harm.

U.S. Department of Labor

OSHA® Occupational Safety and Health Administration

DTSEM OSHA 3790-05 2015

Fig 4.5 (continued)

ity to use a respirator; a PLHCP, supervisor, or the respirator program administrator observes that the employee is having a medical problem during respirator use, and they inform the employee of their observation; information from the respiratory protection program, including observations made during fit testing and program evaluation, indicates a need for employee reevaluation; or a change occurs in workplace conditions (e.g., physical work effort, type of respirator used, protective clothing, or temperature) that may result in a substantial increase in the physiological burden placed on an employee.

The employer must obtain a written opinion from the PLHCP regarding whether the employee is medically able to wear a respirator. The opinion must identify any limitations on the employee's use of the respirator, as well as the need for any follow-up medical evaluations that are necessary to assist the PLHCP in making a recommendation about respirator use. The employee must also receive a copy of the PLHCP's written opinion. In some circumstances, it may be appropriate for the PLHCP to approve the person to use a positive pressure respirator instead of a negative pressure respirator. The employer must provide the employee with a powered air-purifying respirator (PAPR) if information from the medical evaluation indicates that the employee can use a PAPR but not a negative pressure respirator. Approval for the use of self-contained breathing apparatus (SCBA) may require more extensive medical evaluation.

Here is an example of a recommendation form that the PLHCP provides to the employer (Fig. 4.6):

After the employee receives medical clearance, the employee can be fit-tested with the respirator(s) that will be used for protection. The fit test used depends on the type of respirator and the relative workplace exposure level. There are both qualitative and quantitative fit tests:

- Qualitative fit test: A worker is exposed to an atmosphere ("tent") containing an odorant, irritant, or taste agent and then asked to breathe normally and deeply, move the head from side to side and up and down, grimace, bend at the waist, and talk. The wearer reports any noticeable odor or taste agent that leaks into the mask.
- Quantitative fit test: Quantitative fit test (QNFT) methods generate a numerical assessment of respirator fit.

Employees must also receive training on the proper use of the respirator for which they have been fit tested. Every time a respirator is put on, a fit check should be conducted (also referred to as a user seal check) to be sure the respirator forms a complete seal around the face, and air cannot leak in or out along the edges. There are two types of fit checks: "Positive pressure" refers to the user breathing out and exerting positive pressure on the respirator, and "negative pressure" refers to the user breathing in and exerting negative pressure on the respirator. The fit check must be performed before using a respirator in the field and may also be performed periodically while in the field.

- Positive pressure check: Cover the exhalation valve with your hand and exhale gently into the facepiece. If a slight positive pressure is built up inside the facepiece without any evidence of leakage, the fit is satisfactory. This method is the most widely used to check proper fit in the field.
- Negative pressure check: Close off the air inlet valves (cover the cartridges with your hands), inhale gently to collapse the facepiece slightly, and hold your breath for 10 s. If the facepiece remains slightly collapsed and no leakage is detected, the respirator fits properly. It may be difficult to get a good seal when trying to cover the inlet valves (cartridges).

Most respirator styles will not protect a person with a beard or other facial hair because the respirator will not seal properly against the face. If the person has facial hair, use a powered particulate respirator (TC-21C) that constantly pumps air through a cartridge or canister into a loose-fitting helmet- or hood-like head covering. The positive outward pressure caused by the steady outflow of air prevents contaminants from enter-

Respirator Medical Clearance Form

Empolyee's Name_____________________Date of Birth____________

Employer's Name_____________________Employer's phone number____________

Type of respirator use requested (circle): Disposable, Negative pressure, PAPR, Airline, SCBA

The above referenced employee was evaluated on _______(date) for medical fitness to wear a respirator in the performance of his/her job.

A. The employee is given medical clearance to use the following respirator(s):

______N,R,P disposable respirator (filter mask, non-cartridge type ex. N-95)

______Negative pressure air-purifying (cartridge) respirator (either half or full face)

______Powered air purifying (PAPR) respirator (either half or full face)

______Supplied air (air line) respirator

______Self contained breathing apparatus (SCBA)

When using respirators, the employee is approved to perform the following:

_____ Normal job duties

______Escape only

______Restricted duties (describe)____

B. The employee is not given medical clearance for respirator use because more information is needed:

_____1. A medical examination including physical evaluation and other tests as deemed appropriate by a licensed health care professional is needed to make a decision.

_____2. The following additional information is needed for review (specify what)"

Fig. 4.6 Health recommendation form for respirator use

Comments:____

This respirator clearance is valid (based on PLHCP opinion) for:

___1 year from date of evaluation

___2 years from date of evaluation

___Until a change occurs in employee's medical condition

Signature of Physician or Licensed Health Care Professional

Print Name

Name of Clinic (if different)____________________________________

Street Address____

City/State/Zip code____

Phone number____

Remember to provide a copy to the individual and to the employer

Fig. 4.6 (continued)

ing the headpiece. The purified air circulating over the user's head, face, and neck also provides some cooling. Because those loose-fitting respirators do not have to form a seal on the face, they do not need a medical or fit test. Not all loose-fitting respirators move the air at the same rate. Most pesticide-handling tasks require a minimum airflow rate of 4 cubic feet per minute. If performing physically strenuous work, workers should use a respirator with an airflow rate of at least 6 cubic feet per minute. If wearing a respirator that filters out dust and mists, workers should change the filter or respirator when it is getting hard to breathe through the respirator or if the filter gets torn, damaged, or wet. Workers should not use a filtering facepiece dust/mist mask if the pesticide soaks the mask. In this case, they should use a full-face respirator.

If wearing a respirator that removes vapors and gases, the cartridge or canister should be changed immediately if one notes a taste or smells pesticide or if the pesticide burns or stings the nose or throat. Workers should follow the manufacturer's instructions on when to replace filters, cartridges, and canisters even if no problem is noticed. If there are no instructions, workers should contact the cartridge manufacturer or adopt a change-out schedule that avoids cartridge "breakthrough" and the symptoms indicated above. Generally, most cartridges are limited to less than 8 h of use. However, canisters generally provide more than 8 h of protection. To ensure the integrity of the seal between the facemask and the cartridge, workers should make sure the manufacturer of the cartridge is also the manufacturer of the facemask.

Hearing Protection

Occupational hearing loss is one of the most pervasive problems in today's occupational environment, affecting workers in manufacturing, construction, transportation, agriculture, and the military. Occupational hearing loss can occur when you are exposed to loud noise or ototoxic chemicals while at work. At the present exposure limits established by OSHA, one in four will develop permanent hearing loss as a result of their occupational exposure to these hazards. Exposure to loud noise and ototoxic chemicals can lead to more than just hearing damage. Research shows that hearing loss is associated with cognitive decline and heart problems. Hearing loss and tinnitus can also impact mental health, which may result in depression, anxiety, and a feeling of isolation and sadness. Hearing loss can impact safety at home and on the job. The sound of a smoke detector, the warning beep as a forklift backs up, and the engine of an oncoming car may be missed. Workers with hearing loss are more likely to get injured on the job. Working in a noisy job if pregnant can increase stress levels, which can impact the health of a developing fetus. Despite decades of OSHA-mandated hearing protection device use, noise-induced hearing loss (NIHL) remains highly prevalent.

Ototoxic Chemicals

Exposure to certain chemicals can cause damage to different parts of the ear, especially the inner-ear hair cells. These chemicals are called ototoxicants or "ototoxic chemicals" (NIOSH (a) 2023). Exposure to ototoxic chemicals can cause hearing loss. Sometimes, exposure to chemicals can make ears more sensitive to the harmful effects of noise. Examples of chemicals that damage hearing are:

- Solvents (e.g., toluene, styrene, xylene, ethylbenzene, and trichloroethylene)
- Metals and compounds (e.g., mercury compounds, lead, and organic tin compounds)
- Asphyxiants (e.g., carbon monoxide, hydrogen cyanide and its salts, and tobacco smoke)
- Nitriles (e.g., 3-butenenitrile, cis-2-pentenenitrile, and acrylonitrile)
- Pharmaceuticals (e.g., certain antineoplastic drugs)
- Pesticides

Exposure to other workplace hazards (such as noise) and other individual factors (such as age and smoking status) also influence the effect chemicals have on hearing.

Noise

Decibels (dB) are a scale for measuring noise and the A-weighted noise level or dBA is used to predict hearing risk (NOISH (c) 2023). Noise is considered loud (hazardous) when it reaches 85 dBA or higher. Most hearing loss occurs slowly over time. Symptoms of hearing loss include:

- Having difficulty hearing when there is background noise
- Thinking people are mumbling when they talk to you
- Needing to ask others to repeat themselves often
- Suffering from tinnitus (an annoying buzzing, rushing, or ringing noise in your ears or in your head)

Personal Hearing Protection Devices (HPDs)

In the absence of feasible engineering or administrative controls, personal hearing protection devices (HPDs, also referred to as hearing protectors) remain the only means of preventing hazardous noise levels from damaging one's hearing. All HPDs sold in the United States are evaluated in a test laboratory and labeled with a noise reduction rating (NRR). However, studies have repeatedly demonstrated that the NRR does not accurately predict noise reduction performance for an individual in the workplace. Research shows that most workers achieve less than half of the sound attenuation predicted by the NRR. The difference between the NRR and actual worker attenuation varies widely across different types of protectors and ear canal sizes and shapes. Personal hearing protector fit-testing can determine how much noise reduction an individual receives and ensure that each worker is sufficiently protected from excessive noise.

Hearing protection comes in many styles, materials, colors, and sizes (Fig. 4.7). The main types of hearing protectors include (NIOSH (National Institute for Occupational Safety and Health) 1996):

- Earplugs: Devices which slide snugly into the ear canal. Earplugs can be formable (such as foam, which expands to fit the contour of the canal), preformed (which is already shaped to fit most ears), or custom (which uses an impression of the worker's ear to make a device uniquely fitted to that person).
- Earmuffs: Devices that completely surround the outer ear and are held in place by a headband or attached to a hard hat.
- Canal caps: Devices that cover the entrance to the ear canals and are held in place by a lightweight band.

In choosing an HPD, the noise exposure level is the most basic consideration. The majority of workers need 10 dB or less of a sound reduction to bring their exposure down to a safe level. When fitted correctly, almost any HPD can reduce noise by 10 dB. Keep the following guidelines in mind (NIOSH (d) 2023):

- Aim for just enough noise reduction to bring exposure down to 75–85 dBA.
- Avoid overprotection. Too much sound reduction can make workers feel isolated and less aware of their surroundings. Workers might take off their hearing protectors to hear someone speak or listen to equipment.
- Provide double hearing protection (earmuffs over earplugs) for workers exposed to noise levels of 100 dBA or greater or impulse sounds.
- Fit test workers to make sure their hearing protectors are providing the right level of noise reduction.

The correct use of personal hearing protection has a critical impact on hearing loss prevention. Workers must recognize the importance of wearing their hearing protectors whenever they are exposed to hazardous noise. Following manufacturers' instructions and use of hearing protection correctly is just as important as wearing a hearing protector consistently. The differences between the maximum protection theoretically possible and the protection usually obtained in the "real world" are influenced by many factors. A worker's failure to correctly insert an earplug or adjust an earmuff is among the main reasons responsible for diminished real-world hearing protection. Thus, even if the worker has been issued a correctly sized hearing protector and trained in its use and care, it is quite possible that he or she could receive little or no effective hearing protection because of faulty fit. Workers must wear their hearing protection correctly, or they will greatly reduce its ability to prevent harmful noise from damaging their hearing.

Monitor Worker Hearing

Regular testing of workers' hearing is the most effective means of ascertaining that hearing loss is being prevented. Audiometry is a hearing test that measures the lowest level of sound a person can hear (called thresholds) across a range of frequencies (pitches). An audiogram is a graph of hearing thresholds at various frequencies in each ear. Thresholds that are 25-dB hearing level or better (lower) are considered normal for adults. Noise exposure initially affects hearing most at frequencies around 3000–6000 Hz, creating a "notch" in the audiogram, characteristically at 4000 Hz. NIOSH recommends annual audiometric testing for workers exposed to noise above the recommended exposure level (REL) of 85 dBA. Figure 4.8 is an example of a questionnaire to use in evaluation of workers with noise exposure.

Results of annual hearing tests should be compared with results from the baseline hearing test to check for significant threshold shift (STS). NIOSH considers a 15-dB change in hearing

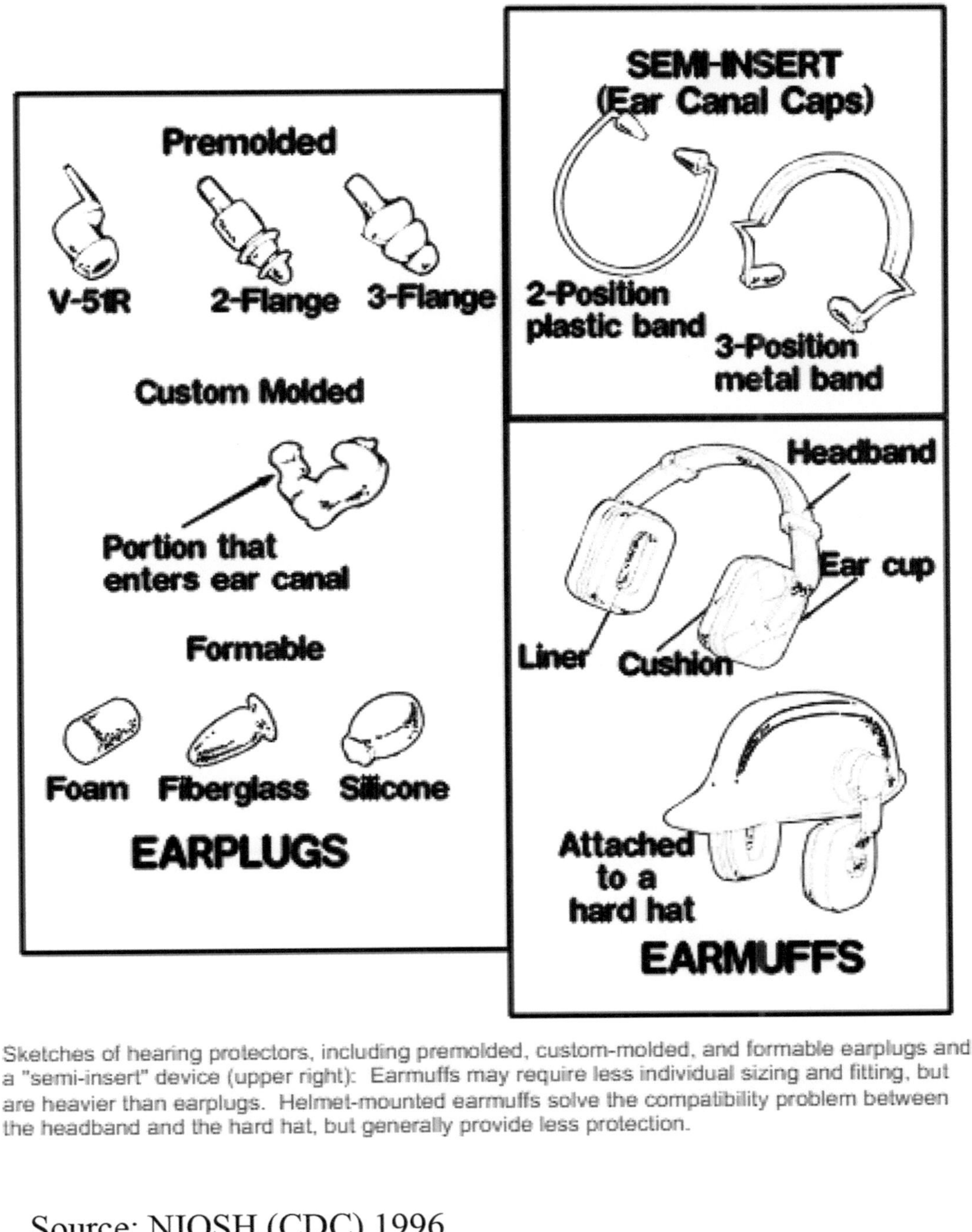

Fig. 4.7 Example of hearing protection devices. (Source: NIOSH (National Institute for Occupational Safety and Health) 1996)

Audiometric and Identification Information

Name ______________________________

Soc. Sec. # ____-__-____ Birth Date __/__/__ Gender M F (Circle)

Empl No: ____________ Job Code ____________ Dept No ____________

Test Date __/__/__ Time __:__ Test Type _____ Time since last exposure _____ h

Exposure Level ___ dBA

Hearing Protector Activity

Yes _____ No _____

Issue _____

Reissue _____

Training _____

Retraining _____

Hearing Protector Used (Circle)

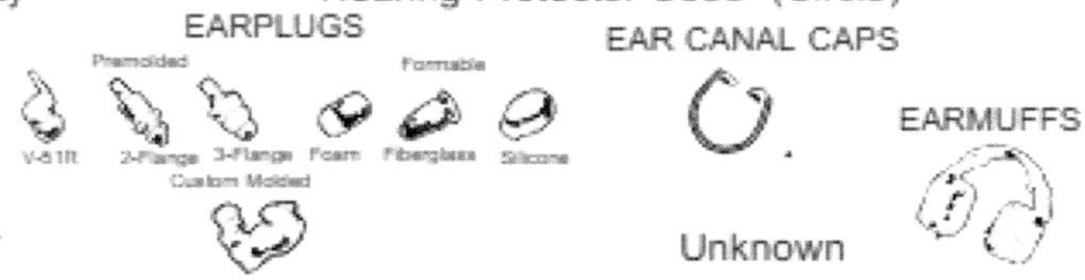

Self-Reported Employee Histories

(Y/N) Medical History

____ Diabetes
____ Ear Surgery
____ Head Injury
____ High Fever
____ Measles
____ Mumps
____ Hypertension
____ Ringing in Ears
____ Ear Infection
____ Other

(Y/N) Hobby & Military History

____ Hunt/Shoot
____ Car racing
____ Motorcycles
____ Other Loud Vehicles
____ Loud Music/Band
____ Power Tools
____ Other Noisy Hobbies
____ Military Service
____ Fire Weapon
____ Other

(Y/N) Additional Information

____ Noisy 2nd Job
____ Noisy Past Job
____ Exposure to Solvents
____ Exposure to Metals
____ Difficulty Hearing
____ Hearing Aid
____ Recent Change in Hearing
____ See Physician About Ears
____ See Prior Histories
____ Other

Audiogram

Test Frequency

	500	1000	2000	3000	4000	6000	8000
Right Ear							
Left Ear							

Audiometer ____________________

Exhaustive Cal. Date __/__/__

Tester Identificaiton ___-__-____

Review Identification ___-__-____

Serial Number ____________________

Biological Cal. Date __/__/__

Test Reliability (Good, Fair, Poor) __

Audiogram Classification Code __ __ __

Comments ______________________________

Source: NIOSH (CDC) 1996

Fig. 4.8 Questionnaire evaluating worker. (Source: NIOSH (National Institute for Occupational Safety and Health) 1996)

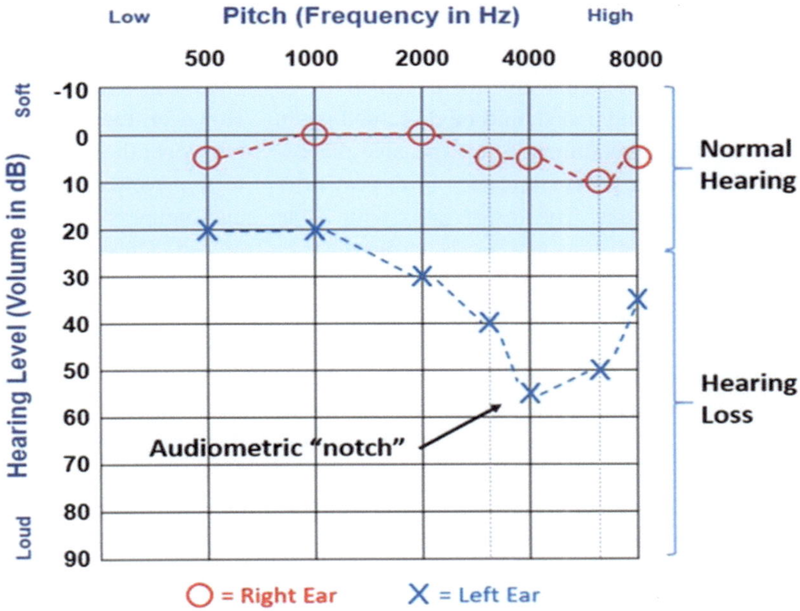

Fig. 4.9 Audiogram demonstrating noise-induced hearing loss

threshold at any frequency to represent an STS. If an STS is noted during an annual hearing test, the worker should be retested within 30 days to confirm. Like the baseline audiogram, workers should have at least a 12-hour quiet period before a confirmation test to tell whether the shift was temporary or permanent.

Workers who develop an STS—whether temporary or permanent—should be notified, and steps should be taken to prevent further damage to hearing. These steps could include refitting with hearing protection, additional training on noise exposure, or if possible, reassignment to a quieter area.

Figure 4.9 is an example of an audiogram demonstrating an individual with an asymmetric noise-induced hearing loss (in this case, a right-handed farmer who liked to shoot guns but without consistent use of hearing protection). The audiogram shows normal hearing thresholds (<25 dBA) in the right ear. The left ear shows normal low-frequency thresholds and mild-to-moderate hearing loss in the higher frequencies with a notch (4000 Hz) consistent with noise exposure.

Maintaining Personal Protective Equipment

When finished with an activity involving handling chemicals or if exposed to them, workers should clean the outside of the PPE as much as practical before removing it. They can start by washing the outside of the gloves with detergent and water while wearing them, and washing the outside of other chemical-resistant items before removing the gloves. This practice helps avoid contacting the contaminated part of the items while removing them, thus keeping the inside surface from becoming contaminated. If any other clothes have pesticides on them, change them also. Workers need to determine whether contaminated items should be disposed of or cleaned for reuse. Some cities/counties have household hazardous waste disposal sites or collection days. It is also a good idea to check with the County Cooperative Extension Center for local disposal alternatives.

Disposables

Disposable PPE items are not designed to be cleaned or reused and should be discarded when they become contaminated. Inexpensive disposables may be a good choice for brief pesticide-handling activities. The instructions with some coated nonwoven suits and hoods permit the user to wear them more than once if each use period is short and not much pesticide gets on them. When reusing these items, workers should be ready to change them whenever there are signs (such as holes in the material or obvious deterioration) that pesticides could be getting through the material or the inside surface is contaminated. Dust/mist masks, prefilters, canisters, filtering, and vapor-removing cartridges cannot be cleaned and are disposable items.

Reusables

Some PPE items, such as rubber and plastic suits, gloves, boots, aprons, capes, and headgear, are designed to be cleaned and reused several times. Reusable items should be washed thoroughly between uses and inspected for signs of wear or abrasion. Contaminated gloves, boots, respirators, or other PPE should never be washed in streams, ponds, or other bodies of water. Workers can check for rips and leaks by filling the PPE item with water to form a "balloon" and/or holding transparent items up to the light. Even tiny holes or thin places can allow large quantities of chemicals to penetrate the material and reach the skin. Workers should discard any PPE item that shows signs of wear. Even if there are no obvious signs of wear, workers or their employers should replace reusable chemical-resistant items regularly—the ability of a chemical-resistant material to resist pesticides decreases each time an item is worn. Pesticides can move through the protective layer in the same way helium leaks out of a balloon, slowly but steadily. A good rule of thumb is to discard gloves that have been worn for about 5–7 workdays. Extra-heavy-duty gloves, such as those made of butyl or nitrile rubber, may last as long as 10–14 days. Footwear, aprons, headgear, and protective suits may last longer than gloves because they generally receive less exposure to chemicals and less abrasion from rough surfaces. However, they should be replaced regularly and whenever they show any signs of wear. Most protective eyewear and respirator bodies, facepieces, and helmets are designed to be cleaned and reused. These items can last many years if they are of good quality and are maintained correctly.

Workers should launder fabric coveralls and work clothing after each day's use but should not attempt to launder clothing made of cotton, polyester, cotton blends, denim, and canvas if these items are drenched or saturated with concentrated pesticides. Always discard any such contaminated clothing or footwear at a household hazardous waste collection site if one is available.

Washing and Drying PPE

Workers should always wash pesticide-contaminated items separately from the family laundry (NPIC 2023). Otherwise, pesticide residues may be transferred to the other laundry and harm the user or his/her family. Be sure that people who clean or maintain the PPE and other work clothes know they can be harmed by touching these pesticide-contaminated items. Instruct them to wear gloves and an apron and work in a well-ventilated area, if possible, and avoid inhaling steam from the washer or dryer. The manufacturer's instructions should be followed for cleaning chemical-resistant items. If the manufacturer instructs a person to clean the item but gives no detailed instructions, follow these guidelines:

1. Wash only a few items at a time so there is plenty of agitation and water for dilution.
2. Wash in a washing machine, using a heavy-duty liquid detergent and hot water for the wash cycle. Set your washer to the longest wash cycle and two rinse cycles.
3. Use two entire machine cycles to wash items that are moderately contaminated.
4. Run the washer through at least one additional cycle without clothing, using detergent and

hot water, to clean the machine before any other laundry is washed.

Some chemical-resistant items that are not flat, such as gloves, footwear, and coveralls, must be washed twice—once to clean the outside of the item and a second time after turning the item inside out. Some chemical-resistant items, such as heavy-duty boots and rigid hats or helmets, can be washed by hand using hot water and a heavy-duty liquid detergent. When hand-washing, the washer should always wear gloves. If possible, the washed items should be hung outside to dry for at least 24 h in an area with plenty of fresh air. When the items are exposed to clean air and sunlight, most remaining residues move to the surface of the fabric and evaporate or break down. The worker or employer may consider buying two or more sets of PPE so they can leave one set airing while wearing the other set. Do not hang items in enclosed living areas—chemical residues that remain in the items may evaporate and expose people or animals in the area. If it is not possible to hang fabric items to dry, a clothes dryer may be used. Over time, however, the dryer may become contaminated with pesticide residues. After cleaning reusable items, they can be placed in a plastic bag or clothing hamper away from personal clothes and the family laundry.

Maintaining Eyewear and Respirators

Workers should wash goggles, face shields, shielded safety glasses, respirator bodies, and facepieces after each day of use, and wear gloves while doing so.

1. Use detergent and hot water to remove any contaminants (such as residual pesticides) under running water with a soft brush.
2. Sanitize them by soaking for at least 2 min in a mixture of 2 tablespoons of chlorine bleach in 1 gallon of hot water.
3. Rinse thoroughly to remove the detergent and bleach.
4. Dry the items thoroughly or hang them in a clean area to dry.

Workers should pay particular attention to headbands and replace headbands made of absorbent materials with chemical-resistant headbands. After each day of use, workers should inspect all headbands for signs of wear or deterioration and replace them as needed. Respirators and eyewear should be stored in an area where they are protected from dust, sunlight, extreme temperatures, excessive moisture, and pesticides or other chemicals. A sturdy plastic bag with a zip closure works well for storage of both the respirator and the cartridges. If stored improperly, cartridges will continue to collect impurities from the air, causing them to lose their effectiveness. Workers should inspect their respirators before each use and repair or replace any part that shows signs of wear or deterioration. Workers or their employers should maintain an inventory of replacement parts for the respirators owned and not use substitutes or incompatible brands. If a respirator is kept for emergency use or as a backup, it should be inspected at least monthly and before use.

If a worker removes their respirator between handling activities, they should follow these guidelines:

- Wipe the respirator body and facepiece with a clean cloth.
- Seal the respirator (except for any prefilters) in a sturdy airtight container such as a plastic bag with a zip container.
- Remove contaminated prefilters before placing the canisters and cartridges in a zip-closeable plastic bag to avoid contaminating the canisters and cartridges. Prefilters do not lose their effectiveness when exposed to air.

At the end of every workday and after wearing a reusable respirator, workers should be sure to:

- Remove the prefilter. Most filters should be discarded.
- Take off the cartridges or canisters. Discard them, or if they are still usable, replace their caps and seal them in an airtight container, such as a plastic bag with a zip closure.
- Clean and store the respirator as directed above.

- Discard disposable respirators according to manufacturer's instructions. Do not try to clean them.

It is important that workers handle respirators with the same care that is given to other protective equipment and clothing.

References

ANSI (American National Standards Institute). ANSI/ISEA Z87.1–2020: current standard for safety glasses. 2020.

ATS (American Thoracic Society). Respiratory protection guidelines. Am J Respir Crit Care Med. 1996;154:1153–65.

CDC (Centers for Disease Control and Prevention). Warning signs and symptoms of heat-related illness. Last reviewed: September 1, 2017. https://www.cdc.gov/disasters/extremeheat/warning.html. Accessed 29 Apr 2024.

Geddie JE. A guide to respiratory protection. North Carolina Department of Labor; 2015. https://www.uncp.edu/sites/default/files/2019-07/ig44.pdf

NCAI (North Carolina Agromedicine Institute). Respiratory protection. 2024. https://www.ncagromedicine.org/program-respiratory.php.

NIOSH. A strategy for assigning new NIOSH skin notations. Current Intelligence Bulletin 61. August 2017. DHHS (NIOSH) Publication No. 2009–147.

NIOSH. Eye protection. DHHS (NIOSH) Publication No 2022–136. Last Reviewed August 31, 2022. https://www.cdc.gov/niosh/docs/2022-136/default.html.

NIOSH (a). Noise and occupational hearing loss. January 12, 2023. https://www.cdc.gov/niosh/topics/noise/chemicals.html.

NIOSH (b). Hierarchy of controls. Last Reviewed January 17, 2023. https://www.cdc.gov/niosh/topics/hierarchy/default.html.

NIOSH (c). Understand noise exposure. Last Reviewed May 3, 2023. https://www.cdc.gov/niosh/topics/noise/preventoccunoise/understand.html.

NIOSH (d). Provide hearing protection. Last Reviewed May 3, 2023. https://www.cdc.gov/niosh/topics/noise/preventoccunoise/provide.html.

Franks JR, Stephenson MR, Merry CJ, editors. Preventing occupational hearing loss—a practical guide. NIOSH (National Institute for Occupational Safety and Health); 1996. October. DHHS (NIOSH) Publication No. 96-110

NPIC. (National Pesticide Information Center). How can I wash out pesticides from dirty work clothes? Last updated October 31, 2023. http://npic.orst.edu/faq/dirtyclothes.htm. Accessed 24 Apr 2024.

OSHA. Respiratory protection. OSHA Technical Manual (OTM) Section VIII: Chapter 2. January 20, 1999. https://www.osha.gov/otm/section-8-ppe/chapter-2#medeval.

OSHA. 1915 Subpart I App A. Non-mandatory guidelines for hazard assessment, Personal Protective Equipment (PPE) selection, and PPE training program. 47 FR 16986, Apr. 20, 1982; 61 FR 26321, May 24, 1996; 67 FR 44544, July 3, 2002. https://www.osha.gov/laws--regs/regulations/standardnumber/1915/1915SubpartIAppA.

OSHA. 1910.134(e) https://www.osha.gov/pls/oshaweb/owadisp.show_d ocument?p_id=12716&p_table=STANDARDS [63 FR 1152, Jan. 8, 1998; 63 FR 20098, April 23, 1998; 71 FR 16672, April 3, 2006; 71 FR 50187, August 24, 2006; 73 FR 75584, Dec. 12, 2008; 76 FR 33606, June 8, 2011; 84 FR 50755, Sept. 26, 2019].

OSHA. Personal protective equipment. OSHA 3151-02R 2023. 2023.

OSHA. (Occupational Health and Safety Administration). OSH Act of 1970. 1970. https://www.osha.gov/laws-regs/oshact/section5-duties.

Proctor NH. Toxicological concepts-setting exposure limits. In: Proctor and Hughes' chemical hazards of the workplace, 5th ed. by Hathaway GJ, Proctor NH. Wiley. 2004;3–10.

US EPA. Agricultural Worker Protection Standard (WPS). Last Updated February 22, 2024. https://www.epa.gov/pesticide-worker-safety/agricultural-worker-protection-standard-wps.

US EPA (Environmental Protection Agency). Exposure factors handbook: 2011 edition. September 2011. EPA/600/R-09/052F.

5 Organophosphates and Carbamates

Dalia Alwasiyah

Introduction

Cholinergic agents, also called anticholinesterases, include organophosphates and carbamates. These agents are used as insecticides but also as chemical warfare agents, sometimes called nerve agents. Cholinergic agents have been used in many terrorist attacks and assassinations. In the Tokyo subway attacks in 1994, Sarin, an organophosphate, was used (Wiener and Hoffman 2004). Novichok agents, which are organophosphates, were reported to be used to poison multiple opponents of the Russian government. (Noga and Jurowski 2023; Wiener and Hoffman 2004). More recently, Kim Jong-nam, the North Korean leader's half-brother, was murdered with VX (Zhen 2017). Military personnel exposed to low levels of Sarin in the 1991 Gulf War developed a chronic illness known as Gulf War illness (Haley et al. 2022).

Exposure to these agents can cause significant morbidity and possible long-term effects.

Therefore, it is important to understand the toxicity of these agents and their management. In 2019, pesticides accounted for around 4% of US poison center exposures, and cholinergic agents comprised 4% of pesticide exposures (Gummin et al. 2020).

There are many organophosphates and carbamates (Tables 5.1 and 5.2). One can assume that if a pesticide's name starts or ends in "phos" or "thion," it might be an organophosphate. On the other hand, most carbamates' names end in "carb." Many of these are no longer registered in the United States, but patients may still have these pesticides either obtained from outside the country, or remnants of these pesticides that were once registered may be found in barns or sheds.

D. Alwasiyah (✉)
North Carolina's Poison Center, Charlotte, NC, USA

W. J. Meggs, R. L. Langley (eds.), *Farm Toxicology*, https://doi.org/10.1007/978-3-031-80441-0_5

Table 5.1 Examples of organophosphates (Roberts 2013a)

Highly toxic	Highly toxic but no longer registered in the United States	Moderately toxic	Moderately toxic but no longer registered in the United States
azin***phos***-methyl carbopheno***thion*** chlorfenvin***phos*** couma***phos*** demeton dialifor dicroto***phos*** dioxa***thion*** disulfoton Ethyl 4-nitrophenyl phenylphosphonothioate ethyl para***thion*** fenami***phos*** fensulfo**thion** fono***fos*** fosthietan isofen***phos*** methamido***phos*** methida***thion*** methyl para***thion*** mevin***phos*** monocroto***phos*** phorate phosphamidon sulfotep terbu***fos***	bomyl chlormephos chlorthiophos cyanofenphos dimefox endothion famphur fenophosphon mephosfolan mipafox phosfolan prothoate schradan tetraethyl pyrophosphate	acephate bensulide chlorpyrifos crotoxyphos demeton-S-methyl diazinon dichlofenthion dichlorvos ethion ethoprop fenitrothion fenthion malathion merphos naled oxydemeton-methyl phosalone phosmet pirimiphos-methyl profenofos propetamphos ronnel temephos tetrachlorvinphos trichlorfon	bromophos-ethyl bromophos chlorphoxim crufomate cyanophos cythioate edifenphos etrimfos formothion heptenophos iodofenphos isoxathion leptophos methyl trithion dimethoate oxydeprofos phenkapton phenthoate phoxim pirimiphos-ethyl propyl thiopyrophosphate pyrazophos pyridaphenthion quinalphos sulprofos thiometon triazophos

Table 5.2 Examples of carbamates (Roberts 2013b)

Highly toxic	Highly toxic but no longer registered in the United States	Moderately toxic	Moderately toxic but no longer registered in the United States
aldicarb carbofuran formetanate methiocarb methomyl oxamyl	aminocarb bendiocarb cloethocarb isolan	carbaryl propoxur	bufencarb dimetan dioxacarb isoprocarb pirimicarb promecarb trimethacarb

Examples of Organophosphate and Carbamate Pesticides

The following are examples of highly toxic organophosphates with an LD_{50} of less than 50 milligrams per kilogram (mg/kg) that are still registered in the United States (Roberts 2013a):

azinphos-methyl
carbopheno***thion***
chlorfenvin***phos***
couma***pho***s
demeton
dialifor
dicroto***phos***
dioxa***thion***
disulfoton

Disulfoton can accumulate in plants and can be detected in fruits (Roberts 2013a).

Examples of moderately toxic organophosphates with LD_{50} greater than 50 mg/kg but less than 500 mg/kg that are still registered in the United States include:

acephate
bensulide
chlorpyrifos
crotoxyphos
demeton-S-methyl
diazinon

The following are examples of highly toxic carbamates with an LD_{50} of less than 50 mg/kg that are still registered in the United States:

aldicarb
carbofuran
formetanate
methiocarb
methomyl
oxamyl

Carbaryl and propoxur are moderately toxic carbamates with LD_{50} greater than 50 mg/kg but less than 500 mg/kg and are still registered in the United States.

Routes of Exposure

Organophosphates and carbamates are efficiently absorbed by inhalation and ingestion. Symptoms occur rapidly after inhalation and ingestion. Dermal exposures can have a delayed presentation. Also, dermal toxicity can vary. Agents with a higher toxicity have a higher chance of dermal absorption and subsequent systemic toxicity. For example, parathion, a highly toxic organophosphate, has oral and dermal LD_{50} that are very similar (Eddleston et al. 2005; Heide 2010; Roberts 2013a).

The route of exposure determines the type of symptoms. With inhalation exposures, you will expect to see more respiratory symptoms, and with oral exposures, you will see more gastrointestinal symptoms (Eddleston 2019; Heide 2010; Roberts 2013a; Wiener and Hoffman 2004).

The time of onset of symptoms depends on the toxicity of the substance and the amount exposed; the higher the toxicity or the larger the amount of exposure, the sooner the symptoms occur. In addition, inhalational exposures present faster than other routes (Eddleston 2019).

One organophosphate worth mentioning is fenthion. Fenthion is moderately toxic and life-threatening symptoms can be delayed up to 30 hours (Eddleston et al. 2005).

Mechanism of Action

Organophosphates and carbamates block the breakdown of the neurotransmitter acetylcholine by inhibiting acetylcholineesterase and other similar compounds in the body including butyrylcholinesterase (Heide 2010).

Initially, organophosphates and carbamates bind to acetylcholinesterase. This bond can break down or become permanent. The process of the bond becoming permanent is called aging. Aging is unique to organophosphates. The lack of aging in carbamates may make the clinical course shorter and less severe (Heide 2010).

Once aging has occurred, acetylcholinesterase is permanently nonfunctional, and the generation of new acetylcholinesterase molecules is needed for the restoration of acetylcholinesterase function (Heide 2010; Roberts 2013a).

The inhibition of acetylcholineesterase leads to excess acetylcholine in the neuromuscular junction. This causes a cholinergic response, both nicotinic and muscarinic (Eddleston 2019; Heide 2010).

Clinical Effects

Clinical effects of organophosphate and carbamate toxicity include the acute cholinergic toxidrome, the intermediate syndrome, organophosphate-induced delayed neuropathy (OPIDN), and organophosphorus ester-induced chronic neurotoxicity (OPICN) (Eddleston 2019; Heide 2010; Roberts 2013a).

Acute Clinical Effects

Acute toxicity is a result of muscarinic and nicotinic stimulation. In some patients, muscarinic activation predominates, and in others, the nicotinic activation predominates (Heide 2010; Roberts 2013a).

Muscarinic effects that can be seen can be remembered with the mnemonic "DUMBELS" (Robb et al. 2024):

D: Defecation
U: Urinary incontinence
M: Miosis
B: Bronchorrhea, bronchospasms, and bradycardia
E: Emesis
L: Lacrimation
S: Salivation

Nicotinic effects can be remembered with the mnemonic Monday, Tuesday, Wednesday, Thursday, and Friday (Robb et al. 2024):

Mydriasis/muscle cramps
Tachycardia
Weakness
Twitching
Hyperglycemia/hypertension
Fasciculations

Other possible effects that can occur in the acute setting include electrocardiogram changes. Sinus tachycardia, QT prolongation, nonspecific S-T findings, and ventricular dysrhythmias have been reported. It is unclear if these changes are more related to hypokalemia, acidosis, shock, as a side effect atropine or if they are from direct organophosphate effects (Laudari et al. 2014; Liu et al. 2012; Paul and Bhattacharyya 2012; Saadeh et al. 1997).

Hypertension or hypotension can occur depending on muscarinic vs nicotinic predominance (Roberts 2013a).

Muscular fasciculations, weakness, and paralysis can occur. Seizures and coma occur mostly with severe organophosphate (OP) poisoning but also predominate in children (Sofer et al. 1989).

Death in the acute setting is due to respiratory failure, which is caused by central respiratory depression, muscle weakness, bronchorrhea, and bronchoconstriction (Sungur and Güven 2001).

Laboratory changes that can occur in the acute phase include hypokalemia, leukocytosis, ketosis, hyperglycemia, and elevated amylase (Moon et al. 2016; Sahin et al. 2002). An elevated amylase can occur with or without elevation of lipase or clinical signs of pancreatitis, and it is most associated with oral organophosphate poisonings (Sahin et al. 2002). An elevated amylase can be a marker of severe organophosphate poisoning (Lee et al. 1998).

The clinical effect of cholinergic agents is different in children than in adults. They tend to lack the classic muscarinic effects, and their symptoms tend to be more neurologic. The most common features in children include miosis, sialorrhea, muscle weakness, and depressed mental status (Lifshitz et al. 1999; Sofer et al. 1989; Zwiener and Ginsburg 1988).

Seizures are more likely to occur in children than in adults. Seizures occur in up to 70% of patients who are children, compared to less than 5% in adults (Hayes et al. 1978; Levy-Khademi et al. 2007; Wiener and Hoffman 2004; Zwiener and Ginsburg 1988).

Respiratory complications are common in children, with up to 50% of patients requiring intubation (Zwiener and Ginsburg 1988).

Given the lack of classic muscarinic effects in children, these cases tend to be misdiagnosed. One study showed that 80% of patients with cholinergic agent poisoning transferred to their center were initially misdiagnosed (Zwiener and Ginsburg 1988).

Differential Diagnosis of Organophosphate and Carbamate Poisoning

- Asthma and respiratory infections
- Gastroenteritis
- Meningitis
- Opiate overdose
- Myasthenia gravis
- Guillain-Barre syndrome (GBS)
- Botulism

Acute cholinergic toxicity can resemble asthma and respiratory infections with its respiratory symptoms. With vomiting and diarrhea, it can resemble gastroenteritis. Altered mental status and leukocytosis can resemble meningitis. Depressed mental status and miosis can look like an opiate overdose. Weakness can resemble myasthenia gravis, GBS, and botulism.

Other toxicities like nicotinic agents or other cholinergic drugs may present with a similar picture.

The key to differentiating these is obtaining a thorough exposure history and inquiring about the patient's occupational and environmental history (Heide 2010).

Laboratory Diagnosis

Cholinesterase levels have limited utility in managing acute cholinergic poisonings because at most facilities, their turnaround time is prolonged. However, they can be useful for confirming exposure and monitoring treatment. They can also be useful in chronic exposures.

When ordering and interpreting cholinesterase levels, one needs to consider that they are indirect measures of cholinesterase levels in the neuronal synapse.

Red blood cell (RBC) cholinesterases are more reflective of neuronal cholinesterase but are not readily available in all settings. Butyrylcholinesterases, also known as pseudocholinesterase, are more readily available. However, they are less accurate than RBC cholinesterases at reflecting neuronal cholinesterase function (Table 5.3).

After exposure to organophosphates, butyrylcholinesterase levels decrease before RBC cholinesterase, but the decrease of RBC cholinesterases lasts longer than that of butyrylcholinesterase.

In carbamate poisoning, however, RBC cholinesterase inhibition is short-lived and returns to normal within a few days.

Baseline variations in healthy individuals' cholinesterase levels can range up to 40%. Other causes of decrease in cholinesterase levels besides organophosphate poisoning include genetic variations, pregnancy, malnutrition, acute infections, and some drugs (e.g., antimalarial drugs, oral contraceptives, and succinylcholine). Multiple myeloma, spinal issues, and nephrotic syndrome can cause baseline elevations (Kamanyire and Karalliedde 2004; Karalliedde 2002).

Table 5.3 A comparison between RBC cholinesterase and butyrylcholinesterase

	Red blood cell cholinesterase	Serum cholinesterase (butyrylcholinesterase/ pseudocholinesterase)
Accuracy	More	Less
Test availability	Less	More
Onset of decrease	Later	Earlier
Normalization	35–100 days from exposure	28–42 days from exposure
Possible utility	Suspected previous exposure in a patient with normal butyrylcholinesterase	Acute setting

Sample collection and storage errors can make cholinesterase levels inaccurate (Heide 2010; Karalliedde 2002; Midtling et al. 1985).

Another way to confirm or monitor exposure to organophosphates is by analyzing the urine for organophosphate metabolites. These metabolites are called alkyl phosphates. These indicate exposure and not disease. Alkyl phosphates can be used for biological monitoring in the occupational setting, especially if tested at the end of the work shift. They are short-lived and appear for up to 48 hours (Cocker et al. 2002). There are specific markers for certain organophosphates, for example: P-nitrophenol for parathion and P-nitrocresol for fenitrothion (Heide 2010).

Treatment

Treatment in these cases is centered around early aggressive resuscitation and administration of antidotes.

Early respiratory support is crucial as these patients can suffer from respiratory failure from the direct effects of cholinergic agents and aspiration (Eddleston 2019).

These patients will be volume-depleted from all the secretions. So they will need intravenous fluids. If they are hypotensive despite adequate fluid resuscitation, vasopressors might be needed.

Antidotes used for cholinergic poisonings include atropine, oximes, and benzodiazepines. It is recommended to consult with a medical toxicologist or with the poison control center (1-800-222-1222) to assist with the management of exposed patients.

Decontamination

Decontamination is specifically important in these patients. Decontamination should not interfere with patient stabilization. However, all healthcare personnel should wear personal protective equipment (Eddleston 2019; Heide 2010). There are reports of treatment teams becoming symptomatic after managing patients with pesticide poisonings (De Groot et al. 2021; Little and Murray 2004). If the patient is stable enough, assessment and decontamination of the patient should occur outdoors or in an area with separate ventilation (Roberts 2013a; Little and Murray 2004). The patient should be isolated from other patients, staff, and visitors, especially if actively vomiting (Little and Murray 2004). Removing the patient's clothing eliminates 80% of chemical contaminants.

The skin should be decontaminated with soap and water, if possible, because dermal absorption can contribute to further toxicity (Eddleston 2019; Heide 2010).

Gastrointestinal decontamination can be extremely labor intensive in an awake patient, and there are no studies demonstrating a mortality benefit of gastrointestinal decontamination. In fact, there is evidence indicating harm and that respiratory complications outweigh the benefits of gastrointestinal decontamination (Eddleston 2019).

However, if the patient is intubated, there is a low risk for further respiratory complications from gastrointestinal decontamination, and it can be considered in severe oral intoxications if these patients present early. Nasogastric suction can be considered within an hour of ingestion (Eddleston 2019).

Activated charcoal can be considered after intubation as it has been shown to bind organophosphates and carbamates in animal studies, but human studies do not show any mortality benefit from administering activated charcoal. However, there are no studies demonstrating the effect of activated charcoal on the duration of ICU stay and intubation (Eddleston et al. 2008; Moon et al. 2015).

Specific Antidotes

Atropine

Atropine is a muscarinic antagonist. Atropine can be given intravenous, intraosseous, endotracheal, and intramuscular. However, in cholinergic toxicity, the preferred route is intravenous (IV) (Heide 2010; Wiener and Hoffman 2004). Endotracheal administration is not as reliable, and the recommended dose is 2–2.5 times the usual intravenous dose (Heide 2010). Oral atropine has been described in one case series in the ICU, after discontinuation of IV atropine (du Toit et al. 1981). Ophthalmic atropine was reported for pain control from severe miosis due to organophosphate poisoning (Heide 2010).

For IV administration, incremental bolus doses are recommended. Studies demonstrate that doubling the dose rather than repeating the dose causes faster resuscitation and reduces mortality and the requirement for ventilation (Abedin et al. 2012). In adults, the initial dose is between 1 and 6 milligrams (mg) depending on the severity of the case. In children, the initial dose is 0.05–0.1 mg/kg. Patients who ingest pesticides generally require higher doses than patients who are exposed to nerve agents (Heide 2010).

After the initial bolus, if an adequate response is not achieved, then the dose needs to be doubled every 5 min until an adequate response is achieved. Adequate response (atropinization) in the setting of cholinergic poisoning is to reverse bronchorrhea and bronchospasm and provide adequate blood pressure and heart rate for tissue oxygenation. Tachycardia is not a contraindication or a reason to discontinue atropine if the patient still has respiratory secretions. Once an adequate response has occurred, a continuous infusion at 10–20% of loading dose per hour can be started (Abedin et al. 2012; Eddleston 2019).

For out-of-hospital events or in mass casualty situations, auto-injectors can be used. Auto-injectors allow atropine to diffuse into the circulation faster than a regular intramuscular needle and syringe. The MARK I kit is an auto-injector used for adults. Each MARK 1 kit contains 2 mg of atropine and 600 mg of pralidoxime. The initial dose is 1–3 MARK I kits, depending on the severity. If a patient has severe manifestations, you can start with 3 MARK I kits administered back-to-back. Pediatric atropine auto-injectors come in 0.5-mg and 1-mg sizes. The dose is 0.5 mg in children weighing 15–40 pounds (lbs), and in children weighing 40–90 lbs., the dose is 1 mg. Children over 90 lbs. can be given adult doses. The auto-injection doses can be repeated every 10–15 min until appropriate response. If pediatric auto-injectors are not available and a child is symptomatic, one adult atropine auto-injector can be given (Baker 2007; Heide 2010).

Adverse effects are usually mild, and they are anticholinergic (Eddleston et al. 2007; Heide 2010). In a study of children with up to 17 times the recommended doses for their age, no life-threatening events were reported (Amitai et al. 1992). If patients do develop anticholinergic symptoms, physostigmine is contraindicated because it is a cholinergic agent, and it will worsen the patient's cholinergic symptoms (Heide 2010).

Oximes

Pralidoxime (2-PAM) is the only FDA-approved oxime in the United States. Although there are controversies regarding 2-PAM, when the recommended dose of pralidoxime is given, the mortality rate and length of mechanical ventilation are reduced (Eddleston 2019; Heide 2010; Wiener and Hoffman 2004).

Obidoxime is used in Europe and Iran and is associated with hepatotoxicity (Eddleston 2019).

2-PAM binds organophosphate and displaces it from its binding site on the cholinesterase, allowing cholinesterase to regenerate. 2-PAM is most beneficial if given in the first few hours after exposure, before the organophosphate ages, but it is still beneficial if given later. There is strong evidence that 2-PAM is also beneficial in carbamate poisoning when given together with atropine (Eddleston 2019; Heide 2010).

2-PAM can be given intravenously or intramuscularly. After a bolus is given, an infusion is needed because the levels of 2-PAM fall below therapeutic levels at 90–120 minutes after the initial dose. In adults, the intravenous bolus dose is 1 or 2 grams (g) over 15–30 min, and at least 30 mg/kg is needed. Then the infusion is started at 500 mg/h with a minimum of 8 mg/kg/h. In children, the bolus is 20–40 mg/kg, with a max of 1 g, and the infusion is at 10–20 mg/kg/h. The infusion of 2-PAM should be continued until symptoms resolve and the patient no longer requires atropine (Eddleston 2019; Heide 2010).

2-PAM is available in an intramuscular auto-injection as part of the MARK I kit. For mild symptoms, the dose is 600 mg (one MARK I kit), and for severe symptoms, the dose is 1800 mg (three MARK I kits). For persistent symptoms, repeat the dose every 15 min to a maximum total dose of 45 mg/kg; doses may be administered in rapid succession if severe symptoms develop. In children less than 1 year old, 2-PAM auto-injector is generally not recommended; however, in children older than 1 year old, one dose of 600-mg auto-injector can be given (Baker 2007; Eddleston 2019; Eddleston et al. 2007; Heide 2010; Levy-Khademi et al. 2007; Quail and Shannon 2007).

Adverse effects from 2-PAM are mild and are usually associated with high doses or rapid IV infusions. Serious adverse effects are extremely rare, limited to single case reports (Baker 2007; Eddleston 2019; Heide 2010; Jeong et al. 2015; Quail and Shannon 2007; Scott 1986; Wiener and Hoffman 2004).

Benzodiazepines

Benzodiazepines should not be given prophylactically to all patients. The indications for benzodiazepines include seizures, agitation, and to aid with intubation. The benzodiazepine of choice is diazepam as it improves survival and reduces central nervous system (CNS) damage and myocardial dysfunction associated with cholinergic poisonings (Heide 2010; Wiener and Hoffman 2004).

The Intermediate Syndrome

The intermediate syndrome occurs around 24–96 hours after exposure, with an incidence of about 20–68% (Heide 2010; Karalliedde et al. 2006).

Patients with severe acute presentations with pseudocholinesterase <10% of normal are at an increased risk (Karalliedde et al. 2006).

The danger of intermediate syndrome is that the patients appear like they are ready to be extubated or discharged, only to have respiratory failure develop due to muscle paralysis. The muscle paralysis starts in the proximal muscles. Classically, patients are described as unable to lift their necks off the bed. They can also develop cranial neuropathies, with ocular palsies and laryngeal nerve palsies being frequently described (Karalliedde et al. 2006).

These patients have findings suggesting a myopathic process: muscle biopsies showed decreased acetylcholine esterase and myopathic changes. An increase in creatinine kinase and creatinine kinase isoenzyme MM can be seen in these cases. Electromyographic changes are seen even without paralysis being present These patients have normal consciousness and electroencephalograms (Karalliedde et al. 2006).

The intermediate syndrome resolves spontaneously within 1 or 2 weeks. Treatment is supportive with early recognition and respiratory assistance (Heide 2010; Karalliedde et al. 2006).

Organophosphate-Induced Delayed Neuropathy

Organophosphate-induced delayed neuropathy (OPIDN) occurs between 1 and 5 weeks after organophosphate toxicity. It is a distal axonopathy that presents with cramping in extremities, distal paresthesias, diminished tendon reflexes, high stepping gate, foot and wrist drop, spastic ataxia, or quadriplegia. Inhibition of neuropathy target esterases may be the cause (Eddleston et al. 2005; Heide 2010).

It occurs after acute exposures, but these acute exposures do not have to result in a cholinergic toxidrome or show a decrease in RBC cholinesterase levels (Lotti and Moretto 2005). OPIDN occurs mostly with organophosphates, but there are reports of OPIDN with carbamate exposures (Lotti and Moretto 2005).

Definitive diagnosis of OPIDN is by electromyogram and nerve biopsies. An electromyogram will show signs of denervation. A nerve biopsy will show axonal degenerations (Heide 2010; Lotti and Moretto 2005).

There is no strong evidence to suggest development of OPIDN from repeated low-level exposure (Lotti and Moretto 2005).

No specific treatment is needed, and the prognosis varies. Sensory recovery is better than motor recovery. Paralysis and ataxia tend to be permanent. When recovery occurs, it occurs over several months (Heide 2010; Lotti and Moretto 2005).

An important historical disaster to mention is Ginger Jake paralysis, which occurred in 1930. During prohibition, the ethanolic extract of Jamaican ginger, aka the Jake, was an alcohol substitute. People who drank the Jake developed triorthocresyl phosphate poisoning, presenting as OPIDN. The paralysis was termed Ginger Jake paralysis, and the associated gait impairment was termed "Jake walk" or "Jake leg" (Wax 2019).

Chronic Clinical Effects

Organophosphate exposure has been linked to neuropsychological effects such as difficulties with cognition, memory, concentration, and mood (Munoz-Quezada et al. 2016). These effects might be due to central nervous system damage from hypoxia or seizures rather than a direct organophosphate effect. Studies linking neuropsychiatric effects to exposure to organophosphates are confounded by exposure to mixed pesticides, and these effects cannot be attributed to organophosphates alone (Heide 2010; Roberts 2013c).

Maternal exposure to organophosphates during pregnancy can have negative effects on neonatal primitive reflexes and early childhood neurobehavioral function. There is conflicting evidence regarding childhood exposure and negative effects on intelligence quotient and increasing the risk of attention deficit disorders (Roberts 2013c).

Cholinergic agents have been linked to cancer, but there is no cholinergic pesticide that has been proven to cause human cancer. Some cholinergic pesticides like tetrachlorvinphos and parathion have been proven to cause cancer in animals. Both agents have been classified as possible human carcinogens by the International Agency for Research on Cancer (IARC 2017).

Malathion and diazinon are classified as probable carcinogens to humans (IARC 2017). Malathion has been linked to thyroid, breast, and ovarian cancer in postmenopausal women, in addition to non-Hodgkin's lymphoma and prostate cancer. However, a recent risk assessment by the U.S. Environmental Protection Agency (EPA) stated that there was insufficient epidemiologic evidence to suggest that a clear associative or causal relationship exists between malathion exposure and adverse health outcomes (U.S. EPA 2024).

Suggested Surveillance for Occupational Exposure

Recommendations for patients chronically exposed to cholinergic agents in the occupational setting include:

- A baseline medical exam, specifically a neurological exam.
- Renal and liver function, because they impact the metabolism of organophosphate and carbamates.
- Baseline cholinesterase levels. Three separate measurements are needed to account for baseline fluctuations.

- Surveillance exams can be performed at 6-month to one-year intervals.
- Cholinesterase levels can be repeated as needed if patients develop signs or symptoms.

  - If the patient's cholinesterase levels are at 30–60% of their baseline or at 50–70% of the normal reference, continue monitoring levels every 6 months (Kamanyire and Karalliedde 2004).
  - If levels are less than 30% of their baseline or 50% of normal reference, removal from work and analysis of working conditions is recommended (Kamanyire and Karalliedde 2004).

References

Abedin MJ, Sayeed AA, Basher A, Maude RJ, Hoque G, Faiz MA. Open-label randomized clinical trial of atropine bolus injection versus incremental boluses plus infusion for organophosphate poisoning in Bangladesh. J Med Toxicol. 2012;8(2):108–17. https://doi.org/10.1007/s13181-012-0214-6.

Amitai Y, Almog S, Singer R, Hammer R, Bentur Y, Danon YL. Atropine poisoning in children during the Persian Gulf crisis. A national survey in Israel. JAMA. 1992;268(5):630–2.

Baker MD. Antidotes for nerve agent poisoning: should we differentiate children from adults? Curr Opin Pediatr. 2007;19(2):211–5.

Cocker J, Mason H, Garfitt S, Jones K. Biological monitoring of exposure to organophosphate pesticides. Toxicol Lett. 2002;134(1–3):97–103.

De Groot R, Van Zoelen GA, Leenders MEC, Van Riel AJHP, De Vries I, De Lange DW. Is secondary chemical exposure of hospital personnel of clinical importance? Clin Toxicol. 2021;59(4):269–78. https://doi.org/10.1080/15563650.2020.1860216.

du Toit PW, Müller FO, van Tonder WM, Ungerer MJ. Experience with the intensive care management of organophosphate insecticide poisoning. S Afr Med J. 1981;60(6):227–9.

Eddleston M. Chapter 11 Insecticides: organic phosphorous compounds and carbamates. In: Flomenbaum N, editor. Goldfrank's toxicologic emergencies. 11th ed. New York: McGraw-Hill Education; 2019.

Eddleston M, Eyer P, Worek F, Mohamed F, Senarathna L, von Meyer L, et al. Differences between organophosphorus insecticides in human self-poisoning: a prospective cohort study. Lancet. 2005;366(9495):1452–9. https://doi.org/10.1016/S0140-6736(05)67598-8.

Eddleston M, Singh S, Buckley N. Organophosphorus poisoning (acute). BMJ Clin Evid. 2007;2007:2102.

Eddleston M, Juszczak E, Buckley NA, Senarathna L, Mohamed F, Dissanayake W, Hittarage A, Azher S, Jeganathan K, Jayamanne S, Sheriff MR, Warrell DA, Ox-Col Poisoning Study collaborators. Multiple-dose activated charcoal in acute self-poisoning: a randomised controlled trial. Lancet. 2008;371(9612):579–87. https://doi.org/10.1016/S0140-6736(08)60270-6.

Gummin DD, Mowry JB, Beuhler MC, Spyker DA, Brooks DE, Dibert KW, et al. 2019 Annual report of the American Association of Poison Control Centers' National Poison Data System (NPDS): 37th annual report. Clin Toxicol (Phila). 2020;58(12):1360–541. https://doi.org/10.1080/15563650.2020.1834219.

Haley RW, Kramer G, Xiao J, Dever JA, Teiber JF. Evaluation of a gene-environment interaction of PON1 and low-level nerve agent exposure with gulf war illness: a prevalence case-control study drawn from the U.S. Military Health survey's national population sample. Environ Health Perspect. 2022;130(5):57001. https://doi.org/10.1289/EHP9009.

Hayes MM, van der Westhuizen NG, Gelfand M. Organophosphate poisoning in Rhodesia. A study of the clinical features and management of 105 patients. S Afr Med J. 1978;54(6):230–4.

Heide, E. A. d. Agency for toxic substances and disease registry case studies in environmental medicine cholinesterase inhibitors: including pesticides and chemical warfare nerve agents. 2010, October 17, 2010. Retrieved from https://www.atsdr.cdc.gov/csem/cholinesterase/docs/cholinesterase.pdf.

IARC. Some organophosphate inescticide and herbicides. IARC Monographs on the Evaluation of Carcinogenic Risks to Humans Volume 112; 2017. Retrieved from https://monographs.iarc.who.int/list-of-classifications.

Jeong TO, Lee JB, Jin YH, Yoon JC. Respiratory arrest caused by accidental rapid pralidoxime infusion. Clin Toxicol. 2015;53(4):412.

Kamanyire R, Karalliedde L. Organophosphate toxicity and occupational exposure. Occup Med (Lond). 2004;54(2):69–75. https://doi.org/10.1093/occmed/kqh018.

Karalliedde L. Cholinesterase estimations revisited: the clinical relevance. Eur J Anaesthesiol. 2002;19(5):313–6. https://doi.org/10.1017/s0265021502000510.

Karalliedde L, Baker D, Marrs TC. Organophosphate-induced intermediate syndrome: aetiology and relationships with myopathy. Toxicol Rev. 2006;25:1–14.

Laudari S, Patowary BS, Sharma SK, Dhungel S, Subedi K, Bhattacharya R, et al. Cardiovascular effects of acute organophosphate poisoning. Asia Pacific J Med Toxicol. 2014;3(2):64–7. https://doi.org/10.22038/apjmt.2014.3045.

Lee WC, Yang CC, Deng JF, Wu ML, Ger J, Lin HC, et al. The clinical significance of hyperamylasemia in organophosphate poisoning. J Toxicol Clin Toxicol. 1998;36(7):673–81. https://doi.org/10.3109/15563659809162615.

Levy-Khademi F, Tenenbaum AN, Wexler ID, Amitai Y. Unintentional organophosphate intoxication in children. Pediatr Emerg Care. 2007;23(10):716–8. Retrieved from https://journals.lww.com/pec-online/fulltext/2007/10000/unintentional_organophosphate_intoxication_in.7.aspx.

Lifshitz M, Shahak E, Sofer S. Carbamate and organophosphate poisoning in young children. Pediatr Emerg Care. 1999;15(2):102–3. Retrieved from https://journals.lww.com/pec-online/fulltext/1999/04000/carbamate_and_organophosphate_poisoning_in_young.6.aspx.

Little M, Murray L. Consensus statement: risk of nosocomial organophosphate poisoning in emergency departments. Emerg Med Australas. 2004;16(5–6):456–8. https://doi.org/10.1111/j.1742-6723.2004.00649.x.

Liu SH, Lin JL, Weng CH, Yang HY, Hsu CW, Chen KH, et al. Heart rate-corrected QT interval helps predict mortality after intentional organophosphate poisoning. PLoS One. 2012;7(5):e36576. https://doi.org/10.1371/journal.pone.0036576.

Lotti M, Moretto A. Organophosphate-induced delayed polyneuropathy. Toxicol Rev. 2005;24(1):37–49. https://doi.org/10.2165/00139709-200524010-00003.

Midtling JE, Barnett PG, Velasco AR, Romero P, Clements CL, O'Malley MA, et al. Clinical management of field worker organophosphate poisoning. West J Med. 1985;142(4):514.

Moon J, Chun B, Song K. An exploratory study; the therapeutic effects of premixed activated charcoal-sorbitol administration in patients poisoned with organophosphate pesticide. Clin Toxicol (Phila). 2015;53(2):119–26. https://doi.org/10.3109/15563650.2014.1001516.

Moon JM, Chun BJ, Cho YS. Hyperglycemia at presentation is associated with in hospital mortality in non-diabetic patient with organophosphate poisoning. Clin Toxicol. 2016;54(3):252–8. https://doi.org/10.3109/15563650.2015.1128544.

Munoz-Quezada MT, Lucero BA, Iglesias VP, Munoz MP, Cornejo CA, Achu E, et al. Chronic exposure to organophosphate (OP) pesticides and neuropsychological functioning in farm workers: a review. Int J Occup Environ Health. 2016;22(1):68–79. https://doi.org/10.1080/10773525.2015.1123848.

Noga M, Jurowski K. What do we currently know about Novichoks? The state of the art. Arch Toxicol. 2023;97(3):651–61. https://doi.org/10.1007/s00204-022-03437-5.

Paul UK, Bhattacharyya AK. ECG manifestations in acute organophosphorus poisoning. J Indian Med Assoc. 2012;110(2):98–107-108. Retrieved from http://europepmc.org/abstract/MED/23029843.

Quail MT, Shannon MW. Pralidoxime safety and toxicity in children. Prehosp Emerg Care. 2007;11(1):36–41.

Robb EL, Regina AC, Baker MB. Organophosphate toxicity. In: StatPearls. Treasure Island: StatPearls Publishing; 2024. Copyright © 2024, StatPearls Publishing LLC.

Roberts JR. Chapter 5, organophosphate insecticides. In: Recognition and management of pesticide poisonings. 6th ed; 2013a. Retrieved from https://www.epa.gov/sites/default/files/documents/rmpp_6thed_ch5_organophosphates.pdf.

Roberts JR. Chapter 6. N-methyl carbamate insecticides. In: Recognition and management of pesticide poisonings. 6th ed; 2013b. Retrieved from https://www.epa.gov/sites/default/files/documents/rmpp_6thed_ch6_carbamates.pdf.

Roberts JR. Chapter 21. Chronic effects. In: Recognition and management of pesticide poisonings. 6th ed; 2013c. Retrieved from https://www.epa.gov/pesticide-worker-safety/pesticide-poisoning-handbook-section-v-chronic-effects.

Saadeh AM, Farsakh NA, al-Ali MK. Cardiac manifestations of acute carbamate and organophosphate poisoning. Heart. 1997;77(5):461. https://doi.org/10.1136/hrt.77.5.461.

Sahin I, Onbasi K, Sahin H, Karakaya C, Ustun Y, Noyan T. The prevalence of pancreatitis in organophosphate poisonings. Hum Exp Toxicol. 2002;21(4):175–7. https://doi.org/10.1191/0960327102ht234cr.

Scott R. Repeated asystole following PAM in organophosphate self-poisoning. Anaesth Intensive Care. 1986;14(4):458–60.

Sofer S, Tal A, Shahak E. Carbamate and organophosphate poisoning in early childhood. Pediatr Emerg Care. 1989;5(4):222–5. https://doi.org/10.1097/00006565-198912000-00005.

Sungur M, Güven M. Intensive care management of organophosphate insecticide poisoning. Crit Care. 2001;5(4):211–5. https://doi.org/10.1186/cc1025.

U.S.EPA. Malathion: revised human health risk assessment for registration review. 2024. Retrieved from https://www.regulations.gov/document/EPA-HQ-OPP-2009-0317-0161.

Wax PM. Toxicologic misfortunes and catastrophes in history. In: Nelson LS, Howland MA, Lewin NA, Smith SW, Goldfrank LR, Hoffman RS, editors. Goldfrank's toxicologic emergencies. 11th ed. New York: McGraw-Hill Education; 2019.

Wiener SW, Hoffman RS. Nerve agents: a comprehensive review. J Intensive Care Med. 2004;19(1):22–37. https://doi.org/10.1177/0885066603258659.

Zhen, W. Kim Jong-nam killed by VX nerve agent, say Malaysian police. 2017. Retrieved from https://www.theguardian.com/world/2017/feb/24/kim-jong-nam-north-korea-killed-chemical-weapon-nerve-agent-mass-destruction-malaysian-police.

Zwiener RJ, Ginsburg CM. Organophosphate and carbamate poisoning in infants and children. Pediatrics. 1988;81(1):121. Retrieved from http://pediatrics.aappublications.org/content/81/1/121.abstract

Organochlorine Pesticides 6

Ricky L. Langley and Dalia Alwasiyah

Introduction

Organochlorine pesticides (OCPs) comprise various chemical compounds containing carbon, hydrogen, and chlorine. They have been mainly used as insecticides. The toxicity of OCPs varies by their molecular size, volatility, and the effects on the central nervous system, which can be either stimulation or depression, depending upon the dose and the xenobiotic (Wong 2022). The basic characteristics of OCPs are their environmental persistence, low polarity, low aqueous solubility, and high lipid solubility (Jayara et al. 2016).

According to the U.S. Environmental Protection Agency (EPA), persistent organic pollutants (POPs) are manmade organic chemicals that remain in the environment for years or decades and are of concern because they often remain toxic for decades or longer after release to the environment. There are three broad classes of POPs: organochlorine pesticides, polychlorinated dibenzo-p-dioxins (dioxins), and polychlorinated dibenzo-p-furans (furans) and polychlorinated biphenyls (PCBs) (USEPA 2023).

R. L. Langley (✉)
Department of Biological Sciences,
North Carolina State University,
Raleigh, NC, USA
e-mail: rllangley@ncsu.edu

D. Alwasiyah
North Carolina's Poison Center, Charlotte, NC, USA

Organochlorine pesticides were first introduced in the 1940s. They were widely used by troops in World War 2 and were found to prevent typhus and malaria by controlling their arthropod vectors. Organochlorine pesticides also found wide use in structural buildings, especially as termite control agents (Holland 2019) and in fire ant eradication. In 1962, Rachael Carson wrote the book *Silent Spring,* where she discussed the detrimental effects of pesticides on the environment, especially from DDT (Wikipedia 2024). DDT was responsible for the near-extinction of the American bald eagle (Colborn 1991, USFWS (Fish and Wildlife Services) 2024). Because of their environmental persistence and concern for biomagnification, the EPA banned most uses of these chemicals during the 1970s and 1980s in the United States, and many European countries also banned the use of the OCPs. Only three OCPs retain EPA approval for limited use in the United States: dicofol, endosulfan, and lindane (Roberts and Reigart 2013a). However, many developing countries still produce and/or use organochlorines, especially for malaria control.

Intentional and unintentional exposures to OCPs may result in severe poisoning. Due to their environmental persistence, food ingestion is often a source of exposure to low levels of OCPs, which rarely cause acute symptoms; however, there is concern that long-term exposure may lead to the development of various chronic illnesses. These fat-soluble chemicals are most

W. J. Meggs, R. L. Langley (eds.), *Farm Toxicology*, https://doi.org/10.1007/978-3-031-80441-0_6

commonly absorbed through the ingestion of fatty foods.

Examples

The following are examples of organochlorine pesticides that are used in various countries:

- Aldrin
- Benzene hexachloride (BHC) (also referred to as hexachlorobenzene (HCB))
- Chlordane
- Chlorobenzilate
- Chlorfenethol
- Chloropropylate
- Dichlorodiphenyltrichloroethane (DDT) [para, para isomer]
- Dichlorodiphenyldichloroethane (DDE) [para, para isomer]
- Dicofol
- Dieldrin
- Endosulfan
- Endrin
- Heptachlor
- beta-Hexachlorocyclohexane (beta-HCH)
- Isobenzan
- Isodrin
- Methoxychlor
- Mirex
- trans-Nonachlor
- Oxychlordane
- Toxaphene
- 2,4,5-Trichlorophenol
- 2,4,6-Trichlorophenol

Based on the WHO classification of pesticide toxicity from oral LD_{50} studies in rats, a hazardous rating has been established (Table 6.1; see Toxicology primer chapter) 6.1.

Table 6.1 Toxicity and environmental half-life of select organochlorine pesticides

Chemical name	Toxicity	Environmental half-life
Aldrin	High	4–7 years
BHC	Acute hazard unlikely	3–6 years
Chlordane	Moderate	10 years
Chloropropylate	Acute hazard unlikely	~2 months
1,4-dichlorobenzene	Moderate	<2 months
DDD Dichloro-diphenyldichloroethane	Acute hazard unlikely	5–10 years
DDE	Slight	10 years
DDT	Moderate	2–15 years
Dicofol	Moderate	2 months
Dieldrin	High	9 months
Endosulfan	High	1–5 months
Endrin	High	1 day to 12 years
Heptachlor	High to moderate	2 years
Isobenzan	High	2.8 years
Isodrin	High	0.5–6 years
Lindane	Moderate	15 months
Methoxychlor	Acute hazard unlikely	<3 months
Mirex	Acute hazard unlikely	10 years
Toxaphene	Slight	11 years

Adapted from Jayara et al. (2016)

Mechanism of Action

Organochlorines are often classified into four groups (Holland 2019). These four groups are based on similarities in chemical structures and similar toxicities (Table 6.2).

1. Dichlorodiphenyltrichloroethane (DDT) and related analogs
2. Cyclodienes
3. Hexachlorocyclohexane
4. Mirex and chlordecone

DDT and its analogs such as DDD, methoxychlor, dicofol, chlorfenethol, ethylan, and chlorobenzilate are poorly absorbed transdermally unless dissolved in organic solvents. Due to their low volatility, inhalation toxicity is also unlikely to occur. They prolong the opening of sodium channels and inhibit Ca^{2+}-ATPase.

Cyclodienes and lindane bind to the picrotoxin binding site of the GABA receptors, causing decreased GABA activity. Examples of cyclodi-

Table 6.2 Mechanism of action

	DDT and analogs	Cyclodienes	Hexachlorocyclohexane	Mirex and chlordecone
Route of absorption	Oral Inhalation	Oral Inhalation Transdermal	Oral Inhalation Transdermal	Oral Inhalation Transdermal
Mechanism of action	Prolonged opening of sodium channels Inhibits Ca^{2+}-ATPase	GABA-Gamma-aminobutyric acid antagonists	GABA antagonists	Mechanism not understood
Examples	DDT Methoxychlor Dicofol Chlorobenzilate	Aldrin Dieldrin Endrin Chlordane Endosulfan Heptachlor Isobenzan Dienochlor Toxaphene	Lindane	Dechlorane Kepone

enes include aldrin, dieldrin, endosulfan, endrin, chlordane, heptachlor, dienochlor, and toxaphene. Toxaphene can also affect ATPases in the brain, kidneys, and liver. Most have been banned by the EPA for use in the United States. Isobenzan was never registered in the United States. Endosulfan has been involved in many serious or fatal poisonings in recent years (Yavuz et al. 2007; Moses and Peter 2010; Roberts and Reigart 2013a).

Routes of Exposure

Lindane is well-absorbed dermally. Factors that increase absorption include loss of skin integrity, thin skin, heat, and occlusive dressing. Toxicity can occur from a single topical application, especially in children (Holland 2019; Lee and Groth 1977). However, toxicity occurs more commonly with repeated exposures. Systemic toxicity can occur even with appropriate use of topical lindane (Hall and Hall 1999; Munk and Nantel 1977). Lindane also volatilizes when heated. In the past, toxicity occurred by inhalation of home lindane vaporizers though these are no longer used.

OCPs are absorbed from the gastrointestinal tract, by the lungs, and through the skin in varying degrees dependent upon the specific OCP. Factors that increase absorption include loss of skin integrity, thin skin, heat, and occlusive dressing. Organochlorines are all metabolized by the liver; some of them like chlordane have the potential to affect the metabolism of other medications, which leads to altered drug effects. For example, they can reduce the efficacy of oral contraceptives (Garrettson et al. 1984). Once absorbed, many are stored in fatty tissue (including the brain and liver) due to their lipophilicity. Most OCPs are, to some degree, dechlorinated, oxidized, and then conjugated (Roberts and Reigart 2013a). In a few OCPs, the metabolite may be more toxic than the parent compound, such as heptachlor to heptachlor epoxide, aldrin to dieldrin, and chlordane to oxychlordane (Holland 2019). OCPs undergo biliary excretion. Some unmetabolized OCPs are reabsorbed in the intestine via the enterohepatic and enteroenteric circulation. Various OCPs that are slowly metabolized, leading to fat storage, such as DDT, DDE, beta-HCH, dieldrin, heptachlor epoxide, and mirex, may be excreted in breast milk. Some OCPs may cross the placental barrier (Roberts and Reigart 2013a; Jayara et al. 2016).

Clinical Effects

Acute Clinical Effects

All organochlorines reduce the seizure threshold. Lindane and cyclodienes cause seizures without warning signs. All organochlorines can cause cardiac arrhythmias due to myocardial sensitization.

The following clinical signs are frequently noted in different groups of the OCPs:

DDT and analogs cause:

- Tremors are the most commonly seen neurologic sign.
- Seizures and altered mental status only occur after large intentional exposures.
- Nausea and vomiting frequently occur.
- Paresthesias and hyperesthesias of the face, mouth, and extremities may be reported.
- Headache, dizziness, myoclonus, and weakness are often noted.

Lindane causes:

- Seizures: The larger the exposure, the sooner the seizures develop. With oral exposures, seizures can occur in minutes. Seizures can be multiple; status epilepticus can occur.
- Myoclonus and rhabdomyolysis also occur.

Cyclodienes cause:

- Multiple seizures that may be recurrent up to days following exposures. Recovery is complete, provided no hypoxia and complications occur from the intensive care unit stay. Endosulfan is notorious for causing status epilepticus and death. Mortality from endosulfan is around 30%.
- Hyperthermia, hypotension, rhabdomyolysis, and renal impairment are common.

Differential Diagnosis of Acute Presentation

Signs such as seizures, fever, and altered mental status from OCP poisoning can resemble meningitis and encephalitis.

Alcohol and sedative–hypnotic withdrawals have a similar presentation.

Strychnine toxicity with myoclonus can be similar, but in organochlorine poisonings, the patients are more likely to have altered mental status, whereas with strychnine, the patients have "awake" seizures.

These cases can appear like nicotinic toxicity with seizures, rhabdomyolysis, and renal impairment.

Other conditions to consider include central nervous system (CNS)–stimulant ingestions and overdoses, camphor toxicity, picrotoxin toxicity, sodium monofluoroacetate toxicity, hypoxemia, and idiopathic epilepsy (Wong 2022).

Chronic Effects

Chronic effects that occur from prolonged exposure or as persistent symptoms after acute exposure (Roberts and Reigart 2013b) include tremors and ataxia.

OCPs may adversely affect infant neurodevelopment. In utero exposure may lead to attention deficit hyperactivity disorder (ADHD) and autism spectrum disorder. Idiopathic intracranial hypertension can also occur.

There are various studies of patients with Parkinson's disease who may have been exposed (usually occupational) to pesticides. In adults, most studies note an association of parkinsonism with exposure to pesticides in general rather than organochlorines specifically. However, this remains an area of research interest.

The reproductive effects of OCPs are of continued concern. Fertility and endocrine disruption have been shown in animals, but human studies are lacking. DDT, DDE, and endosulfan have been shown to have estrogenic activity (Roberts and Reigart 2013b). A study from China (Guo et al. 2014) showed that prenatal exposure to OCPs caused a decrease in the birth weight of infants. With DDT, there is limited evidence of an association between maternal exposure and cryptorchidism and hypospadias in male offspring (Chen et al. 2008), but it has not been confirmed in other studies. One study of workers at a pesticide facility showed that they had oligospermia and decreased sperm motility, specifically from exposure to chlordecone (Cannon et al. 1978).

Studies in animals show that OCPs can disrupt the endocrine system. In humans, DDE has been linked to precocious puberty in a study of immigrant females in Belgium (Krstevska-Konstantinova et al. 2001), and a negative correlation with the duration of lactation has been reported in females exposed to DDE (Rogan and Ragan 2007). Hypothyroidism in female spouses of farmers who worked with organochlorines has been described (Goldner et al. 2010).

Because of their endocrine disruption effects, studies have looked at possible associations with hormone-responsive cancers in humans. Studies evaluating prostate cancer show some association, but there may be other confounding factors leading to this association (Roberts and Reigart 2013b). There is also some association of DDT with breast cancer, but multiple recent meta-analyses showed no increased risk (Park et al. 2014).

There is an association of DDT with childhood asthma (Karmaus et al. 2001; Sunyer et al. 2005).

Hexachlorobenzene is an organochlorine used as a seed-protectant fungicide. Toxicity occurs from chronic low-level exposure. The biggest poisoning outbreak occurred in Turkey from 1955–1959 when grains that were supposed to be used for agriculture were used for baking. This occurred primarily in children between 6–16 years and resulted in porphyria cutanea tarda with a mortality of 10%. This is a disease of disrupted porphyrin metabolism. These children had photosensitivity, with hemorrhagic bullae developing in sun-exposed areas, loss of appetite, painful hepatomegaly, and anemia. Pembe yara is another disease with 95% mortality rate that affects infants. At that time, it affected children between 2 months and 5 years of age in some villages. It occurred in infants of mothers with porphyria cutanea tarda. These infants had fevers, diarrhea, vomiting, and lesions on hands and feet that were papules and later became sores with central darkness. These patients had anorexia, muscle atrophy, anemia, and hepatomegaly. Death usually occurred from secondary pulmonary infections (Courtney 1979).

Laboratory Evaluation

Organochlorines are stored in fat and their level increases with age, but levels in fat do not correlate with illness. Serum levels of organochlorine-exposed population are higher than nonexposed but do not necessarily correlate with adverse health effects (however, serum levels of lindane correlate with clinical picture). Serum levels can be used for confirmation of exposure but, usually, are not rapidly available and are only performed by a few laboratories. Screening serum and urinary toxicology panels, if intentional exposure is suspected, are recommended. If mixed pesticide exposure is a concern, then plasma and serum cholinesterase should be considered if the patient has additional cholinergic symptoms. If possibility of aspiration or pulmonary symptoms are present, a chest X-ray should be done. If the history of exposure is unclear and the patient has neurologic symptoms, then a head computer tomography scan and lumbar puncture should be considered to rule out infection or other central nervous system conditions (Wong 2022).

Treatment

Decontamination should occur as per any other chemical exposure. Nasogastric suction can be considered if patients present early. Activated charcoal is contraindicated due to the risk of seizures unless the patient is intubated.

There is no specific antidote for organochlorine poisoning. Treatment is mainly supportive (Roberts and Reigart 2013a; Holland 2019; Wong 2022). Continuous cardiac monitoring is indicated. Use epinephrine and sympathomimetics with caution because myocardial sensitization to catecholamines may increase the risk of dysrhythmias. Beta-blockers are reported to control ventricular dysrhythmias.

For seizures, you want to use high doses of benzodiazepines and escalate to phenobarbital, if needed. Rhabdomyolysis should be considered in patients with prolonged convulsions.

These substances undergo biliary excretion, and enhanced elimination can occur with the use of cholestyramine. Cholestyramine has been used successfully in chlordecone poisoning and has been shown to decrease seizures and mortality in animals. The dose for adults is 4 g four times a day and in children 240 mg/kg/24 h divided into three doses, every 8 h. Sucrose polyester can be used instead of cholestyramine (Wong 2022). A medical toxicologist or the poison control center (1-800-222-1222) should be consulted for the management of these poisonings.

References

Cannon SB, Veazey JM Jr, Jackson RS, Burse VW, Hayes C, Straub WE, Landrigan PJ, Liddle JA. Epidemic kepone poisoning in chemical workers. Am J Epidemiol. 1978;107(6):529–37.

Chen JJ, Zhang G, Wasnick R, Priebe C, Roelof B, Steinhardt GF, et al. Maternal burden of organochloro-compounds associated with undescended testes. J Urol. 2008;179(4S):97, abstract 276

Colborn T. Epidemiology of Great Lakes bald eagles. J Toxicol Environ Health. 1991;33(4):395–453. https://doi.org/10.1080/15287399109531537.

Courtney KD. Hexachlorobenzene (HCB): A review. Environ Res. 1979;20(2):225–66. https://doi.org/10.1016/0013-9351(79)90001-X.

Garrettson LK, Guzelian PS, Blanke RV. Subacute chlordane poisoning. J Toxicol Clin Toxicol. 1984;22(6):565–71. https://doi.org/10.3109/15563658408992585.

Goldner WS, Sandler DP, Yu F, Hoppin JA, Kamel FL, Levan TD. Pesticide use and thyroid disease among women in the Agricultural Health Study. Am J Epidemiol. 2010;171(4):455–64.

Guo H, Jin Y, Cheng Y, Leaderer B, Lin S, Holford T, Qiu J, Zhang Y, Shi K, Zhu Y, Niu J, Bassig B, Xu S, Zhang B, Li Y, Hu X, Chen Q, Zheng T. Prenatal exposure to organochlorine pesticides and infant birth weight in China. Chemosphere. 2014;110:1–7. https://doi.org/10.1016/j.chemosphere.2014.02.017.

Hall RC, Hall RC. Long-term psychological and neurological complications of lindane poisoning. Psychosomatics. 1999;40(6):513–7. https://doi.org/10.1016/S0033-3182(99)71191-6.

Holland MG. Insecticides: organic chlorines, pyrethrins/pyrethroids, and insect repellents. In: Nelson LS, Howland MA, Lewin NA, Smith SW, Goldfrank LR, Hoffman RS, editors. Goldfrank's toxicologic emergencies. 11th ed. New York: McGraw-Hill Education; 2019.

Jayara R, Megha P, Sreedev P. Organochlorine pesticides, their toxic effects on living organisms and their fate in the environment. Interdiscip Toxicol. 2016;9(3–4):90–100.

Karmaus W, Kuehr J, Kruse H. Infections and atopic disorders in childhood and organochlorine exposure. Arch Environ Health. 2001;56(6):485–92.

Krstevska-Konstantinova M, Charlier C, Craen M, Du Caju M, Heinrichs C, de Beaufort C, Plomteux G, Bourguignan JP. Sexual precocity after immigration from developing countries to Belgium: evidence of previous exposure to organochlorine pesticides. Hum Reprod. 2001;16(5):1020–6.

Lee B, Groth P. Scabies: transcutaneous poisoning during treatment. Pediatrics. 1977;59(4):643.

Moses V, Peter JV. Acute intentional toxicity: Endosulfan and other organochlorines. Clin Toxicol (Phila). 2010;48(6):539–44. https://doi.org/10.3109/15563650.2010.494610.

Munk ZM, Nantel A. Acute lindane poisoning with development of muscle necrosis. Can Med Assoc J. 1977;117(9):1050–4.

Park JH, Cha ES, Ko Y, Hwang MS, Hong JH, Lee WJ. Exposure to dichlorodiphenyltrichloroethane and the risk of breast cancer: a systematic review and meta-analysis. Osong Public Health Res Perspect. 2014;5(2):77–84. https://doi.org/10.1016/j.phrp.2014.02.001.

Roberts JR, Reigart JR. Chapter 7. Organochlorines. In: Recognition and management of pesticide poisonings. U. S. Environmental Protection Agency (EPA); 2013a. p. 63–9. Accessed 22 Feb 2021.

Roberts JR, Reigart JR. Chapter 21. Chronic effects. In: Recognition and management of pesticide poisonings. U.S. Environmental Protection Agency (EPA); 2013b. p. 212–38. Accessed 22 Feb 2021.

Rogan WJ, Ragan NB. Some evidence of effects of environmental chemicasl on the endocrine system in children. Int J Hyg Environ Health. 2007;210(5):659–67.

Sunyer J, Torrent M, Munoz-Ortiz L, Ribas-Fito N, Carrizo D, Grimalt J, Anto JM, Cullinan P. Prenatal dichlorodiphenyldichloroethylene (DDE) and asthma in children. Environ Health Perspect. 2005;113(12):1787–90.

USEPA (Environmental Protection Agency). Serum persistent organic pollutants. Report on the Environment https://www.epa.gov/report-environment. Updated On September 13, 2023.

USFWS (Fish and Wildlife Services). Eagle Management. https://www.fws.gov/program/eagle-management. Accessed 17 Feb 2024.

Wikipedia. Silent Spring. Last edited on 16 February 2024. Available at: https://en.wikipedia.org/wiki/Silent_Spring. Accessed 19 Feb 2024.

Wong ML. Organochlorine Pesticide Toxicity. May 14, 2022. Medscape. https://emedicine.medscape.com/article/815051-overview?form=fpf. Accessed 16 Feb 2024.

Yavuz Y, Yurumez Y, Kücüker H, Ela Y, Yüksel S. Two cases of acute endosulfan toxicity. Clin Toxicol. 2007;45(5):530–2. https://doi.org/10.1080/15563650701365909.

Nicotine and Neonicotinoid Insecticides

7

Jason B. Hack

Nicotine Insecticides

Introduction

Nicotine insecticides belong to the class of natural pesticides. Nicotine has a complex biochemistry, pharmacology, and toxicology and is used in nature for defensive purposes by many plants against herbivorous animals and insects. These plants include *Nicotiana tabacum*, *N. glauca*, and *N. rustica* (Solanaceae), and are also found in a number of plant families like Lycopodiaceae, Crassulaceae, Leguminosae, Chenopodiaceae, and Compositae. It is also found in trace amounts naturally in several solanaceous food plants, including potatoes, tomatoes, eggplant as well as peppers. Millions of people worldwide have and continue to exploit plant-derived nicotine for its psychoactive effects for millennia.

Use in Agriculture

Tobacco extracts have been used to repel and kill insects since the 1690s. Tobacco smoke has been used for insect fumigation since this time. The most notorious commercial nicotine-containing insecticide product was "Black Leaf 40" (nicotine sulfate 40%), which was associated with poisonings and deaths, although the FDA banned its sale in 1992. Currently, nicotine products have only very limited use in the United States but are still used elsewhere in the world—primarily in Asia.

Mechanism of Action

Nicotine is a naturally occurring plant alkaloid, found in certain species as noted above, that has addictive, central nervous system, and stimulant effects. It causes effect in the brain, ganglia, and at the level of the nerves. Nicotine acts as an agonist at the nicotinic cholinergic receptors in the autonomic ganglia, at neuromuscular junctions, in the adrenal medulla, and in the brain (Taillebois et al. 2018). It causes stimulation in low doses and ganglionic blockage in high doses. Humans are very sensitive to nicotine and its related molecules.

Nicotine's central nervous system (CNS) and cardiovascular (CV) stimulating activities are mediated through the release of several neurotransmitters, including acetylcholine, dopamine, norepinephrine, and serotonin. Centrally, nicotine stimulates the chemoreceptor trigger zone, thereby inducing severe nausea and vomiting in some sensitive people not used to the chemical (a predominant symptom in green

J. B. Hack (✉)
Department of Emergency Medicine, Brody School of Medicine, East Carolina University, Greenville, NC, USA
e-mail: hackj20@ecu.edu

W. J. Meggs, R. L. Langley (eds.), *Farm Toxicology*, https://doi.org/10.1007/978-3-031-80441-0_7

tobacco sickness). Its dose-dependent effects cause peripheral vasoconstriction that can result in tachycardia and elevated blood pressure.

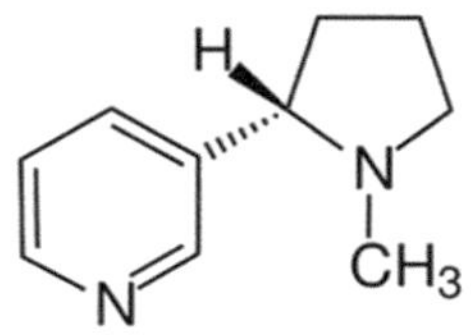

Routes of Exposure

Nicotine is well-absorbed and is distributed throughout the body. Toxicity can occur with dermal (spray, splash, or contact with green tobacco leaves), oral (mucous membrane exposure), gastrointestinal (GI) (ingestion), or pulmonary (vapor, droplet, dust, or smoke) exposures.

Toxicity

Cigarette smokers absorb approximately 1 mg of nicotine per dose (Solarino et al. 2010a). The adult fatal dose has been reported to be 60 mg (Solarino et al. 2010b. Moriya and Hashimoto 2005) or 0.5–1 mg/kg (CDC 2003).

Severity of symptoms after exposure and total fatal dose depend on many factors and, without controlled studies, likely vary from patient to patient. Because of the sensitivity to nicotine, even a small exposure can cause both central and peripheral stimulation and arousal, resulting in increased heart rate, blood pressure, and CNS activation.

Acute overdoses generally present with profound CNS, CV, and GI symptoms (Lavoie and Harris 1991).

Ocular findings include miosis, initially followed by mydriasis.

Gastrointestinal symptoms often predominate and include nausea and vomiting, salivation, abdominal pain, and diarrhea (CDC 2003).

Pulmonary findings include increased bronchial secretions (bronchorrhea), shortness of breath, and respiratory failure.

Cardiovascular symptoms may include hypertension or hypotension, tachycardia or bradycardia.

Central nervous system symptoms include confusion, dizziness, tremors, altered mental status, seizure, coma, depressed reflexes, large muscle body fasciculations and weakness, and ultimately, paralysis.

Death can result from respiratory muscle paralysis, seizures, and coma (Solarino et al. 2010a, b).

Treatment

Treatment includes immediate and thorough decontamination by removal of any contaminated clothing, copious irrigation of any areas of exposed skin, and consideration of gastrointestinal decontamination for large intentional ingestions.

There is no antidotal therapy. Nicotine and cotinine levels can be sent for confirmation of exposure (they will also be present if the patient is a tobacco user). Treatment after exposure is supportive and directed at the encountered symptoms—antiemetics for nausea and vomiting, medications to support cardiovascular and pulmonary alterations (e.g., atropine for bradydysrhythmias or pulmonary secretions), intubation and supplemental oxygen for respiratory insult or arrest, benzodiazepines for agitation or seizures, and fluid resuscitation and vasopressor medications for hypotension.

Neonicotinoid Insecticides

Introduction

Neonicotinoids or "neonics" are a class of natural insecticides derived from nithiazine molecules that target nicotinic acetylcholine receptors. Their name means "new-nicotine-like" insecticides. These groups have nitromethylene, nitroimine, or cyanoimine groups attached to the core nicotine structure. The first commercially produced neonicotinoid, imidacloprid, was developed in 1994.

Use in Agriculture

Because they are effective at very low doses and have limited mammalian toxicity, broad-spectrum activity, low application rates, upward systemic movement in plants (from seeds to flowers), and versatile application methods, this class of insecticides is the most widely used in the world. Neonicotinoid insecticides are used as replacements for highly toxic-to-humans organophosphate and carbamate insecticides. Neonicotinoid insecticides include first-generation insecticides (e.g., imidacloprid, nitenpyram, acetamiprid, and thiacloprid); and second-generation insecticides (e.g., thiamethoxam, clothianidin, dinotefuran, sulfoxaflor, and cycloxaprid) (Tomizawa and Casida 2005). They are very persistent in the exposed plants and soil where they are applied.

Mechanism of Action

Neonicotinoids share a mechanism of action with the nicotinergic insecticides and primarily work at neuronal nicotinic acetylcholine receptors (NAChR, receptors that are stimulated and, ultimately, result in the development of insect paralysis and death).

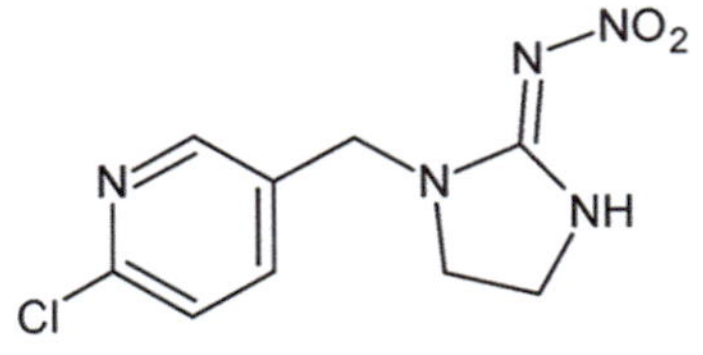

Figure 1. Chemical structure of imidacloprid.
doi:10.1371/journal.pone.0005127.g001

Toxicity

Because of its low toxicity in humans, symptoms are usually absent or mild with unintentional dermal exposures. Intentional exposures (as in self-poisoning) of typically larger doses have resulted in a constellation of symptoms including nausea, vomiting, headache, dizziness, abdominal pain, and diarrhea—most of which resolved with only supportive care (Mohamed et al. 2009). Long-term effects of human exposure are largely unknown [Chapter from the book: *Poisoning: From Specific Toxic Agents to Novel Rapid and Simplified Techniques for Analysis*].

Environmental Concerns

There is concern that the use of neonicotinoids is associated with injury to beneficial and non-pest insects like bees and butterflies (Forister et al. 2016). Because these chemicals are absorbed by treated plants (or treated seeds) systemically and can persist for an entire growing season, they are present in the nectar and pollen that the plant produces. This has direct effects on the beneficial insect populations in environments where they are being used—especially bees and butterflies. It has been shown to have sublethal effects on bees' foraging and colony performance (Muth and Leonard 2019). The decimation of these pollinating animal numbers can have a direct impact on harvests of pollinator-dependent food plants.

In bees, the effects of neonicotinoids are similar to those of nicotine in humans. Not only is the pesticide detrimental to their health, but bees also tend to prefer it to their own food source. Honeybees and bumblebees will preferentially choose to drink sucrose solution spiked with neonicotinoids compared to solution without (Yang et al. 2008).

Bees that are exposed to neonicotinoids can experience problems with their central nervous systems, often resulting in impaired memory, movement, and even death. For this reason, the chemicals are banned in many parts of Europe and are under increased scrutiny in the United States.

Treatment

Dermal and mucosal exposures should be decontaminated as soon as possible. Gastric irrigation may be considered in patients who present early with massive ingestions, as long as the airway is properly protected and the patient is not vomiting.

Activated charcoal should be used very cautiously or not at all as vomiting (like in nicotine poisoning) is a prominent feature after neonicotinoid insecticide exposure, and charcoal may hamper endoscopic evaluation among patients with corrosive injuries.

Patients should be monitored closely for adverse respiratory effects, especially hypoventilation and respiratory failure. Atropine has been used to assist with management of symptoms such as profuse sweating and excessive pulmonary secretions.

Due to possible irritant and corrosive effects of the solvent that the product is dissolved in, patients with significant symptoms suggestive of upper-airway injury like hoarseness and stridor, chest/abdominal pain, or gastrointestinal injury should be evaluated for tissue injury. Techniques of investigating include CT scanning for perforation, direct visualization by endoscopic evaluation of the airway (e.g., vocal cords), or proximal GI tract (esophagus and gastric endoscopy).

References

Centers for Disease Control and Prevention (CDC). Nicotine poisoning after ingestion of contaminated ground beef-Michigan, 2003. MMWR Morb Mortal Wkly Rep. 2003;52(18):413–6. PMID: 12807090.

Forister ML, Cousens B, Harrison JG, Anderson K, Thorne JH, Waetjen D, Nice CC, De Parsia M, Hladik ML, Meese R, van Vliet H, Shapiro AM. Increasing neonicotinoid use and the declining butterfly fauna of lowland California. Biol Lett. 2016;12(8):20160475. https://doi.org/10.1098/rsbl.2016.0475.

Lavoie FW, Harris TM. Fatal nicotine ingestion. J Emerg Med. 1991;9:133–6.

Mohamed F, Gawarammana I, Robertson TA, Roberts MS, Palangasinghe C, et al. Acute human self-poisoning with imidacloprid compound: a neonicotinoid insecticide. PLoS One. 2009;4:e5127.

Moriya F, Hashimoto Y. A fatal poisoning caused by methomyl and nicotine. Forensic Sci Int. 2005;149:167–70.

Muth F, Leonard AS. A neonicotinoid pesticide impairs foraging, but not learning, in free-flying bumblebees. Sci Rep. 2019;9(1):4764.

Solarino B, Rosenbaum F, Riesselmann B, Buschmann CT, Tsokos M. Death due to ingestion of nicotine-containing solution: case report and review of the literature. Forensic Sci Int. 2010a;195:e19–22.

Solarino B, Rießelmann B, Buschmann CT, Tsokos M. Multidrug poisoning involving nicotine and tramadol. Forensic Sci Int. 2010b;194:e17–9.

Taillebois E, Cartereau A, Jones AK, Thany SH. Neonicotinoid insecticides mode of action on insect nicotinic acetylcholine receptors using binding studies. Pestic Biochem Physiol. 2018;151:59–66.

Tomizawa M, Casida JE. Neonicotinoid insecticide toxicology: mechanism of selective action. Annu Rev Pharmacol Toxicol. 2005;45:247–68.

Yang EC, Chuang YC, Chen YL, Chang LH. Abnormal foraging behavior induced by sublethal dosage of imidacloprid in the honey bee (Hymenoptera: Apidae). J Econ Entomol. 2008;101:1743–8.

Pyrethrums and Pyrethroid Insecticides

8

Jason B. Hack

Pyrethrins

Pyrethrum, which is a natural product derived directly from the *Tanacetum cinerariaefolium* (chrysanthemum) plant, is among the first commercially produced anti-pest products. It was first used for body lice in the 1800s.

The flowers were produced for sale in Armenia, then Dalmatia (Yugoslavia) until the First World War, Japan until the Second World War, and East Africa since—most of the world's current production comes from Kenya, Tanzania, Rwanda, and Ecuador (Casida 1980; Matsuo 2019).

Terminology

Pyrethrum extracts are chemicals that come directly from the plant—it contains insecticidal esters—that are referred to as **pyrethrins**. These **pyrethrin** molecules can be altered to create **pyrethroids**, which are synthetic structures that are designed to have attributes to make them more attractive (have enhanced insecticidal characteristics) for commercial use (Davies, 2007).

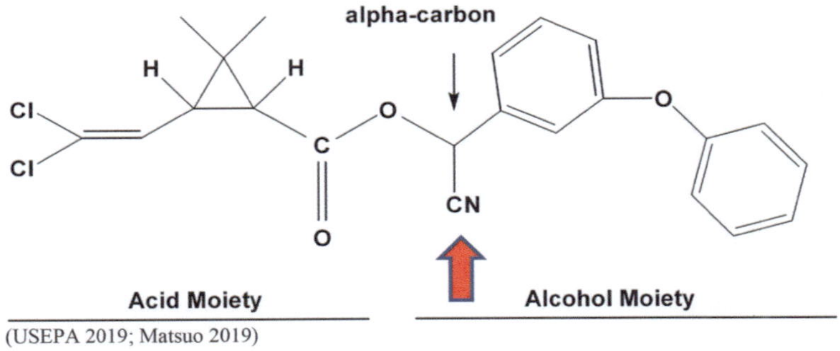

(USEPA 2019; Matsuo 2019)

Structure of pyrethrin (USEPA 2019; Matsuo 2019)

J. B. Hack (✉)
Department of Emergency Medicine, Brody School of Medicine, East Carolina University, Greenville, NC, USA
e-mail: hackj20@ecu.edu

W. J. Meggs, R. L. Langley (eds.), *Farm Toxicology*, https://doi.org/10.1007/978-3-031-80441-0_8

The typical pyrethroid structure includes a chrysanthemic acid linked to an aromatic alcohol through an ester linkage (see illustration). There are two broad classes, which are based on the molecular structures and linkages between them. Pyrethroid molecules that lack the alpha-cyano group are referred to as type I, or first-generation. Pyrethroids with the alpha-cyano group are referred to as type II, or second-generation—this CN group enhances the insecticidal activity and molecular stability and results in clinical differences of exposures between groups (Matsuo 2019; USEPA 2019).

In general, there are two distinct toxicity syndromes described in rats following pyrethroid exposure from these two classes of pyrethroids. The T-syndrome (fine tremors) is associated with type I pyrethroids and characterized by aggressive sparring, increased sensitivity to external stimuli, and fine whole-body tremors. The CS-syndrome (choreoathetosis and salivation) is associated with type II pyrethroids and characterized by initial pawing and burrowing, salivation, and choreoathetosis (USEPA 2019).

Table 8.1 Available pyrethrins

Allethrin
Bioallethrin
D-Allethrin
Esbiothrin
Bifenthrin
Cyclethrin
Cyfluthrin, C. beta
Cyhalothrin, C lambda, C. gamma
Cypermethrin
Cypermethrin, C. alpha, C. beta, C. zeta
Cyphenothrin
Deltamethrin
Esfenvalerate
Fenvalerate
Fenfluthrin
Fenpropathrin

This table is a modification from: USEPA Office of Pesticide Programs' Re-Evaluation of the FQPA Safety Factor for Pyrethroids: Updated Literature and CAPHRA Program Data Review. July 1, 2019

Manufacture

Allethrin was the first synthetic derivative of pyrethrum, produced commercially in 1949. Since its release, successive isosteric structural modifications have been made to enhance the molecule's diverse characteristics. These adjustments targeted enhancing the effectiveness and usefulness in the control of both household insect pests and for agricultural use, making them one of the most important classes of crop protection chemicals currently available. These synthetic pyrethrins are more potent, cheaper, and more stable than natural pyrethrins.

As such, there are at least 30 synthetic pyrethrins available for use in the home and on crops—a result of these structural manipulations, which has made them commercially attractive. First-generation pyrethroids include bifenthrin, permethrin, and d-phenothrin, and second-generation pyrethroids include cypermethrin, fenvalerate, cyfluthrin, and deltamethrin (see Table 8.1). These products share attributes including being very effective in knocking down insects (stopping their locomotion), limiting insect resistance, and having no significant persistence in air and soil and limited mammalian toxicity (so much so that early pyrethrins were once labeled as "nontoxic to humans and pets" (Narahashi 2007; Casida et al. 1983)). The latter quality is very important for use as proven safety and effectiveness for the treatment of home pests (lice, fleas, flies, roaches, and mosquitoes) and in agriculture environments (grain storage, use on edible products before harvest, feed animal housing, vegetable fields, and greenhouses) both increase their commercial base. Pyrethrins also play a role in global health and are sprayed in passenger aircraft to prevent the spread of disease-carrying insect vectors from one country to the next and are sprayed in large urban areas to control insect vectors of disease (e.g., mosquitoes that spread the West Nile virus) without significant human health or ecotoxicological consequences (Krieger et al. 2010). In many commercial products of pyrethroids and pyrethrins, they are combined with additional agents to increase their persistence and potency (Anadón et al. 2009; Leone 2007; USEPA 2019). Pyrethrin-based shampoo or cream products used for lice or scabies typically have large LD50s-which varys depending on the specific compounds, additives and endogenous mammalian hydrolysis of pyrethrins to inactive components.

If symptoms do occur, they are most commonly of low toxicity and present with allergic-like symptoms. Massive exposures result in more pronounced symptoms and, rarely, death (Bradberry 2005). Dermatitis can result from prolonged exposures or high concentration, characterized by irritation, itching, urticaria, and transient numbness or tingling in the exposed area. Ocular symptoms of irritation, redness, and tearing occur with direct exposure (frequently described after exposure to pyrethrin-containing shampoos or creams, most commonly described in children); corneal injury and visual disturbances have also been described. Mucosal symptoms with oral exposures include swelling, irritation, and salivation. Inadvertent oral or dermal exposure to high-dose pyrethrins (like a taste or a splash) can cause a temporary numbness of the tongue, lips, or skin. Gastrointestinal symptoms include abdominal pain, nausea, and vomiting. Pulmonary symptoms include respiratory distress, wheezing, coughing, and bronchospasm. Neurologic symptoms may include temporary numbness and tingling in the exposed skin and mucosa, incoordination, "stuttering," altered mental status, seizures, and coma with massive exposures have all been described.

Differential diagnosis for these exposures includes events resulting in similar allergic manifestations including, Hymenoptera stings, medication reactions, disulfiram reactions, and anaphylaxis.

Treatment

Pyrethrins are typically quickly metabolized and excreted by exposed humans—treatment is mainly directed as decontamination and supportive. Copious irrigation of exposed skin and mucous membranes, removal of contaminated clothing, and movement to fresh air are primary maneuvers. Treatment of pulmonary symptoms is directed at alleviating wheezing and bronchospasm and includes inhaled beta agonists, systemic steroids, and intubation as needed for severe cases. There have been cases where vitamin E (alpha-tocopherol) oil has been used for paresthesia among individuals dermally exposed to synthetic pyrethroids. The mode of action of vitamin E appears to be the selective block of pyrethroid-modified Na channels as was shown in situ in rat cells (Song and Narahashi 1995). Neurologic symptoms are generally treated with supportive care.

References

Anadón A, Martínez-Larrañaga MR, Martínez MA. Use and abuse of pyrethrins and synthetic pyrethroids in veterinary medicine. Vet J. 2009;182(1):7–20. https://doi.org/10.1016/j.tvjl.2008.04.008. Epub 2008 Jun 6. PMID: 18539058.

Bradberry SM, Cage SA, Proudfoot AT, Vale JA. Poisoning due to pyrethroids. Toxicol Rev. 2005;24(2):93–106. https://doi.org/10.2165/00139709-200524020-00003. PMID: 16180929.

Casida JE. Pyrethrum flowers and pyrethroid insecticides. Environ Health Perspect. 1980;34:189–202. https://doi.org/10.1289/ehp.8034189.

Casida JE, Gammon DW, Glickman AH, Lawrence LJ. Mechanisms of selective action of pyrethroid insecticides. Annu Rev Pharmacol Toxicol. 1983;23(1):413–38. https://doi.org/10.1146/annurev.pa.23.040183.002213.

Davies TG, Field LM, Usherwood PN, Williamson MS. DDT, pyrethrins, pyrethroids and insect sodium channels. IUBMB Life. 2007;59(3):151–62. https://doi.org/10.1080/15216540701352042. PMID: 17487686.

Krieger RI, et al. Hayes' handbook of pesticide toxicology, vol. 1. Elsevier; 2010.

Leone PA. Scabies and pediculosis pubis: an update of treatment regimens and general review. Clin Infect Dis. 2007;44 Suppl 3:S153–9. https://doi.org/10.1086/511428. PMID: 17342668.

Matsuo N. Discovery and development of pyrethroid insecticides. Proc Jpn Acad Ser B Phys Biol Sci. 2019;95(7):378–400. https://doi.org/10.2183/pjab.95.027.

Narahashi T, Zhao X, Ikeda T, Nagata K, Yeh JZ. Differential actions of insecticides on target sites: basis for selective toxicity. Hum Exp Toxicol. 2007;26(4):361–6. https://doi.org/10.1177/0960327106078408.

Song JH, Narahashi T. Selective block of tetramethrin-modified sodium channels by (+/−)-alpha-tocopherol (vitamin E). J Pharmacol Exp Ther. 1995;275(3):1402–11. PMID: 8531109.

USEPA Office of Pesticide Programs' Re-Evaluation of the FQPA Safety Factor for Pyrethroids: Updated Literature and CAPHRA Program Data Review. July 1, 2019.

Herbicides

9

William J. Meggs

Introduction

Herbicides are the most widely used class of pesticides worldwide, greatly exceeding the amounts applied of insecticides, fungicides, bactericides, and other pest control classes (see Table 9.1).

Of the herbicides used, glyphosate dominates use, followed by atrazine and then 2,4-dischlorophenoxyacetic acid (2,4-D), as seen in Fig. 9.1.

The herbicides used have different mechanisms of action and varying degrees of plant specificity (Roberts & Reigart 2013). Table 9.2 lists the major herbicides available with brand names, uses, and modes of action.

Table 9.1 Class of pesticides. Statistica 2023

Class	Use in 1000 metric tons
Herbicides	1732.3
Fungicides and bactericides	816.38
Insecticides	757.54
Others	229.15

W. J. Meggs (✉)
Brody School of Medicine, East Carolina University, Greenville, NC, USA
e-mail: meggsw@ecu.edu

W. J. Meggs, R. L. Langley (eds.), *Farm Toxicology*, https://doi.org/10.1007/978-3-031-80441-0_9

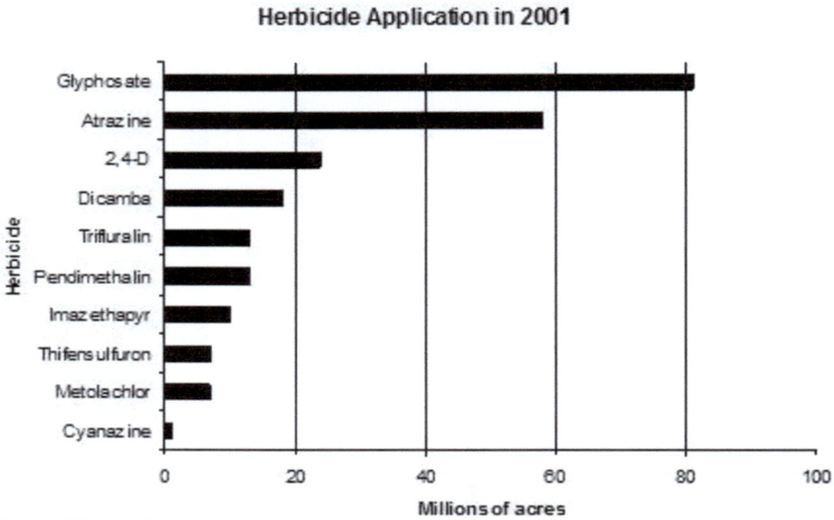

Source EPA 2023.

Fig. 9.1 Herbicide application in 2001. (Source Environmental Protection Agency 2023)

Table 9.2 Herbicides with brand names, use, and mechanism of plant toxicity. Environmental Protection Agency 2023

Herbicide	Common application	Mode of action
Amino acid inhibitors		
Glyphosate *Roundup, Ultra, Rodeo, TouchDown Pro, Accord*	Applied primarily to genetically engineered, glyphosate-resistant varieties of soybeans, corn, canola, and cotton. Also applied to control woody plants. Because of its broad spectrum and relatively low toxicity to animals, it is used in horticulture and in the control of aquatic macrophytes	Applied to the foliage and transported with sugars to metabolic sites where they inhibit amino acid production. Effects will manifest in two or more weeks as discoloration of foliage and deformations in new growth
Imazethapyr *Pursuit*	Applied to control weeds in alfalfa, barley, soybeans, and wheat	Same as glyphosate
Thifensulfuron *Beacon, Pinnacle, and Harmony*	Applied to control weeds in small grains, soybeans, and corn and in conifer and hardwood plantations	Same as glyphosate
Photosynthesis inhibitors		
Atrazine *Aatrex and Atrazine* Cyanazine*Bladex/DuPont*	Applied to crops such as corn, soybeans, and sorghum, particularly for conservation tillage	These broad-spectrum herbicides are applied to the soil and carried to the leaves by transpiration. They inhibit photosynthesis
Synthetic auxin and growth regulators		
2,4-D Dicamba *Banvel, Clarity, Vanquish, and Veteran*	Applied to broad-leaved weeds in corn, small grains, sorghum, pastures, and rangeland. Urban use is on lawns and grassy rights of way. They are also applied for control of broad-leaved trees when planting conifers	These synthetic growth hormones are applied to the foliage of dicots and transported to meristems, causing uncontrolled growth. Effects can be observed as discoloration of foliage and deformations in new growth. They are fast-acting: Effects on foliage are visible within minutes of application

(continued)

Table 9.2 (continued)

Herbicide	Common application	Mode of action
Cell division inhibitors		
Trifluralin *Treflan and others*	Applied to control grasses and broad-leaved weeds in crops such as beans, peanuts, cotton, and tobacco	These herbicides are applied to the soil to control target vegetation before emergence by inhibiting root growth
Pendimethalin *Prowl, Pentagon, Pendulum, and Stomp*		
Metolachlor *Dual, Dual Magnum, and Pennant Magnum*	Applied preplanting to control annual grasses and broad-leaved weeds among crops such as corn and soybeans	This herbicide is applied to the soil to control target vegetation by inhibiting or disrupting cell division in shoots

Glyphosate

Glyphosate is used extensively for weed control on lawns, crops, and in forestry. It is marketed with numerous brand names including Roundup®, Glyphomax®, and Glypro®. An estimated 280 million pounds are used annually in the United States, making it the most-used herbicide. In addition to technical grade glyphosate, different formulations have other ingredients including surfactants that may add to toxicity (Martins-Gomes 2022). The formulations are irritants and corrosives (ATSDR 2023).

Exposures can be dermal, inhalational, ocular, and by ingestion. Ingestion can be unintentional in small children and, in many cases, intentional in older age groups. In large ingestions, the corrosive effects on the gastrointestinal tract, from the mouth downward, can be severe. In addition, surfactants in the preparations have been associated with myocardial depression (Nincevic et al. 2017). In a review of 93 cases of acute exposure (Talbot et al. 1991), accidental dermal exposure was asymptomatic. Accidental oral ingestion had only had mild oral discomfort. Intentional ingestions were severe, with gastrointestinal erosions, dysphagia, sore throat, and gastrointestinal hemorrhage. In another study, accidental exposure was asymptomatic after dermal contact with spray, while mild oral discomfort occurred after accidental ingestion. Intentional ingestion resulted in erosion of the gastrointestinal tract, throat pain, dysphagia, and gastrointestinal hemorrhage (Craig 2018; Bradberry et al. 2004).

In the evaluation of a potential exposure case, specific levels of glyphosate are unlikely to be helpful in the acute setting and can only be obtained from reference laboratories.

Treatment is supportive. There are no specific antidotes. In severe exposures, maintain the airway and support respiration and circulation. Consultation with a gastroenterologist for endoscopic evaluation can be helpful to determine the extent of damage. Surgical consultation is also prudent in cases where surgical intervention may be indicated.

Chlorophenoxy Herbicides

2,4-dischlorophenoxyacetic acid, commonly known as 2,4-D, is widely used, with an estimated 46 million pounds used annually in the United States. Various salts of 2,4-D are marketed under different brand names. The pure form of 2,4-D has low toxicity from inhalation, skin contact, and ingestion, but the acid and salt forms can be irritating to the eyes and skin. Ingestion is associated with gastrointestinal symptoms of nausea, vomiting, diarrhea, and abdominal pain. Rhabdomyolysis with muscle weakness, metabolic acidosis, and renal failure have been reported after ingestions of large quantities. Neurotoxic effects that may be noted include hypertonia, hyperreflexia, nystagmus, miosis, hallucinations, fasciculation, and paralysis, seizure, and coma. Liver failure has also been reported (ATSDR 2020; Bradberry et al. 2000; National Poison Information Center (NPIC); O'Malley 2018).

Occupational inhalational exposures have been associated with transient gastrointestinal and peripheral neuropathies. Acute ingestions have been associated with progressive neuropathies.

There is no antidote, so treatment is supportive care. Activated charcoal should be considered for early presentations after ingestion if it can be safely given. Alkalinization of the urine with sodium bicarbonate given as boluses or IV infusion may be of help (Bradberry et al. 2000). One method of urinary alkalinization is accomplished by adding two or three ampules (44 mEq or 50 mEq ampules) of sodium bicarbonate to a one-liter bag of D5W infusion that is infused at 100–200 mL/hour with a targeted urine pH between 7.0 and 8.0. Consultation with a medical toxicologist or poison center (800-222-1222) is highly recommended.

Dipyridyl Herbicides: Diquat and Paraquat

Dipyridyl herbicides are used for weed control and to defoliate crops such as soybeans to facilitate mechanical harvesting. While both diquat and paraquat have significant human toxicity, paraquat uniquely causes potentially fatal delayed pulmonary fibrosis after ingestion but not with inhalational exposures. The brand Roundup QuikPro is a mixture of glyphosate and diquat. Topical and inhalational exposures from both compounds are strong irritants to the skin, eyes, and the airway. Even small-volume ingestions can be highly toxic with corrosive injury to the gastrointestinal tract, with mucosal ulcerations. Fluid sequestration, electrolyte abnormalities, and shock have been reported (Geller 2018; Chandra et al. 2021; Jones and Vale 2000; Centers for Disease Control (CDC 2018)). Acute renal failure can occur with diquat and paraquat ingestions. After paraquat ingestions, pulmonary fibrosis occurs after days or weeks and has a high case-fatality rate. Specific levels are available from reference labs and have prognostic significance but are generally not available in the acute setting.

Acute management involves rapid replacement of fluid and electrolyte losses. No specific antidotes are available though a combination of glucocorticoids and cyclophosphamide has been reported to ameliorate pulmonary fibrosis from paraquat ingestions. Decontamination of ocular and skin exposures is essential. Copious irrigation of eyes with normal saline using a Morgan lens is recommended. Skin should be decontaminated with soap and water, with large volumes of water used. Multiple doses of activated charcoal should be given as soon as possible. Hemodialysis is of questionable benefit. Consultation with a medical toxicologist or poison center (+800-222-1222) is highly recommended.

Atrazine

Atrazine and cyanazine are representative of the triazine class of herbicides. Atrazine is the most widely used of this class and is considered to be of low acute toxicity. It has the potential to cause eye, skin, and airway irritation, particularly with direct contact (Hanson et al. 2020; Pathak & Dikshit 2011). Human experience with acute toxicity of triazines is limited to case reports with coingestants. In a case of prometryn with ethanol poisoning, emesis, somnolence, and anion gap metabolic acidosis that resolved with hemodialysis were reported (Brvar et al. 2008). A fatality occurred after ingestion of a herbicide preparation containing atrazine, aminotriazole, ethylene glycol, and formaldehyde. Coma, metabolic acidosis, circulatory collapse, and gastrointestinal hemorrhage occurred in this case (Pommery et al. 1993). An unwitnessed fatality occurred after ingesting a herbicide containing ametryn, xylene, and cyclohexanone (Takayasu et al. 2010). These cases illustrate that herbicide preparations are often mixtures with uncertain toxicity from the primary active ingredients.

Chronic Effects

Glyphosate is classified as "probably carcinogenic to humans" (Group 2A) by the International Agency for Research on Cancer (IARC 2016).

The classification is based on "limited evidence of cancer in humans (from real-world exposures that actually occurred) and sufficient evidence of cancer in experimental animals (from studies of 'pure' glyphosate)" (IARC 2016).

Paraquat has been linked to Parkinson's disease (PD). Low-level and chronic paraquat exposure has been reported to be epidemiologically associated with the prevalence of Parkinson's disease in humans (Kalia and Lang 2015; Tanner et al. 2011). An animal study of paraquat exposure has demonstrated a link and established the mechanism as the induction of neuroinflammation in the midbrain (Tong et al. 2022).

Atrazine is a known endocrine disrupter in adult and larval stage amphibians, young fish, developing alligators, and both male and female peripubertal rats (Kucka et al. 2012). The Agriculture Health Study (Rusiecki et al. 2004) "did not find any clear associations between atrazine exposure and any cancer analyzed. However, further studies are warranted for tumor types in which there was a suggestion of trend (lung, bladder, non-Hodgkin lymphoma, and multiple myeloma."

References

ATSDR. Glyphosate. https://wwwn.cdc.gov/TSP/ToxProfiles/ToxProfiles.aspx?id=1488&tid=293. Accessed 25 Nov 2023.

ATSDR. Toxicological profile for 2,4-dichlorophenoxyacetic acid (2,4-D). Atlanta: Agency for Toxic Substances and Disease Registry (US); 2020.

Bradberry SM, Proudfoot AT, Vale JA. Glyphosphate poisoning. Toxicol Rev. 2004;23(3):159–67.

Bradberry SM, Watt BE, Proudfoot AT, Vale JA. Mechanisms of toxicity, clinical features, and management of acute chlorophenoxy herbicide poisoning: a review. J Toxicol Clin Toxicol. 2000;38(2):111–22.

Brvar M, Okrajsek R, Kosmina P, Staric F, Kaps R, Kozelj G, Bunc M. Metabolic acidosis in prometryn (triazine herbicide) self-poisoning. Clin Toxicol (Phila). 2008;46(3):270–3.

CDC. Paraquat. 2018. https://emergency.cdc.gov/agent/paraquat/basics/facts.asp#. Accessed 26 Nov 2023.

Craig S. Glyphosate. In: Olson KR, et al., editors. Poisoning & drug overdoses. 7th ed. McGraw Hill; 2018. p. 257–8.

Chandra A, Shah KA, Mahato S, Bhattacharjee MS, Mandal T. Paraquat poisoning. BMJ Case Rep. 2021;14(11):e246585.

Environmental Protection Agency. 2023. https://www.epa.gov/caddis-vol2/herbicides. Accessed 29 Nov 2023.

Geller RJ. Paraquat and diquat. In: Olson KR, et al., editors. Poisoning & drug overdoses. 7th ed. McGraw Hill; 2018. p. 361–4.

IARC. Monogram on glyphosate. 2016. https://www.iarc.who.int/wp-content/uploads/2018/11/QA_Glyphosate.pdf. Accessed 18 Jan 2024.

Jones GM, Vale JA. Mechanisms of toxicity, clinical features, and management of diquat poisoning: a review. J Toxicol Clin Toxicol. 2000;38(2):123–8.

Kalia LV, Lang AE. Parkinson's disease. Lancet. 2015;386:896–912.

Kucka M, Pogrmic-Majkic K, Fa S, et al. Atrazine acts as an endocrine disrupter by inhibiting cAMP-specific phosphodiesterase-4. Toxicol Appl Pharmacol. 2012;15:19–26.

Martins-Gomes C, Silva TL, Andreani T, Silva AM. Glyphosate vs. glyphosate-based herbicides exposure: a review on their toxicity. J Xenobiot. 2022;12(1):21–40.

Hanson W, Strid A, Gervais J, Cross A, Jenkins J. Atrazine fact sheet. National Pesticide Information Center, Oregon State University Extension Services; 2020. http://npic.orst.edu/factsheets/atrazine.html. Accessed 14 Jan 2024.

Nincevic Z, Nincevic J, Gabelica M, et al. Severe glyphosate—surfactant herbicide poisoning; successful treatment-case report. MOJ Addict Med Ther. 2017;4(1):202–4.

O'Malley MA. Glyphosate. In: Olson KR, et al., editors. Poisoning & drug overdoses. 7th ed. McGraw Hill; 2018. p. 257–8.

Pathak RD, Dikshit AK. Atrazine and human health. Int Jour Ecosyst. 2011;1:14–23.

Pommery J, Mathieu M, Mathieu D, Lhermitte M. Atrazine in plasma and tissue following atrazine-aminotriazole-ethylene glycol-formaldehyde poisoning. J Toxicol Clin Toxicol. 1993;31(2):323–31.

Roberts JR, Reigart JR. Recognition and management of pesticide poisonings. 6th ed. Office of Pesticide Programs. U.S. Environmental Protection Agency; 2013. English edition: https://www.epa.gov/pesticide-worker-safety/recognition-and-management-pesticide-poisonings.

Rusiecki JA, De Roos A, Lee WJ, Dosemeci M, Lubin JH, Hoppin JA, Blair A, Alavanja MC. Cancer incidence among pesticide applicators exposed to atrazine in the Agricultural Health Study. Natl Cancer Inst. 2004;96:1375–82.

Statistica. 2023. https://www.statista.com/statistics/1263206/global-pesticide-use-by-type/. Accessed 19 Jan 2024.

Takayasu T, Ishida Y, Kimura A, Nosaka M, Kawaguchi M, Kondo T. Postmortem distribution of ametryn in the blood and organ tissues of an herbicide-poisoning victim. J Anal Toxicol. 2010;34(5):287–91.

Talbot AR, Shiaw MH, Huang JS, Yang SF, Goo TS, Wang SH, Chen CL, Sanford TR. Acute poisoning with a glyphosate-surfactant herbicide ('Roundup'): a review of 93 cases. Hum Exp Toxicol. 1991;10(1):1–8.

Tanner CM, Kamel GW, Ross JA, et al. Rotenone, paraquat, and Parkinson's disease. Environ Health Perspect. 2011;119:866–72.

Tong T, Duan W, Xu Y, et al. Paraquat exposure induces Parkinsonism by altering lipid profile and evoking neuroinflammation in the midbrain. Environ Int. 2022;169:107512.

Vo K. Paraquat and diquat. In: Olson KR, et al., editors. Poisoning & drug overdoses. 7th ed. McGraw Hill; 2018. p. 364–5.

Fungicides

10

H. Thomas Cusick III

Introduction

Even with the availability of fungicides, plant fungi (molds, mildews, and blights) destroy over 100 million tons of crops annually worldwide, worth an estimated $60 billion. That amount of food could otherwise help feed 600 million people. Some book authors and movie writers imagine dystopian futures where the worldwide food chain has collapsed due to fungal disease, and a look at history shows that such a scenario is not unprecedented. Beginning around 1845, a blight began spreading across northern Europe, decimating the potato crop for years. Affected potatoes turned black and were inedible. Ireland was particularly affected because that single food so dominated their diet. During this so-called Great Famine, an estimated 1 million Irish men, women, and children died due to starvation, and millions more left their home country because of the famine. This one blight forever changed Ireland and the Irish people.

Fungicides are a class of pesticides that overlap in some ways with algaecides and antibacterial agents. However, because of the plant-like characteristics of fungi, fungicides are distinct because they must kill (or at least inhibit the growth of) the fungi without adversely affecting the host plant or crop (Gupta 2018; O'Malley 2014). Fungicides discussed in this chapter have been divided into classes that share similar chemical characteristics, as depicted in Table 10.1. Elemental sulfur may be the original fungicide since its use dates back to as early as 1803 (Gupta 2018). Inorganic mercury- or copper-based fungicide and thiocarbamate were once very common, but their use has declined since the mid-twentieth century. Captan, chlorothalonil, and organic fungicides account for 90% of current use (Gupta 2018). Most of the approximately 150 available fungicides currently used are recently developed synthetic organic compounds that have low toxicity to humans (Gupta 2018; O'Malley 2014).

Occupational fungicide exposure can occur during production, seed treatment, plant application, or harvest. Fungicides are typically applied as a spray or dust, and they often leave a film on the seed or plant's surface (O'Malley 2014). Crop treatment is often done repeatedly during the season, and since the plant is coated, exposure can occur not only during application but also any time the plant is handled. Most fungicides act locally, which means they need to be frequently reapplied, further increasing the opportunities for worker exposure. Individuals at the highest risk of occupational fungicide exposure include not just field workers but also employees in seed-treatment facilities, nurseries, and greenhouses.

H. Thomas Cusick III (✉)
Duke University, Durham, NC, USA

Concentra Urgent Care, Durham, NC, USA

W. J. Meggs, R. L. Langley (eds.), *Farm Toxicology*, https://doi.org/10.1007/978-3-031-80441-0_10

Table 10.1 Examples of common fungicides in use worldwide

Fungicide class	Examples
Strobilurin compounds	Azoxystrobin, pyraclostrobin, trifloxystrobin, picoxystrobin, kresoxim-methyl
Triazole compounds	Triadimefon, triadimenol, myclobutanil, propiconazole, thiazopyr, imazalil, flutriafol, terazole
Substituted aromatics (substituted benzenes)	Chloroneb, chlorothalonil, dicloran, hexachlorobenzene (HCB), pentachloronitrobenzene (PCNB)
Phthalimido compounds (thiophthalimide compounds)	Captan, folpet, captafol
Thiocarbamate compounds (dithiocarbamate compounds)	Thiram, ziram, ferbam, propamocarb, metam-sodium, maneb, zineb, nabam, mancozeb
Copper compounds	Copper sulfate, copper lime dust, copper hydroxide, cupric oxide, cuprous oxide, copper oxychloride, etc.
Sulfur	Elemental sulfur crude lime sulfur
Organomercury compounds	Methyl mercury, methoxyethyl mercury, phenyl mercuric acetate
Organotin compounds	Triphenyl tin, fentin hydroxide, fentin chloride, fentin acetate
Cadmium compounds	Cadmium chloride, cadmium sulfate, cadmium succinate
Miscellaneous organic fungicides	Anilazine, fluazinam, iprodione, metalaxyl, triforine, dodine, benomyl, cycloheximide, etridiazole, thiabendazole, edifenphos

Classes of Fungicides

Strobilurin Compounds

Strobilurins are newer fungicides, only developed in and used since the 1990s. Common examples include azoxystrobin, pyraclostrobin, trifloxystrobin, picoxystrobin, and kresoxim-methyl. They have low or minimal systemic toxicity, and they also appear to be less irritating than many other fungicides (O'Malley 2014). Short-term and self-limited toxic effects, primarily irritation of the eyes and upper and lower respiratory tracts, as well as irritant contact dermatitis have been reported from pyraclostrobin (Centers for Disease Control and Prevention (CDC) 2008, Wang et al. 2022). For example, over two dozen field workers in Iowa were accidentally sprayed with pyraclostrobin during an aerial application in 2007, and while most had symptoms (eye or respiratory-tract irritation or chest pain) acutely, all were treated and released from a local emergency room after their symptoms resolved (Centers for Disease Control and Prevention (CDC) 2008). There is a report of death after one patient intentionally ingested an unknown amount of pyraclostrobin and suffered respiratory arrest (Nendick et al. 2022).

Triazole Compounds

The triazoles are structurally related to some antifungals used in medicine such as ketoconazole (O'Malley 2014). Examples of triazole fungicides include triadimefon, triadimenol, myclobutanil, propiconazole, thiazopyr, imazalil, flutriafol, and terazol. While they may cause eye irritation, dermal effects are not common, although propiconazole and imazalil have been reported as possible causes of irritant or contact dermatitis (Penagos 2002; Penagos et al. 2004). Ingestion of propiconazole has been reported to cause a toxic chorea (Paul et al. 2017). The Environmental Protection Agency (EPA) classifies triadimefon and terazol as possible and probable carcinogens, respectively (O'Malley 2014).

Substituted Aromatics

Also known as substituted benzenes, examples of substituted aromatic fungicides include chloroneb, chlorothalonil, dicloran, pentachloronitrobenzene (PCNB), and hexachlorobenzene (HCB). These fungicides have been used in various forms for decades, although some (e.g., HCB) have been removed from use in the United States (Roberts and Reigart 2013). HCB as a seed treatment was the cause of an outbreak of toxic porphyria in Turkey in the 1950s (Gupta 2018). Thousands of people were affected, hundreds died, and the survivors suffered chronic effects (Peters et al. 1982). There are even studies suggesting negative effects on the children who were exposed to HCB in utero (Ribas-Fito et al. 2007).

Some of these compounds, for example, chloroneb and chlorothalonil, can cause skin and mucous membrane irritation. Chlorothalonil has been cited to cause irritant and allergic contact dermatitis (Lenson et al. 2011; Lensen et al. 2007; Penagos 2002; Penagos et al. 2004), occupational asthma (Draper et al. 2003), at least one case of an immediate anaphylactoid reaction to direct contact (Dannaker et al. 1993), and another case of diabetic ketoacidosis after ingestion (Fernandez-Garcia et al. 2014). HCB and chlorothalonil are listed by the EPA as probable carcinogens (O'Malley 2014).

Phthalimido Compounds (Sometimes Called Thiophthalimides)

Phthalimido fungicides are widely used and include captan, folpet, and captafol. Each can cause skin, eye, and respiratory-tract irritation (Roberts and Reigart 2013). Captan and captafol have been associated with either immediate or delayed allergic reactions and contact dermatitis (Ajayi et al. 2023; O'Malley 2014). Captan has been suggested to cause olfactory impairment in farmers (Shrestha et al. 2020), and captafol has been reported to both exacerbate underlying asthma and cause occupational asthma (Royce et al. 1993). One case of captafol ingestion caused numerous systemic pathologic signs and symptoms (e.g., headache, weakness, chest pain, and T-wave inversion) that resolved within a few days with supportive care (Roberts and Reigart 2013). One case study and another case-control study concluded that occupational exposure to captan was associated with a diagnosis of multiple myeloma (Packard et al. 2019; Pahwa et al. 2012), while another prospective cohort study listed it as associated with age-related macular degeneration (Montgomery et al. 2017). The EPA and International Agency for Research on Cancer (IARC) consider them to be probable human carcinogens based upon mice and rat studies (O'Malley 2014).

Thiocarbamate Compounds (Including Ethylenebis-Dithiocarbamates, or EBDC)

The thiocarbamates (also called dithiocarbamates) include thiram, ziram, ferbam, propamocarb, and metam-sodium. They are related to disulfiram (Antabuse), and alcohol ingested after exposure may lead to an Antabuse-like reaction, with symptoms similar to a hangover, including nausea, vomiting, flushing, dizziness, headache, or chest or abdominal discomfort (O'Malley 2014). Thiram, ziram, and ferbam are irritating to the skin, eyes, and mucous membranes (Roberts and Reigart 2013). Thiram has also caused contact dermatitis and inhalational lung injury (Siwiec et al. 2019). It is a component of latex and may be the cause of latex sensitization. Metam-sodium must be used outdoors because when it decomposes in water, it releases an irritating gas that can cause pulmonary edema (Roberts and Reigart 2013). There is a case report of a death due to cardiopulmonary arrest after an intentional ingestion of an unknown amount of propamocarb (Nendick et al. 2022).

The EBDC compounds include maneb, zineb, nabam, and mancozeb. (Zineb is no longer available in the United States.) They can all cause skin, eye, and respiratory-tract irritation (Roberts and Reigart 2013), and both maneb and zineb have been linked to chronic skin diseases, possibly by sensitization (Cole et al. 1997; Nater et al. 1979). A few systemic poisonings have been reported in case studies, including hemolytic anemia caused by zineb (Roberts and Reigart 2013), acute renal failure and metabolic acidosis due to maneb (Koizumi et al. 1979; Taymez et al. 2023), and neurological symptoms due to maneb and zineb (Israeli et al. 1983; de Tollenaer et al. 2006). One case of toxic epidermal necrolysis and systemic symptoms was reported after mancozeb exposure (Zakharov et al. 2016). Maneb and mancozeb both contain manganese (Mn); Parkinson-like symptoms have been reported after chronic exposure to maneb, and animal studies suggest that mancozeb may also produce similar effects in the brain (Domico et al. 2006; Ferraz et al. 1988). Furthermore, the EPA has listed mancozeb and zineb as probable human carcinogens due to thyroid cancer in animals exposed to these chemicals (O'Malley 2014).

Copper Compounds

Copper–arsenic compounds have been discontinued in the United States due to the arsenic component, but they were used as wood preservatives as recently as 2003 (Roberts and Reigart 2013). Numerous other organic and inorganic copper-containing fungicides are available, and copper sulfate is particularly common. They can cause irritation to the skin, eyes, or respiratory tract, and soluble versions are corrosive to the mucous membranes and cornea (Roberts and Reigart 2013). Ingestion can cause gastric irritation (Barceloux 1999), and systemic poisoning may cause methemoglobinemia, especially in patients with glucose-6-phosphate dehydrogenase (G6PD) deficiency (Yang et al. 2004). Early signs and symptoms of acute copper poisoning include a metallic taste, nausea, vomiting, epigastric pain, and (in more severe cases) hematuria, hematemesis, and melanotic stools. Later, patients may develop jaundice, hepatomegaly, hemolysis, acute renal failure, and circulatory collapse (Agarwal et al. 1993). In addition to supportive care, methylene blue may be used to treat severe methemoglobinemia. One case report documented death likely due to ingestion of a copper fungicide (Otter and Cantrell 2021). Chronic copper toxicity primarily affects the liver (Barceloux 1999).

Sulfur

Elemental sulfur and crude lime sulfur are commonly used fungicides and have low toxicity (Roberts and Reigart 2013) but also a low potency; sulfur must be used more often with high application rates. It is commonly used in organic farming (Gupta 2018). Elemental sulfur does not directly cause acute skin irritation or dermatitis, but workers have reported mild skin symptoms, which are likely due to transformation from the elemental form to more active oxide forms (O'Malley 2014). Sulfur dioxide (SO_2) and sulfuric acid (H_2SO_4) cause irritation, and sulfite compounds can cause allergic reactions.

Organomercury Compounds

The mercurial fungicides include various compounds based on methyl mercury, methoxyethyl mercury, or phenyl mercuric acetate. They used to be very common seed treatments and paint preservatives, but due to their significant toxicity, they are no longer used in the United States (O'Malley 2014; Roberts and Reigart 2013). Absorption can occur across the skin and through the gut, and mercury is concentrated in the nervous system and red blood cells. Early symptoms include a metallic taste, numbness, tingling, tremors, headache, fatigue, mood changes, and poor concentration, with more severe neurological symptoms, gastrointestinal bleeding, and acute renal failure developing later and with more severe poisoning (Agarwal et al. 1993; Bakir et al. 1980). Mercury exposure can cause permanent neurological disorders or be fatal (Gupta 2018), and in addition to decontamination and supportive treatment, exposed patients may require chelation therapy (Roberts and Reigart 2013).

Organotin Compounds

Examples of organotin fungicides include triphenyl tin, fentin hydroxide, fentin chloride, and fentin acetate. They cause irritation to the skin, eye, and respiratory tract in occupational exposures, and more severe poisonings cause diffuse gastrointestinal and neurological damage and sometimes, death (Roberts and Reigart 2013). Most organotin fungicides have been discontinued in the United States.

Cadmium

Cadmium compounds (including cadmium chloride, cadmium sulfate, and cadmium succinate) and mixtures of cadmium with other fungicides have been discontinued in the United States as fungicides (Roberts and Reigart 2013). They are very irritating to the respiratory and gastrointestinal tracts, sometimes causing symptomatic pneumonitis (metal fume fever), renal impairment, or hemorrhagic pulmonary edema (Ando et al. 1996). Occupational exposure to cadmium can still occur from other sources of this potentially toxic metal.

Miscellaneous Organic Fungicides

Anilazine can cause skin irritation, but no systemic symptoms have been reported (Roberts and Reigart 2013). Fluazinam has been reported as a cause of occupational asthma (Draper et al. 2003). Iprodione, metalaxyl, and triforine do not exhibit significant acute dermal or systemic toxicity (Roberts and Reigart 2013), but iprodione is classified by the EPA as a likely carcinogen (O'Malley 2014). Dodine causes skin, eye, and gastrointestinal symptoms in animal studies, but symptoms in humans have not been reported (Roberts and Reigart 2013). Benomyl, cycloheximide, and etridiazole are not used in the United States, and no human systemic poisonings have been reported (Roberts and Reigart 2013), but benomyl has been associated with allergic contact dermatitis (Penagos et al. 2004). Thiabendazole is used as a fungicide, but it is used in medicine as an antiparasitic at higher doses than would occur in an occupational exposure (Roberts and Reigart 2013). Edifenphos is an organochlorine fungicide listed as highly hazardous by the World Health Organization (WHO), and there are case reports of death due to respiratory arrest after intentional ingestion (Nendick et al. 2022).

Medical Considerations

Fungicide exposure can occur during production, seed treatment, during the spraying or dusting of plants and crops, or during harvest. Like many drugs or chemicals, fungicides can cause harm through skin or eye contact, through inhalation, or through ingestion. The latter is primarily a problem with intentional ingestion.

Many fungicides, with a significant-enough exposure, can cause irritation to a worker's skin, airways, eyes, and/or mucous membranes. Like any other chemical exposure, removing the worker from the exposure or removing the irritating product from the worker is the primary (and often, only) required treatment. Symptoms caused by irritation should resolve quickly and fully. Patients with ongoing dermatitis or asthmatic symptoms can be treated and controlled similar to any other patient with these symptoms; these workers may need to be permanently removed from the offending chemical. To confirm hypersensitivity from a fungicide, patch-testing or (rarely) an inhalation challenge may be required.

Most organic fungicides cannot be easily tested for in body fluids, but copper, mercury, and cadmium levels can be measured in the blood and/or urine (Roberts and Reigart 2013). Similar to any chemical exposure, medical testing and treatment in an acutely symptomatic worker exposed to fungicides will be guided by the presenting symptoms. Contaminated skin, eyes, or clothing should be washed, flushed, or removed as appropriate. Patients with accidental or intentional ingestions may require admission and even intensive care treatment. Monitoring for methemoglobinemia in patients with copper poisoning should be performed, and treatment with methylene blue should be considered, especially if the methemoglobin levels are high (e.g., >30%) or the patient is cyanotic. Mercury levels can be measured if acute exposure is suspected, and chelation therapy may be considered in acute mercury poisoning.

Conclusion

Fungicides are very important for worldwide food-crop production, and while newer chemicals are safer than the older options, their use is increasing. This means worker exposure will also increase. Most fungicides used in the

United States either do not cause acute symptoms or only cause self-limited irritation that resolves with the removal of the exposure. Some workers may develop dermatitis or asthma, requiring removal from the job where the exposure occurs. With the exception of intentional high-dose ingestion, which often requires inpatient treatment, most fungicide exposures are not life-threatening. Future research will likely focus more on long-term chronic health effects of fungicide exposure, including cancer, reproductive effects, and neurologic disorders.

Acknowledgments Duke and Concentra were my two employers at the time I helped write this chapter.

References

Agarwal SK, Tiwari SC, Dash SC. Spectrum of poisoning requiring haemodialysis in a tertiary care hospital in India. Int J Artif Organs. 1993;16(1):20–2.

Ajayi A, Hall M, Yiannias JA, Killian JM, Davis MDP, Youssef MJ, Cantwell HM, Drage LA, Sokumbi O. Trends in patch testing of black patients: the Mayo Clinic experience (January 1, 2011, to December 31, 2020). Dermatitis. 2023;34(2):113–9.

Ando Y, Shibata E, Tsuchiyama F, Sakai S. Elevated urinary cadmium concentrations in a patient with acute cadmium pneumonitis. Scand J Work Environ Health. 1996;22(2):150–3.

Bakir F, Rustam H, Tikriti S, Al-Damluji SF, Shihristani H. Clinical and epidemiological aspects of methylmercury poisoning. Postgrad Med J. 1980;56(651):1–10.

Barceloux DG. Copper. J Toxicol Clin Toxicol. 1999;37(2):217–30.

Centers for Disease Control and Prevention (CDC). Acute pesticide poisoning associated with pyraclostrobin fungicide—Iowa, 2007. Morb Mortal Wkly Rep. 2008;56(51):1343–5.

Cole DC, Carpio F, Math JJ, Leon N. Dermatitis in Ecuadorean farmworkers. Contact Derm. 1997;37(1):1–8.

Dannaker CJ, Maibach HI, O'Malley M. Contact urticaria and anaphylaxis to the fungicide chlorothalonil. Cutis. 1993;52(5):312–5.

de Tollenaer SM, Buysse C, van den Anker JN, Touw DJ, de Hoog M. Life threatening central nervous system manifestations and hypothermia due to maneb intoxication in a child: a case report. Ther Drug Monit. 2006 Dec;28(6):813–5.

Domico LM, Zeevalk GD, Bernard LP, Cooper KR. Acute neurotoxic effects of mancozeb and maneb in mesencephalic neuronal cultures are associated with mitochondrial dysfunction. Neurotoxicology. 2006;27(5):816–25.

Draper A, Cullinan P, Campbell C, Jones M, Newman TA. Occupational asthma from fungicides fluazinam and chlorothalonil. Occup Environ Med. 2003;60(1):76–7.

Fernandez-Garcia JC, Arrebola JP, Gonzalez-Romero S, Soriguer F, Olea N, Tinahones FJ. Diabetic ketoacidosis following chlorothalonil poisoning. Occup Environ Med. 2014;71(5):382.

Ferraz HB, Bertolucci PH, Pereira JS, Lima JG, Andrade LA. Chronic exposure to the fungicide maneb may produce symptoms and signs of CNS manganese intoxication. Neurology. 1988;38(4):550–3.

Gupta PK. Toxicology of fungicides. In: Gupta RC, editor. Veterinary toxicology. 3rd ed. Academic Press; 2018. p. 569–80.

Israeli R, Sculsky M, Tiberin P. Acute intoxication due to exposure to maneb and zineb. A case with behavioral and central nervous system changes. Scand J Work Environ Health. 1983;9(1):47–51.

Koizumi A, Shiojima S, Omiya M, Nakano S, Sato N, Ikeda M. Acute renal failure and maneb (manganous ethylenebis [dithiocarbamate]) exposure. JAMA. 1979;242(23):2583–5.

Lensen G, Jungbauer F, Goncalo M, Coenraads PJ. Airborne irritant contact dermatitis and conjunctivitis after occupational exposure to chlorothalonil in textiles. Contact Derm. 2007;57(3):181–6.

Lenson G, Coenraads PJ, Jungbauer F, Schuttelaar M. Contact dermatitis caused by chlorothalonil on imported roses: irritant or contact reaction? Contact Derm. 2011;65(1):50–1.

Montgomery MP, Postel E, Umbach DM, Richards M, Watson M, Blair A, Chen H, Sandler DP, Schmidt S, Kamel F. Pesticide use and age-related macular degeneration in the Agricultural Health Study. Environ Health Perspect. 2017;125(7):077013.

Nater JP, Terpstra H, Bleumink E. Allergic contact sensitization to the fungicide Maneb. Contact Derm. 1979;5(1):24–6.

Nendick E, Mohamed F, Raubenheimer J, Gawarammana I, Buckley NA, Eddleston M. Acute fungicide self-poisoning—a prospective case series. Clin Res. 2022;60(10):1106–12.

O'Malley MA. Pesticides. In: LaDou J, Harrison R, editors. Current occupational & environmental medicine. 5th ed. New York: McGraw-Hill Education; 2014. p. 609–12.

Otter J, Cantrell FL. Death by copper ammonium complex-containing fungicide. Am J Forensic Med Pathol. 2021;42(1):62–3.

Packard E, Shahid Z, Groff A, Patel R, Jain R. Multiple myeloma in an agricultural worker exposed to pesticides. Cureus. 2019;11(5):e4762. https://doi.org/10.7759/cureus.4762.

Pahwa P, Karunanayake CP, Dosman JA, Spinelli JJ, McDuffie HH, McLaughlin JR. Multiple myeloma and exposure to pesticides: a Canadian case-control study. J Agromedicine. 2012;17(1):40–50.

Paul BS, Paul G, Kaur J, Singh G. Chorea as unusual complication of fungicide poisoning. J Postgrad Med. 2017;63(1):53–4.

Penagos HG. Contact dermatitis caused by pesticides among banana plantation workers in Panama. Int J Occup Environ Health. 2002;8(1):14–8.

Penagos H, Ruepert C, Partanen T, Wesseling C. Pesticide patch test series for the assessment of allergic contact dermatitis among banana plantation workers in Panama. Dermatitis. 2004;15(3):137–45.

Peters HA, Gocmen A, Cripps DJ, Bryan GT, Dogramaci I. Epidemiology of hexachlorobenzene—induced porphyria in Turkey: clinical and laboratory follow-up after 25 years. Arch Neurol. 1982;39(12):744–9.

Ribas-Fito N, Torrent M, Carrizo D, Julvez J, Grimalt JO, Sunyer J. Exposure to hexachlorobenzene during pregnancy and children's social behavior at 4 years of age. Environ Health Perspect. 2007;115(3):447–50.

Roberts JR, Reigart JR. Fungicides. In: Recognition and management of pesticide poisonings. 6th ed. United States Environmental Protection Agency Office of Pesticide Programs; 2013. p. 143–60.

Royce S, Wald P, Sheppard D, Balmes J. Occupational asthma in a pesticides manufacturing worker. Chest. 1993;103(1):295–29.

Shrestha S, Umbach DM, Freeman LEB, Koutros S, Alavanja MCR, Blair A, Chen H, Sandler DP. Occupational pesticide use and self-reported olfactory impairment in US farmers. Occup Environ Med. 2020:oemed-2020-106818.

Siwiec J, Siek E, Grzywa-Celinska A, Mackiewicz B, Czekajska-Chehab E. Thiram—toxic inhalational lung injury. Ann Agric Environ Med. 2019;26(4):672–3.

Taymez DG, Caklili OT, Gurbuz H. Severe metabolic acidosis, acute renal failure, and delayed paralysis leading to respiratory depression due to manganese ethylene-bis-dithiocarbamate. Turk J Anaesthesiol Reanim. 2023;51(1):62–4.

Wang Q, Luo N, Lei M, Zhong L, Li C, Hao P. Facial irritant contact dermatitis caused by pyraclostrobin. Clin Cosmet Investig Dermatol. 2022;15:1643–7.

Yang CC, Wu ML, Deng JF. Prolonged hemolysis and methemoglobinemia following organic copper fungicide ingestion. Vet Hum Toxicol. 2004;46(6):321–3.

Zakharov S, Csomor J, Urbanek P, Pelclova D. Toxic epidermal necrolysis after exposure to dithiocarbamate fungicide mancozeb. Basic Clin Pharmacol Toxicol. 2016;118(1):87–91.

Rodenticides

11

Ricky L. Langley

Introduction

Rodenticides, often referred to as "rat poisons," are a class of pesticides used to kill rodents. Rodents are mammals with continuously growing incisors, which require continuous eroding by gnawing. There are over 2000 species of rodents worldwide, and around 5% are considered serious pests. Examples of rodents include rats, mice, squirrels, woodchucks, porcupines, nutria, beavers, and voles. Rodents are responsible for billions of dollars of damage yearly worldwide including eating and contaminating food/plant products such as grains, forestry and nursery damage, damage to ornamental plants, causing property damage such as chewing through cables and irrigation pipes, and chewing through electrical wiring, increasing risks of fires (Witmer et al. 2014).

Rodents bite over 13,000 persons in the United States annually (Langley et al. 2020). In addition, rodents can also transmit various diseases. Worldwide, over 30 diseases, as noted in Table 11.1, have been reported to be transmitted by rodents (CDC (Centers for Disease Control and Prevention) 2023). Rodent exposure can also cause allergies or asthma from proteins in their saliva, fur, and urine.

Rodents multiply rapidly when left on their own. Eradicating rodent populations is challenging. Methods used to control rodents include building physical barriers such as fencing, repairing holes, improving sanitation, and eliminating hiding places. Trapping, natural predators, ultrasound devices, and the use of chemical repellants such as predator scents and pheromones have been used (Hazra et al. 2017). Rodenticides are also widely used, but even these are not completely effective as rodents will avoid some toxic compounds by taste alone (primary bait refusal), will not feed twice on a substance that causes illness (shyness), and learn to avoid certain supplies of food or water if they cause death in other rodents (Hazra et al. 2017).

Finding ideal rodenticides with the following characteristics has been difficult:

- Easy to apply.
- Specific to rodents in toxicity and less toxic to nontarget species (humans and domesticated animals). An example is norbormide.
- Effective in small amounts so that adding it to food or water supply will not cause bait refusal.
- It must kill and not partially sicken rodents who ingest it; otherwise, it may arouse suspicion in the surviving animals and cause bait shyness for future encounters.

R. L. Langley (✉)
Department of Biological Sciences, North Carolina State University, Raleigh, NC, USA
e-mail: rllangley@ncsu.edu

W. J. Meggs, R. L. Langley (eds.), *Farm Toxicology*, https://doi.org/10.1007/978-3-031-80441-0_11

Table 11.1 Diseases directly or indirectly transmitted by rodents to humans

Anaplasmosis	Lyme disease
Angiostrongylus	Lymphocytic choriomeningitis (LCM)
Babesiosis	Moniliformis moniliformis
Borreliosis	Monkeypox
Colorado tick fever	Omsk hemorrhagic fever
Cutaneous leishmaniasis	Plague
Flea-borne (murine) typhus	Powassan virus
Hymenolepis diminuta	Rickettsialpox
Hantavirus	Rat-bite fever
Hantavirus pulmonary syndrome	Salmonellosis
Hemorrhagic fever with renal syndrome	Scrub typhus
La Crosse virus	South American arenaviruses (Argentine hemorrhagic fever, Bolivian hemorrhagic fever, Chapare hemorrhagic fever, Sabiá-associated hemorrhagic fever, and Venezuelan hemorrhagic fever)
Lassa fever	
Leptospirosis	
Lujo hemorrhagic fever	Sylvatic typhus
	Tick-borne relapsing fever
	Tularemia

Integrated pest management that uses a variety of methods is the most effective means to control rodent populations.

Rodenticide Toxicity

Toxicity from rodenticides can result from oral, inhalational, or dermal exposures, depending on the specific rodenticide. In addition, the degree of toxicity can vary by the species of animal exposed. Toxicity will also vary by the concentration of the active ingredient in the product (formulation) used for rodent control. In 2019, there were 8734 cases of human rodenticide exposure reported to poison centers in the United States (Gummin et al. 2020) of which 44% were due to anticoagulants. Bromethalin was the most common non-anticoagulant exposure reported in the United States. However, rodenticide exposures vary by country. For example, according to national poison center data in India, zinc phosphide, barium carbonate, and aluminum phosphide remain the most common cause of household and agricultural rodenticide poisoning, and deaths frequently occur (Peshin et al. 2014).

Rodenticides are often formulated as baits, often with various flavorings added, such as peanut butter, molasses, and fish oil, to attract the rodent (NPIC (National Pesticide Information Center) 2016). Depending on the country, various formulations are available as baits, pellets, powders, liquids, and toxic gas fumigants. Due to their toxicity, many rodenticides have been banned or their use restricted in the United States although they may be available in other countries (both legally and illegally) and exported throughout the world (e.g., aldicarb, also called "Tres Pasitos" in some countries). Tetramine (known as "Dushuquiang" in some countries) is so toxic that it has been banned worldwide, but it may be made illegally.

Rodenticides can be divided into various categories depending on their chemical class, their mode of action, or even their toxicity (BCPC (British Crop Production Council) 1995–2022). By chemical class, rodenticides available in different countries are shown in Table 11.2.

Different rodenticides have different modes of action that result in lethality (Table 11.3). As noted earlier, all mammals share essentially the same enzymes and metabolic processes and may show similar signs of symptoms after exposure.

A clinically helpful categorization of rodenticides utilizes the amount of poison that causes death in 50%of rodents following exposure (lethal dose$_{50}$ or LD_{50}). In the United States, the use of a "signal word" appears on the product label by law and reflects the highest possible toxicity of the product as follows (U.S. EPA 2023):

Table 11.2 Chemical class of rodenticides

Alkaloid (AK)	Halogenated alkanoic acid (HA)
Arsenical (AS)	Indandione (ID)
Botanical (B)	Inorganic (IN)
Calciferol (CA)	Phosphoramidate (PH)
Carbamate (CB)	Pyrimidinamine (PY)
Coumarin (CU)	Thiourea (T)
Fumigant (F)	Unclassified[a] (U)

[a]The unclassified category includes many diverse chemical rodenticides including bromethalin, chloralose, alpha-chlorhydrin, curcumerol, flupropadine, gliftor, mieshaun, norbormide, pyrinuron, silatrane, and tetramine

Table 11.3 Mechanism of action of rodenticides

Disrupts the tricarboxylic (Krebs) cycle	Sodium monofluoroacetate (SMFA), fluoroacetamide, thallium, arsenic
Corrosive and causes chemical burns	Yellow (white) phosphorous
Interferes with oxidative phosphorylation	Thallium, bromethalin, arsenic
Inhibits synthesis of Nicotinamide adenine dinucleotide (NAD) and Nicotinamide adenine dinucleotide + Hydrogen (NADH) and destroys pancreatic beta cells	Pyriminil
Acts as an antagonist of neurotransmitter glycine at the postsynaptic spinal cord motor neuron	Strychnine
Causes vasoconstriction with ischemia	Norbormide
Inhibits potassium diffusion out of cells	Barium carbonate
Combines with sulfhydryl groups, blocking many enzymes and cell-signaling pathways	Arsenic
Blocks reduction of vitamin K–dependent coagulation factors	Warfarins, indanediones
Inhibits cytochrome C oxidase, affecting electron transport	Zn/Al phosphides
Inhibits cholinesterase	Aldicarb
Mobilizes calcium from bones and increases gastrointestinal absorption of calcium	Cholecalciferol
Inhibits the hearts'sodium potassium ATPase from cardioactive glycosides	Red squill

- **Highly toxic**: LD_{50}: 0–50 mg/kg, signal word "**Danger**".
- **Toxic**: LD_{50}: 50–500 mg/kg, signal word "**Warning**".
- **Less toxic**: LD_{50}: 500–5000 mg/kg, signal word "**Caution**".

The World Health Organization (WHO) has developed a list of various pesticides by their toxicity (LD_{50}), as shown in Table 11.4 (WHO (World Health Organization) 2019). Note that most studies of toxicity have been performed in laboratory rodents and may not necessarily reflect the severity of effects in humans. For example, although bromethalin is highly toxic to rodents, rare cases of serious toxicity have been reported in exposed humans. Norbormide is a rat-specific toxicant and is considered to be of low toxicity to humans. Very small amounts of the extremely toxic rodenticides—crimidine, fluoracetamide, sodium fluoroacetate, strychnine, tetramethylene disulfotetramine, thallium sulfate, yellow phosphorus, and zinc phosphide—can cause severe and even fatal poisoning in humans. The anticoagulants, indandiones, and red squill are less hazardous to humans and domestic animals. Some of the newer anticoagulant compounds, termed "second-generation anticoagulants," may cause human toxicity at a much lower dose than conventional "first-generation anticoagulants" and can bioaccumulate in the liver (Roberts and

Table 11.4 Toxicity and chemical class of rodenticides

Highly toxic	Toxic	Less toxic
Alpha-naphthylthiourea (ANTU)(T)	3-chloro-1,2-propanediolol (U)	Red squill (B)
Thallium/thallium sulfate (IN)	Chloralose (U)	
Fluoroacetamide (HA)		
Gophacide (PH)		
Strychnine (AK)		
Al/Zinc/Mg phosphide (IN)		
Yellow phosphorous (IN)		
Arsenic/sodium arsenite (AS)		
Barium carbonate (IN)		
Tetramethylene disulfotetramine (U)		
Pyrinuron (U)		
Brodifacoum (CU)		
Bromadiolone (CU)		
Difethiolone (CU)		
Flocoumafen (CU)		
Bromethalin (U)		
Chlorophacinone (ID)		
Sodium fluoroacetate (HA)		
Ca/H/Na cyanide (F)		
Crimidine (PY)		
Warfarin (CU)		
Cholecalciferol (CA)		
Aldrin (CB)		
Norbormide (U)		
Carbofuran (CB)		

Reigart 2013). Note that many of the highly toxic rodenticides (e.g., tetramine) are banned or not approved for use for rodent control (e.g., aldicarb).

When evaluating human exposures, it is often convenient to classify exposure as either to anticoagulant rodenticides or to non-anticoagulant rodenticides. In 2022, the U.S. EPA proposed interim decisions on a list of 11 rodenticide active ingredients undergoing registration review for use in the United States (U.S. EPA (U.S. Environmental Protection Agency) 2022). The rodenticides under review for use in the United States include:

- First-generation anticoagulants: warfarin, chlorophacinone, and diphacinone
- Second-generation anticoagulants: brodifacoum, bromadiolone, difenacoum, and difethialone
- Non-anticoagulants: bromethalin, cholecalciferol, strychnine, and zinc phosphide

Anticoagulant Rodenticides

Most of the rodenticides used today are anticoagulant compounds that interfere with blood clotting and cause death from excessive bleeding. Deaths typically occur between 4 days and 2 weeks after rodents begin to feed on the bait.

Anticoagulants are classified as coumarins or indandiones, are widely used as rodenticides, and are considered either first- or second-generation agents (Mercer et al. 2022). First-generation anticoagulants, such as warfarin, were developed as rodenticides before 1970. These compounds are much more toxic when feeding occurs on several successive days rather than on 1 day only. Second-generation anticoagulants ("superwarfarins") were developed beginning in the 1970s to control rodents that developed resistance to first-generation anticoagulants. Second-generation anticoagulants also are more likely than first-generation anticoagulants to be able to kill after a single feeding. These compounds remain in ani-

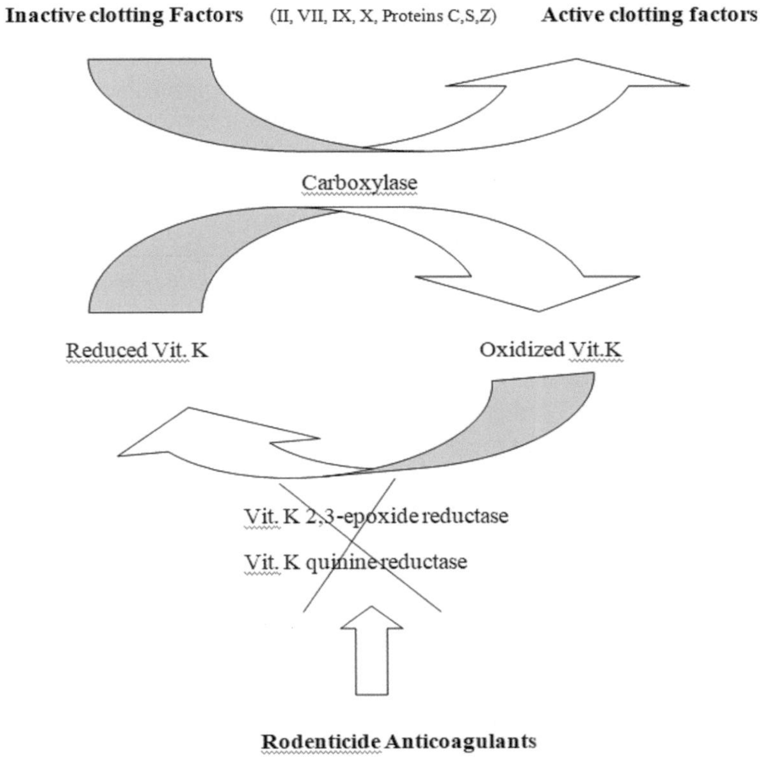

Fig. 11.1 Mechanism of action of rodenticide anticoagulants

mal tissues longer than first-generation rodenticides. Therefore, second-generation products pose greater risks to nontarget species that might feed on bait only once or prey upon animals that have eaten the bait. Due to these risks, in the United States, second-generation anticoagulant rodenticides are no longer registered for direct consumer use and are registered only for the commercial pest control and structural pest control markets. However, the use of these second-generation anticoagulants may not be limited in other countries.

Anticoagulants work by inhibiting the synthesis of vitamin K–dependent clotting factors including factors II, VII, IX, and X and proteins C, S, and Z. Anticoagulants inhibit the enzymes vitamin K 2,3 epoxide reductase and vitamin K quinine reductase, preventing vitamin K from being reduced to its active form (Anderson 2018), as seen in Fig. 11.1. The duration of effect varies for the first- and second- generation anticoagulants. A dose of the first-generation warfarin may last 5–7 days, whereas duration may last from weeks to months for second-generation coumarins.

The agents also increase the permeability of capillaries throughout the body, predisposing to widespread internal hemorrhage.

While most poisonings occur via oral exposure, dermal exposure to the long-acting indandiones has also been reported to cause symptomatic bleeding. Clinical effects of these agents usually begin several days after ingestion because of the long half-life of the factors. Individuals with hepatic dysfunction, bleeding diathesis, or malnutrition may be at greater risk of severe adverse effects. Synthetic cannabinoids, the increasingly popular drugs of abuse, have been found to be contaminated with long-acting anticoagulant rodenticides resulting in coagulopathy and bleeding complications via inhalational exposure (Bahouth et al. 2019).

Primary manifestations include nosebleeds, bleeding gums, hematuria, hematemesis, hematochezia, menorrhagia, melena, subconjunctival hemorrhages, and extensive ecchymoses. Patients may also have symptoms of anemia including fatigue and dyspnea on exertion. For indandiones, headaches, confusion, loss of consciousness, and seizures have been reported that may be secondary to intracranial hemorrhage.

Coumarin or indandione poisoning results in an increase in prothrombin time (PT)/international normalized ratio (INR) levels from reduced plasma prothrombin concentration. PT and INR are reliable tests for the absorption of physiologically significant doses of anticoagulants. Detectable reduction in prothrombin occurs within 24–48 h of ingestion and persists for 1–3 weeks. Blood levels of some second-generation anticoagulants can be measured; however, the test is not immediately available nor does it aid in immediate treatment decisions as does the PT or INR. With superwarfarin ingestion, prolongation of INR and risk of bleeding may persist from several weeks to months. A normal PT/INR at 48 h will rule out significant ingestion (Anderson 2018).

Other useful laboratory tests include complete blood count (CBC), blood type, and cross-match. The partial thromboplastin time (PTT), thrombin time, fibrinogen, and platelet count may be useful in ruling out other causes of bleeding. In a seriously ill patient who is actively bleeding, the differential diagnosis would include conditions noted in Table 11.5.

The approach to treatment will depend upon the presence and severity of bleeding, PT/INR levels, underlying medical conditions, medications, the type of anticoagulant (first- or second-generation) involved, and the fluid status of the patient.

Oral vitamin K_1 (phytonadione) should be given to patients if there is evidence of significant anticoagulation, even if there is no active bleeding (Anderson 2018; Calello 2023; Lung 2023). For minor bleeding (e.g., nose bleed or ecchymosis), oral vitamin K_1 is given. Vitamin K_1 dosage after second-generation anticoagulant exposures is higher and must continue for a longer period of time. For ongoing active bleeding, immediate replacement of active clotting factors with 4-factor prothrombin complex concentrate (4F-PCC), fresh frozen plasma, or fresh whole blood is necessary, as is the administration of vitamin K_1 (Anderson 2018). Do not give vitamin K_3 (menadione or hykinone) or K_4 (menadiol) as neither of these is an antidote for these anticoagulants (Roberts and Reigart 2013). Also, note that there is a risk of anaphylaxis from intravenous administration of vitamin K although this route may be needed in a critically ill patient. Serial monitoring of PT/INR levels should continue until normalized. Optimal management includes a team with hematologist and medical toxicologist support.

Table 11.5 Laboratory evaluation of bleeding disorder

	Rodenticide anticoagulant	Disseminated intravascular coagulation[a]	Hyperfibrinolysis	Liver failure (early)	Liver failure (late)	Thrombotic thrombocytopenic purpura[a]	Uremia	Aspirin or thienopyridine
Bleeding time	Unaltered	↑	± ↑	Unaltered	↑	↑	↑	↑
D-dimer	Unaltered	↑	↑↑	Unaltered	↑	Unaltered	Unaltered	Unaltered
Fibrinogen	Normal	↓	↓	Unaltered	↓	Unaltered	Unaltered	Unaltered
Platelet count	Unaltered	↓	Unaltered	Unaltered	↓	↓↓	Unaltered	Unaltered
PT	↑	↑	↑	↑	↑	Unaltered	Unaltered	Unaltered
aPTT	Normal or ↑	↑	↑	Unaltered	↑	Unaltered	Unaltered	Unaltered

Modified from Hunt (2014)

↑ = prolonged or increased; ↓ = decreased or low; [a] fragmented RBCs may be seen on blood smear

Non-anticoagulant Rodenticides

There are numerous non-anticoagulant rodenticides available worldwide although many have been banned or their use restricted or approved only for use by certified professionals. Many of these agents are highly toxic and responsible for numerous human deaths yearly, especially by suicide.

The following are examples of non-anticoagulant rodenticides. Their clinical effects were abstracted from various sources (Calello 2023; Isackson and Irizarry 2022; Lung 2023; Meier 2018; Osweiler 1996; Roberts and Reigart 2013). It is important to look at the signal words on the pesticide label (if available) as this may give some indication of the toxicity of the product. Always contact the poison center in your region or country for the latest recommendations on treatment if exposure to these agents occurs.

Aldicarb

Highly toxic with LD_{50} in humans of 0.8 mg/kg. It is rapidly absorbed orally.

Mechanism of action (MOA): An extremely potent carbamate cholinesterase inhibitor.

- **Clinical Signs and Symptoms**
  Symptoms after exposure include cholinergic toxidrome, similar to that seen after organophosphorus insecticide poisoning, with salivation, lacrimation, urination, emesis, and diarrhea (SLUDGE) and bronchorrhea, bronchospasm, and bradycardia (Killer BBBs).

Death occurs from severe bronchorrhea and respiratory muscle weakness but usually only when the diagnosis and/or treatment is delayed.

Alpha-Chloralose

Alpha-chloralose is a central nervous system (CNS) depressant and veterinary anesthetic. Reports of severe human toxicity are rare but do occur, usually with massive ingestions.

MOA: Although the exact mechanism of action is unknown, alpha-chloralose can cause excitatory CNS effects when administered at low doses and depressive CNS effects when administered at high doses in both animals and humans. Alpha-chloralose acts like a barbiturate on synaptic transmission in the brain, enhancing the inhibitory effects of gamma-aminobutyric acid type A receptor.

- **Clinical Signs and Symptoms**
  Vomiting, bronchorrhea, metabolic acidosis, and respiratory depression
  CNS depression, coma, and myoclonus
  Death may occur from respiratory failure

Alpha-Naphthylthiourea

Alpha-naphthylthiourea (ANTU) is a selective rodenticide, lethal only to adult Norway rats and some species of dogs.

Toxicity in humans is rarely reported. LD_{50} in humans is estimated at 4 g/kg.

MOA: In target species, disruption of vascular endothelium causes rapid onset of pulmonary edema and pleural effusions.

- **Clinical Signs and Symptoms**
  Sudden onset of whitish, frothy bronchial secretions; pulmonary edema; and hepatotoxicity

Arsenic

Most arsenical pesticides contain the soluble salt arsenic trioxide. It is a highly toxic inorganic compound with an LD_{50} of 14 mg/kg.

MOA: Arsenic impairs cellular respiration by inhibiting mitochondrial enzymes and uncoupling oxidative phosphorylation. It also acts on the Krebs cycle by blocking pyruvate dehydrogenase.

- **Clinical Signs and Symptoms**
  - Gastrointestinal symptoms such as nausea, vomiting, and watery diarrhea over the first 1–3 h.

- May have a garlic odor on the breath and in stools.
- Dehydration and hypotension.
- ECG may show QTc prolongation with subsequent torsades de pointes and cardiac arrhythmias. Shock may develop.
- Acute respiratory distress syndrome.
- Renal injury can lead to proteinuria, hematuria, acute tubular necrosis, and anuria.
- Acute encephalopathy can develop with delirium, coma, and seizures.
- Persistent central nervous system symptoms such as headache, confusion, and memory problems may occur in survivors.

Chronic effects can occur as the sequelae of acute poisoning or the result of chronic longer-term exposure to lower arsenic doses. The clinical effects of chronic toxicity can have an insidious onset and thus be more difficult to diagnose. Arsenic is also a known human carcinogen.

Barium Carbonate

The soluble salts of barium (barium carbonate, sulfide, chloride, chlorate, and nitrate) are highly toxic due to their easy dissolution into ionic barium in the presence of water.

Exposures occur primarily by oral route.

Toxicity has occurred from ingestion of as little as 200 mg of soluble barium.

MOA: Barium competitively inhibits potassium efflux channels, causing sequestration of total body potassium stores in the intracellular compartment. The sodium–potassium adenosine triphosphate (ATP) pump function continues unchanged; however, it causes further potassium influx and severe hypokalemia. The decreased resting potential of cell membranes renders myocardial cells more prone to arrhythmias and causes skeletal muscle paralysis. Vascular smooth muscle may also be affected with hypertension, as is often seen.

- **Clinical Signs and Symptoms**
  - Vomiting, diarrhea, and abdominal pain
  - Generalized weakness, muscle-twitching, and focal or generalized paralysis
  - Hypertension
  - Ventricular arrhythmias that arise from severe hypokalemia
  - Lactic acidosis, usually mild
  - Hypokalemia, often profound
  - ECG findings include diffuse ST-segment depressions, flattened T waves, and U waves

Bromethalin

Very effective single-feeding rodenticide.

LD_{50} for humans has not been established. In animal studies, the LD_{50} ranges from 1.8 mg/kg in the common house cat to 13 mg/kg in a field rabbit, while guinea pigs exposed to a dose greater than 1000 mg/kg demonstrated no signs of toxicity.

MOA: Bromethalin and its more active metabolite, desmethyl-bromethalin, exert their toxic effects by the uncoupling of mitochondrial oxidative phosphorylation, leading to a decrease in the production of adenosine triphosphate (ATP). The lack of ATP causes increased fluid around the neuron myelin sheaths in the brain and spinal cord, with increased intracranial pressure (ICP) subsequently developing.

- **Clinical Signs and Symptoms**
  - Vomiting, nausea, and abdominal pain
  - Drowsiness and lethargy
  - Agitation, hallucinations, ataxia, tremors, coma, and seizures

In a fatal case of bromethalin ingestion in a human, microscopic evaluation of the brain showed vacuolization of the white matter consistent with findings in other animal species.

Cholecalciferol

Cholecalciferol is vitamin D3.

Absorbed orally.

MOA: Alteration in calcium homeostasis. Cholecalciferol causes hypercalcemia by promoting calcium mobilization from bone and increasing intestinal absorption.

Usually, human toxicity involves a chronic ingestion of >50,000 IU daily.

- **Clinical Signs and Symptoms**
  - Calcium concentrations over 11.5 mg/dL cause anorexia, fatigue, disorientation, polyuria, vomiting, nephrocalcinosis, and renal insufficiency

A normal serum calcium concentration at 48 h after exposure precludes the development of toxicity.

Crimidine

A synthetic chlorinated pyrimidine compound.

MOA: Inhibits pyridoxine (vitamin B6), causing gamma-aminobutyric acid (GABA) deficiency.

- **Clinical Signs and Symptoms**
  - Vomiting, seizures, status epilepticus, and pulmonary edema

Elemental Phosphorus

Nonmetallic substance that exists in two common forms, red and white (or "yellow" phosphorus). The red form is not absorbed and has very limited toxicity. The white form, a yellowish, waxy solid, is highly toxic.

The LD_{50} for acute exposure is approximately 1 mg/kg.

Faint garlic odor.

Poses a significant risk of fire and explosion when exposed to air.

Absorbed via the gastrointestinal (GI) tract. Dermal exposure causes burns and systemic effects as well.

MOA: Direct tissue toxicity caused by an exothermic reaction, local production of phosphoric acid leading to tissue corrosion, and formation of phosphorus pentoxide, which reacts with organic molecules. Phosphorus is also caustic to the skin and eyes. In the circulation, phosphorus binds to calcium and can cause life-threatening hypocalcemia. Inhalation of white phosphorus can cause lung irritation and respiratory distress.

- **Clinical Signs and Symptoms**
  It causes significant local as well as systemic toxicity described in three phases as follows:
  - Phase 1 (minutes or hours after the ingestion).
    - Perioral and mucosal burns, nausea, vomiting, and diarrhea.
    - Garlic odor on the breath/vomitus may also be noted.
    - Feces or vomitus may exhibit phosphorescence, sometimes labeled the "smoking stool syndrome."
    - Death in this stage is due to cardiovascular collapse and ventricular dysrhythmia.
  - Phase 2, if present, consists of a latent period of up to several weeks in which symptoms seem to resolve.
  - Phase 3.
    - Liver damage with jaundice and hypoglycemia.
    - Acute kidney injury with renal failure.
    - Damages to the GI tract, heart, and brain may also be noted.

Individual patients may or may not display all phases of toxicity. Overlap of toxic findings between phase 1 and phase 3 or absence of a latent period is common. Monitoring of vital signs as well as electrolytes, especially serum potassium, calcium, and phosphorus, is essential.

Pyriminil (N-3-Pyridylmethyl-N-*P*--Nitrophenyl Urea, PNU, or Vacor)

Highly toxic. Symptoms have occurred with as little as 5 mg/kg exposure and death has been reported after ingestion of less than 3 g.

MOA: Destroys pancreatic beta islet cells, bringing about diabetic ketoacidosis within hours of exposure. A nicotinamide antagonist, it impairs the synthesis of NAD and NADH required for cellular energy metabolism.

- **Clinical Signs and Symptoms**
  - Hyperglycemia.
  - Acidosis.
  - GI hypomotility and bladder atony from autonomic dysfunction.
  - Postural hypotension (may persist for months or indefinitely).
  - Peripheral and cranial neuropathies and pupillary dysfunction.
  - Weakness, anhidrosis, and impotence have been reported.
  - Mental status changes can range from somnolence to delirium.

Red Squill (*Urginea maritime*)

Red squill (*Urginea maritime*) contains two different cardiac glycosides as its active ingredients, scillaren A and scillaren B.

An LD_{50} has not been identified for this compound.

MOA: Similar to digitalis.

U. maritime has a very bitter taste and also acts as a potent emetic, which often prevents toxicity in most animals.

- **Clinical Signs and Symptoms**
  - Although no serious toxicity from red-squill ingestion in humans has been reported, clinical manifestations of acute ingestion might include abdominal pain and vomiting.
  - Hyperkalemia, cardiac arrhythmias, and seizure activity.

Sodium Monofluoroacetate and Fluoroacetamide

Sodium monofluoroacetate (SMFA) is also known as compound 1080. Fluoroacetamide is also known as compound 1081.

Highly toxic rodenticides. SMFA has an LD_{50} of 2 mg/kg.

Fluoroacetamide is chemically and mechanistically similar to SMFA, with a slightly higher fatal dose and a more delayed onset of action.

Absorbed through ingestion, inhalation, ocular exposure, and contact with open wounds.

MOA: Both SMFA and fluoroacetamide irreversibly inhibit the Krebs cycle. The mechanism of action involves the transformation of the parent compound to fluorocitrate, which binds to the enzyme, aconitase, and stops the cycle. As a result, cellular aerobic metabolism ceases, and a variety of enzymatic systems are inhibited including fatty acid oxidation, gluconeogenesis, and the urea cycle. Blocking of the Krebs cycle at this step also causes the accumulation of citrate, which complexes with extracellular calcium, leading to hypocalcemia and worsening metabolic acidosis. As clinical toxicity is due to the fluorocitrate metabolite, a latent period exists after exposure until metabolite formation has occurred. The latent period may range from 30–180 min after SMFA exposure but potentially delayed up to 20 h after fluoroacetamide exposure. With significant exposure, SMFA toxicity has a rapidly deteriorating clinical course; death usually ensues within 72 h and is secondary to persistent shock or cardiac arrhythmias.

- **Clinical Signs and Symptoms**
  - Agitation.
  - Abdominal pain, nausea and vomiting, diarrhea.
  - Respiratory distress.
  - Seizures.
  - Coma.
  - Hypotension that may be refractory to fluid resuscitation and inotropic support.
  - Lactic acidosis, hypokalemia, and hypocalcemia.
  - Arrhythmias including a variety of types such as ventricular tachycardia, supraventricular tachycardia, atrial fibrillation, ventricular fibrillation, and asystole. ECG may show QT-segment prolongation secondary

to hypocalcemia and nonspecific ST- and T-wave abnormalities.

Delayed sequelae may include acute kidney injury, hepatic dysfunction, cerebellar degeneration, cerebral atrophy, and neuropathy.

Strychnine

Highly toxic.

Absorbed via oral, inhalation, or dermal route.

The onset of symptoms from strychnine poisoning usually occurs within 10–20 min of ingestion. However, injection or inhalation may result in more rapid development, and dermal exposure may produce a delayed onset.

MOA: Competitive inhibition of glycine receptors at the postsynaptic and motor neuron levels. Because glycine is an inhibitory neurotransmitter, this receptor blockade leads to a subsequent increase in the downstream firing of muscle fibers and involuntary muscle contraction. Strychnine's effects occur primarily at the level of the spinal cord and may be conscious during muscle spasms. Death usually occurs from respiratory failure and difficulty in ventilating the patient.

- **Clinical Signs and Symptoms**
  - Prodromal signs may include mydriasis, hypervigilance, anxiety, hyperreflexia, clonus, and stiffness of the facial and neck muscles
  - Repetitive facial grimacing (*risus sardonicus*), trismus, and full-body opisthotonus, which can be mistaken for seizure activity
  - Severe and recurring diffuse muscle contractions that last from 30 s to 2 min
  - Conscious with lucid sensorium until hypoxia ensues
  - Rhabdomyolysis, lactic acidosis, and hyperthermia
  - Respiratory failure from spasm of respiratory muscles

Tetramethylenedisulfotetramine (TETS or Tetramine)

Highly toxic with a lethal dose (LD_{50}) of 0.1–0.3 mg/kg in mammals. As little as 7 mg (or a small taste) may be lethal in humans.

MOA: Similar to picrotoxin, tetramine is an irreversible antagonist of the GABA receptor.

The onset of symptoms may begin within 10 min of ingestion or be delayed up to 13 h after exposure.

- **Clinical Signs and Symptoms**
  - Vomiting, headache, dizziness, weakness, and lethargy
  - Perioral paresthesias
  - Tachycardia, palpitations, and cardiac arrhythmias
  - Refractory status epilepticus
  - Liver failure
  - Coagulopathy
  - Rhabdomyolysis
  - Acute kidney injury

Long-term sequelae report that patients may develop chronic seizure disorders, cognitive impairment, and cortical blindness.

Thallium (Thallium Sulfate and Other Thallium Salts

Highly toxic rodenticide (8 mg/kg has caused death in humans).

Absorbed orally, via inhalation, and through intact skin.

MOA: Displacement of potassium in enzyme systems and ion channels, causing global disruption of cellular energy production.

- **Clinical Signs and Symptoms**
  - **Early signs (up to 48 h)**
    - Gastrointestinal symptoms including abdominal pain, vomiting, constipation, and, less commonly, diarrhea are fre-

    quently noted within a few hours of ingestion.
  - Tachycardia, hypertension, and chest pain may also occur.
- **Intermediate signs (2 days to 3 weeks)**
- Neurologic symptoms predominate, later including the following:
  - Ataxia
  - Cranial nerve dysfunction with ptosis and nystagmus
  - Choreoathetosis
  - Cognitive and memory deficiency
  - Delirium
  - Optic neuritis
  - Paresthesias in stocking-glove distribution, which is often painful
  - Psychosis
  - Lethargy and coma

Other common findings include dermatologic signs such as alopecia (often sparing the inner third of the eyebrows and axilla), darkening of hair roots, erythematous changes of the palms and soles, and hyperpigmentation with eczematous skin changes.

Acute liver and kidney injuries may occur, along with anemia and thrombocytopenia. Hyperchloremic metabolic acidosis has been reported.

- **Late signs**
  - Permanent vision defects including optic atrophy with vision loss, central scotomata, cataracts, and blue vision loss.
  - Poisoning victims may die from sudden cardiac death or multi-organ failure weeks after exposure.

Zinc and Aluminum Phosphides

Highly toxic metallic phosphide rodenticides.

Exposure occurs from inhalation of phosphine gas, produced when aluminum or zinc phosphide is exposed to moisture in stored grain, oral ingestion, or dermal contact. Upon ingestion, phosphides are converted by gastric acid to phosphine gas, the primary toxic agent, which is then absorbed from the gastrointestinal tract into the bloodstream.

Phosphine gas is known to have an odor similar to rotten fish.

MOA: Many mechanisms of toxicity have been proposed, but none fully explain the clinical features of poisoning. Toxicity may result from the inhibition of oxidative phosphorylation, free radical production with the promotion of lipid peroxidation, and cholinesterase inhibition.

Phosphide toxicity occurs rapidly, typically within 30 min of exposure. Death often occurs rapidly within the first day of severe phosphide poisoning, regardless of therapy, and typically results from cardiac arrhythmias or refractory shock and cardiac failure.

- **Clinical Signs and Symptoms**
  - Gastrointestinal (GI) irritation marked by nausea, vomiting, retrosternal chest and abdominal pain, and hematemesis.
  - Shock with refractory hypotension caused by direct cardiac toxicity.
  - Cardiac arrhythmias, including bradycardia, supraventricular tachycardia, atrial fibrillation, atrial flutter, and ventricular arrhythmias.
  - Hemorrhagic pulmonary edema with tachypnea, cough, acute respiratory distress syndrome, and respiratory failure.
  - Pericardial and pleural effusions, pancreatitis, adrenal necrosis, and liver damage.
  - Intravascular hemolysis with methemoglobinemia and/or renal failure may occur.
  - Hypokalemia and elevated lactate concentrations.
  - Convulsions and coma.

Risk factors for death after intentional poisoning include dose ($\geq$500 mg of phosphides), hypotension, acidosis, hypoxia, global left ventricular hypokinesis, and left ventricular ejection fraction <40%.

Unknown Poison Exposure

Accidental and/or intentional (suicidal or even homicidal) poisoning may be seen by the rural practitioner. If poisoning is suspected and there is no label on the container or the patient is incapable of answering questions (infant or young child), or the patient has mental incapacities/intoxication, or suicidal attempts and refusal to answer questions), then rodenticides need to be considered as a poison that may be readily available. In all cases, a medical toxicologist should be consulted as quickly as possible as gastric lavage and administration of activated charcoal may decrease absorption of the toxic agent if administered soon after exposure (within 1 h).

All asymptomatic patients with exposure to an unknown rodenticide warrant the following studies (Calello 2023):

- 12-lead ECG and continuous monitoring
- Plain radiographs of the chest and abdomen
- Basic metabolic panel including glucose, electrolytes, calcium, and phosphorus
- Complete blood count
- Liver panel: Alanine aminotransferase (ALT), aspartate aminotransferase (AST), and bilirubin
- Prothrombin time and international normalized ratio (PT and INR) and partial thromboplastin time (PTT)
- Renal panel: Blood urea nitrogen (BUN), serum creatinine, and Estimated Glomerular Filtration Rate (eGFR).
- Venous or arterial blood gas

When the poison is not known, clinical features can help with identification and guide treatment as follows (Calello 2023; Isackson and Irizarry 2022):

- **Cardiovascular toxicity:**
  Arrhythmias, refractory shock, or cardiac arrest: Arsenic, barium carbonate, fluoroacetamide, Zn/Al phosphide, white (yellow) phosphorous, SMFA, thallium, or red squill
- **Neurological toxicity:**
  Seizures: SMFA, fluoroacetamide, tetramine, arsenic, or crimidine.
  Cranial neuropathy, lethargy, or coma: Thallium, arsenic, alpha-chloralose, bromethalin, or pyriminil
- **Musculoskeletal toxicity:**
  Rigidity, opisthotonus, trismus, and facial grimacing (risus sardonicus): Strychnine
- **Hematologic toxicity:**
  Bruising or bleeding: Anticoagulants (first- (warfarin) and second-generation (superwarfarin) compounds)

Changes may be noted on a patient's laboratory tests and electrocardiogram (ECG). Some rodenticides may show up on chest X-ray (CXR) or abdominal X-rays (Table 11.6). Abnormal results can suggest specific rodenticides as follows:

Patients who remain asymptomatic with normal ancillary studies warrant hospital observation for up to 24 h to exclude poisoning from SMFA or fluoroacetamide. Furthermore, all asymptomatic patients should undergo measurement of PT with INR and PTT at approximately 48 h after exposure to identify anticoagulant rodenticide poisoning.

Patients with any symptoms of poisoning or abnormality on ancillary testing warrant hospital admission for observation and supportive care of evolving toxicity. Specific treatment may also be indicated and should be managed with the assistance of a medical toxicologist.

Delayed toxicity in initially asymptomatic patients is most characteristic of poisoning with thallium, arsenic, sodium monofluoroacetate (SMFA), and fluoroacetamide. Thus, exposure to these agents usually warrants hospital admission to a unit with intensive care capability.

Table 11.6 Laboratory/ECG/X-Ray findings suggesting rodenticide poisoning

Finding
Complete blood count
Anemia: Zinc phosphide, arsenic
Basic metabolic panel
Hypoglycemia: Zinc/aluminum phosphide
Hyperglycemia: Pyriminil
Hypocalcemia: Fluoroacetamide, white phosphorous, SMFA
Hypercalcemia: Cholecalciferol
Hypokalemia: Barium carbonate, Zn/Al phosphide
Hyperphosphatemia: White (yellow) phosphorous
Liver/renal panel
Elevated liver enzymes: Arsenic, Zn/Al phosphide, white (yellow) phosphorous, thallium
Elevated creatinine/BUN: Arsenic, Zn/Al phosphide, white (yellow) phosphorous, thallium
Creatine phosphokinase (CPK)
Elevated CPK: Strychnine
Blood gases
Lactic acidosis: SMFA, fluoroacetamide, strychnine
Coagulation profile
Elevated PT and INR: Warfarins, indandiones
Troponin
Elevated: Zn/Al phosphide
Lipase
Elevated: Pyriminil
Cholinesterase
Depressed: Organophosphates, carbamates
Urinalysis
Hematuria: Anticoagulants
ECG
QTc prolongation: Arsenic, fluoroacetamide, SMFA, white (yellow) phosphorous
CXR/abdominal X-rays
Radiopaque: Arsenic, barium carbonate, thallium

Differential Diagnosis of Rodenticide Poisoning

Many conditions can mimic exposure to rodenticides and need to be considered in case of presentation to the practitioner's office or emergency room, especially in young children or persons that may be incapacitated. Important questions to ask the patient/parent/guardian include the following: What were they doing before symptoms started? What underlying medical conditions and medications do they have? Were they working in an agricultural field or harvesting crops that may have recently been treated with a pesticide? Is there a rodent problem, which may have been recently treated by exterminators, or has someone recently used a product (possibly imported or not approved for rodent control) for a rodent or other pest problem? Have they consumed alcohol or an illegal substance recently? Do other family members or friends have similar symptoms? Could they have been bitten by a snake/spider or had a severe reaction to an insect sting? A differential diagnosis to consider in the case of suspected rodenticide poisoning includes the following:

- Gastroenteritis (bacterial, viral, and toxin)
- Hepatitis (viral and alcohol)
- Diabetic ketoacidosis
- Disseminated intravascular coagulopathy
- Hypocalcemia/hypercalcemia
- Hypokalemia
- Snake envenomation coagulopathy
- Organophosphate/carbamate poisoning

Complications of Rodenticide Exposure

Certain rodenticides are so toxic that long-term complications may occur after a poisoning event. Patients should be followed up closely after discharge from the emergency room or hospital to see if they develop these sequelae and are treated appropriately.

- Liver failure: White phosphorous, arsenic, and SMFA
- Kidney failure: Zinc phosphide and SMFA
- Permanent neurologic damage: Arsenic, thallium, and SMFA
- Type 1 diabetes mellitus: Pyriminil
- Hair loss: Thallium
- Hyperpigmentation and keratoses: Arsenic

Unfortunately, some rodenticides may also be carcinogenic, such as arsenic, and patients may have an increased risk of developing cancer years later.

References

Anderson IB. Warfarin and superwarfarins. In: Olson K, editor. Poisoning & drug overdose. 7th ed. New York: McGraw-Hill Companies, Inc; 2018. p. 459–61.

Bahouth MA, Kraus P, Dane K, Montana MP, Tsao W, Tabaac B, Jasem J, Schmidlin H, Einstein E, Streiff MB, Shanbhag S. Synthetic cannabinoid-associated coagulopathy secondary to long-acting anticoagulant rodenticides; observational case series and management recommendations. Medicine (Baltimore). 2019;98(36):e17015.

BCPC (British Crop Production Council). Rodenticides. Copyright 1995–2022. http://www.bcpcpesticidecompendium.org/class_rodenticides.html. Accessed 20 Sept 2023.

Calello DP. Overview of rodenticide poisoning. Last updated July 24, 2023. https://www.uptodate.com/contents/overview-of-rodenticide-poisoning. Accessed 21 Sept 2023.

CDC (Centers for Disease Control and Prevention). How to control wild rodent infestations. Last reviewed January 3, 2023. https://www.cdc.gov/healthypets/pets/wildlife/rodent-control.html. Accessed 24 Sept 2023.

Gummin DD, Mowry JB, Beuhler MC, Spyker DA, Brooks DE, Dibert KW, Rivers LJ, Pham NPT, Ryan ML. 2019 Annual report of the American Association of Poison Control Centers' National Poison Data System (NPDS): 37th annual report. Clin Toxicol (Phila). 2020;58(12):1360–541.

Hazra DK, Karmakar R, Poi R, Bhattacharya S, Mondal S. Rodent menace, their management and role of possible new rodenticide formulations to combat resistance. J Entomol Zool Stud. 2017;5(21):202–6.

Hunt BJ. Bleeding and coagulopathies in critical care. N Engl J Med. 2014;370(9):847–59.

Isackson B, Irizarry L. Rodenticide toxicity. StatPearls Publishing, LLC. Updated 12/04/2022. Available at: https://www.ncbi.nlm.nih.gov/books/NBK554428/. Accessed 1 Oct 2023.

Langley R, Haskell M, Hareza D, et al. Rodent bite injuries presenting to emergency departments in the United States, 2001–2015. J Environ Health. 2020;83(7):18–24.

Lung D. Rodenticide toxicity. Medscape. Updated March 16, 2023. https://emedicine.medscape.com/article/818130-overview?form=fpf. Accessed 2 Oct 2023.

Meier KH. Rodenticides, miscellaneous. In: Olson K, editor. Poisoning & drug overdose. 7th ed. New York: McGraw-Hill Companies, Inc; 2018. p. 405–10.

Mercer MA, Davis JL, Riviere JE, Baynes RE, Tell LA, Jaberi-Douraki M, Maunsell FP, Lin Z. Mechanisms of toxicity and residue considerations of rodenticide exposure in food animals—a FARAD perspective. J Am Vet Med Assoc. 2022;260(5):514–23.

NPIC (National Pesticide Information Center). Rodenticides topic fact sheet. Revised March 2016. http://npic.orst.edu/factsheets/rodenticides.html. Accessed 20 Sept 2023.

Osweiler G. Rodenticides. In: Toxicology. Philadelphia: Williams & Wilkins Media; 1996. p. 275–96.

Peshin SS, Srivastava A, Halder N, Gupta YK. Pesticide poisoning trend analysis of 13 years: a retrospective study based on telephone calls at the National Poisons Information Centre, All India Institute of Medical Sciences, New Delhi. J Forensic Leg Med. 2014;22:57–61.

Roberts JR, Reigart JR. Recognition and management of pesticide poisonings. 6th ed. US EPA Office of Pesticide Programs; 2013. https://www.epa.gov/pesticide-worker-safety/pesticide-poisoning-handbook-complete-document. Accessed 25 Sept 2023

U.S. EPA (U.S. Environmental Protection Agency). Rodent control pesticide safety review. Last updated December 7, 2022. https://www.epa.gov/rodenticides/rodent-control-pesticide-safety-review. Accessed 1 Oct 2023.

U.S. EPA. Label review manual. Last updated March 20, 2023. https://www.epa.gov/pesticide-registration/label-review-manual. Accessed 4 Oct 2023.

Witmer GW, Pitt WC, Howald G. Invasive rodent ecology, impacts, and management with an emphasis on the United States. In: Timm RM, O'Brien JM, editors. Proc. 26th Vertebr. Pest Conf. Published at Univ. of Calif., Davis; 2014. p. 15–20.

WHO (World Health Organization). The WHO recommended classification of pesticides by Hazard and guidelines to classification, 2019 edition. https://www.who.int/publications/i/item/9789240005662. Accessed 5 Oct 2023.

12 Fumigants

Beth Dittman

Introduction to Fumigants

Fumigants are pesticides that are applied as a gas or as a substance that volatilizes into a gas in order to kill pests, including rodents, insects, and fungi. Fumigants can reach and affect pests that are inaccessible to other types of treatment and often do not leave harmful residues behind, which makes fumigation a useful tool for pest control. There are different uses of fumigation, including structural, soil, burrow, and commodity fumigation. In the United States, all fumigants are classified as restricted-use pesticides by the Environmental Protection Agency (EPA), so applicators must be certified or licensed according to their state's regulations in order to be legally credentialed to apply these products.

Soil fumigation is used on a wide variety of crops including potatoes, tomatoes, tobacco, carrots, and strawberries. Fumigants are used to control plant pathogens, nematodes, and weeds and are often applied prior to planting. Soil fumigants may be applied as solids that are then watered into the soil or mechanically incorporated. Liquid formulations can be injected directly or through an irrigation system. Applicators may use tarps to retain the fumigant for a longer period of time and control emissions (Becker et al. 2005).

Commodity fumigation is often used to treat both food and nonfood goods, such as grain, feed, tobacco, wood, and natural fiber products. Treatment of these goods with a fumigant is used to control a variety of pests including invertebrate pests such as insects (beetles and moths) and vertebrate pests like rodents (rats and mice). This allows for long-term storage and transport of goods and prevents the spread of invasive species during import and export.

Structural fumigation may be used to treat indoor and structural pests such as bedbugs, cockroaches, wood-destroying beetles, or termites. Structural fumigation usually relies on tents or tarps to trap gas inside the building, and the fumigant penetrates hard-to-reach areas, such as cracks and crevices where pests may dwell. Fans are often used after fumigation to help dissipate the gas, reducing indoor fumigant levels until it is safe for people to enter. Fumigant gas levels in structures are monitored by gas-detecting devices as specified on the pesticide label. The most commonly used structural fumigant is sulfuryl fluoride, which is odorless, so chloropicrin is often added as a warning agent since it has a sharp, irritating odor (NPIC 2019).

Burrow fumigation is used to treat burrowing pests, often rodents. Even though burrows are in the soil, burrow fumigation is considered non-soil fumigation since it does not directly treat the

B. Dittman (✉)
North Carolina Department of Agriculture and Consumer Services, Structural Pest Control and Pesticides Division, Raleigh, NC, USA
e-mail: Beth.Dittman@ncagr.gov

W. J. Meggs, R. L. Langley (eds.), *Farm Toxicology*, https://doi.org/10.1007/978-3-031-80441-0_12

soil or soil pests but rather targets animals that live in the burrows themselves (CalDPR 2023). Application of burrow fumigants in soils with high porosity may be less effective due to diffusion of the chemical.

Fumigants come in a variety of solid, liquid, and gas formulations, but the solid and liquid formulations are converted to a gaseous form to permeate the entire treatment area. Gas formulations are stored under pressure in metal cylinders, such as carbon dioxide gas often used for treating outdoor burrowing pests. Liquified gases are stored under pressure in metal cylinders as a liquid that turns to gas when exposed to air, such as methyl bromide. Volatile liquids are generally stored as (not-pressurized) liquids at room temperature and turn into gas when exposed to air; for example, chloropicrin can be added to other fumigants to serve as a warning odor. Solids are packaged as pellets or tablets that turn into a gas when exposed to moisture in the air, which is how phosphine gas is often created for fumigant use. Once in a gaseous form, the chemical can penetrate and infiltrate hard-to-reach spaces, such as those between seeds, which makes it very effective for treating pests that are otherwise hard to reach and eradicate. However, this can also create dangerous situations when people enter fumigation areas before they are properly ventilated or if treatment areas are not properly sealed, which allows for vapors to escape to surrounding areas. Fumigants can easily penetrate materials and move beyond the application site, which increases the chance of harm.

The effectiveness of fumigation depends on many environmental factors. For instance, since fumigants exist as or volatilize into gaseous form, temperature plays a role in how quickly the chemical evaporates and diffuses throughout the air. When the temperature is too low, the chemical may not reach a high-enough concentration to be effective against the target pest population. Additionally, at lower temperatures, animal pests have lower respiratory and metabolic rates, which may decrease their susceptibility to the toxicant. When the temperature is too high, the chemical may diffuse too rapidly, which does not allow for sufficient contact time, or it may break down, which decreases effectiveness. Humidity also plays a role as certain fumigants (metal phosphides) are applied as solids that react with moisture in the air to create phosphine gas. Lower humidity will result in slower release of the fumigant, requiring longer treatment times to be effective. However, if the humidity is too high, then the moisture in the air may hinder the diffusion of the fumigant gas molecules and impede penetration of the small areas that need to be treated. Wind is also a consideration for fumigation as increasing windspeeds create difficulty for both tarping and uniform gas diffusion and may carry fumes from the application site. Last, the condition and material of the fumigation site can impact diffusion and effectiveness. Fumigant molecules may adsorb to (stick to the outside of) or absorb into (transfer into) both treated materials and surrounding materials, which impacts the availability of the fumigant to contact the pest to be controlled. Desorption is also an important consideration for how long the treated airspace may contain hazardous levels of chemicals. Temperature affects the rate of absorption, adsorption, and desorption, with lower temperatures increasing adherence to surfaces and higher temperatures encouraging the release, or desorption, of the molecules into the air.

Commonly Used Fumigants (Table 12.1)

Methyl bromide has a wide variety of uses as a fumigant. It can be used to control insects, mites, ticks, microbes, fungi, weeds, and vertebrates (EPA 2020b). Due to its status as an ozone-depleting chemical, its use was phased out, but critical-use exemptions have allowed its continued use to control pests when there is a lack of suitable alternatives. Methyl bromide is used in both soil and non-soil (commodity and structural) fumigation scenarios for many different crop types, including food commodities and non-food commodities. Methyl bromide exists as a gas at room temperature and is not known to be odorous at low concentrations, so exposure to hazardous levels can occur without notice

Table 12.1 Common fumigant chemicals, use sites, and pests controlled

Fumigant	Use sites[a]	Pests controlled[a]
Methyl bromide	Soil (tomatoes, strawberries, peppers, cucumbers, watermelons), commodities (tree fruits, tree nuts, berries, grains, vegetables, cocoa, dried fruits, cheese, processed grains, processed herbs and spices, logs, tobacco, cotton machinery), structures (warehouses, grain elevators, ships, food processing plants)	Nematodes, weeds, plant pathogens, insects, rodents
Chloropicrin	Soil (tobacco, peppers, tomatoes, and cranberries), structures (including residences)	Fungi, weeds, rodents, insects, and nematodes
Sulfuryl fluoride	Structures (including residences), commodities (grains, dried fruits, dried beans)	Insects, rodents
Phosphine	Burrows, commodities (nuts, dried fruits, grains, processed foods, tobacco, wood, paper)	Insects, rodents
1,3-dichloropropene (1,3-D)	Soil (potatoes, tobacco, carrots, onions, cucumbers, peanuts)	Nematodes, pathogens
Methyl isothiocyanate (MITC)	Wood treatment	Fungi
Metam-sodium and metam-potassium	Soil (potatoes, tomatoes, carrots, onions, peanuts, cantaloupes)	Fungi, weeds, insects, and nematodes
Dimethyl disulfide (DMDS)	Soil (tomatoes, peppers, eggplants, cucumbers, squash, melons, strawberries)	Fungi, weeds, and nematodes
Chlorine dioxide	Structures and equipment (hatching facilities and mushroom houses), water systems	Bacteria, fungi, algae
Sulfur dioxide	Commodity (grapes)	Fungi, microbes
Formaldehyde	Commodities (poultry, swine, and citrus operations)	Microbes

[a] This is not a comprehensive list of all use sites or types of pests controlled. Fumigant product label instructions should always be followed

(ATSDR 2020a). Due to its high volatility, methyl bromide disperses into the air once released, unless it is applied in a well-sealed space, such as a container with commodity goods or tarped soil. Methyl bromide can also penetrate many types of materials including some protective materials such as rubber and leather (ATSDR 2020a).

Chloropicrin is commonly used as a soil fumigant but may also be formulated with other fumigants (i.e., methyl bromide or sulfuryl fluoride) to serve as a warning agent due to its irritating odor. Chloropicrin is nonselective and can be used to control a variety of pests including fungi, weeds, insects, and nematodes (EPA 2009a). For use as a soil fumigant, chloropicrin is often injected as a liquid into the soil for both tarped and untarped crops where it quickly volatilizes in the soil, or it may be applied using drip irrigation. Chloropicrin concentrations are often much lower (by an order of magnitude or more) when used as a warning agent compared to the levels when it is used as an active ingredient in the fumigation process (EPA 2009a). At the start of residential structural fumigation, a shallow pan or absorbent material containing chloropicrin is placed in the center of the structure prior to the release of sulfuryl fluoride. Chloropicrin can be heavier than air and will stay along the ground and collect in low-lying areas (NIOSH 2011).

Sulfuryl fluoride is a structural and commodity fumigant used to control animal pests such as termites, cockroaches, bedbugs, rats, and mice. It is the only structural fumigant approved for residential use but only with the use of chloropicrin since sulfuryl fluoride is colorless and odorless (EPA 2023). Sulfuryl fluoride has replaced some uses of methyl bromide, so its use has increased since 2005. Sulfuryl fluoride is a gas at ambient temperature and is heavier than air, so it may accumulate close to the ground.

Metal phosphides are chemicals that include magnesium phosphide and aluminum phosphide that react with moisture in the air to release phosphine gas. Metal phosphide products come in a variety of formulations, such as pellets, tablets, and strips, and are used for food-commodity fumigation to control animal pests and for rodent-burrow fumigation. Phosphine, as a pressurized gas, is used to fumigate nonfood commodities. Metal phosphides and phosphine gas can also be used for structural or space fumigation but are not registered for use as soil fumigants (EPA 2023). Phosphine gas is odorless at lower concentrations but may have a slight garlic odor at higher concentrations. Due to its high toxicity, harmful exposure can occur at levels lower than the odor threshold (ATSDR 2014b). Phosphine gas is denser than ambient air and will often settle close to the ground. Phosphine poses risks due to its flammability and reactivity with water. It can ignite by contact with air (ATSDR 2014b) and must be handled with care.

1,3-dichloropropene (1,3-D) is a soil fumigant used to control nematodes and other soil pests and diseases in vegetables, fruits, nuts, turf, and other nursery crops (Olinger et al. 2007). 1,3-D is formulated as a liquid that can be injected into the soil or applied via drip irrigation. After application to the soil, 1,3-D volatilizes into a gas. 1,3-D can be irritating and has a sweet odor. It dissipates quickly and can be broken down quickly in air, soil, and water (ATSDR 2008).

Metam-sodium, metam-potassium, and dazomet all break down into methyl isothiocyanate (MITC), which is the toxic agent for these pesticide products. Metam-sodium and metam-potassium products are used as soil fumigants for the control of fungi, weeds, insects, and nematodes in agriculture and have additional use sites including turf and ornamental sites, nurseries, and industrial facilities (EPA 2009c). Agriculturally, metam-sodium and metam-potassium are often applied via chemigation or with tractor-drawn equipment. Dazomet is used as a soil fumigant that is similar to metam-sodium, metam-potassium, and MITC. Dazomet granules can be applied to soil on the surface or incorporated into the soil. It breaks down into MITC and several lesser-gaseous degradates that can also diffuse and have pesticidal properties (i.e., formaldehyde, monomethylamine, and hydrogen sulfide) (EPA 2009b). MITC itself is used as an antimicrobial treatment for wood. MITC is highly volatile and has a horseradish-like odor.

Dimethyl disulfide (DMDS) is used as a non-selective soil fumigant to treat for fungi, weeds, insects, and nematodes prior to planting a variety of crop types (EPA 2019). DMDS is a volatile liquid that can be applied to soil in several ways, where it readily volatilizes to gas. DMDS has an irritating sulfurous odor, similar to garlic or decaying matter. DMDS degrades quickly in the environment, which allows for its use without leaving residues on the crops planted after application.

Lesser-used fumigants in agriculture include chlorine dioxide, sulfur dioxide, and formaldehyde. Chlorine dioxide is used to sanitize and disinfect agricultural facilities, such as mushroom houses and poultry operations, and water systems that may be used at these facilities. Chlorine dioxide can also be used as a disinfectant and for odor control in industrial and residential settings and was used to decontaminate buildings after the release of anthrax spores (ATSDR 2004; EPA 2006). Chlorine dioxide has a chlorine-like odor and is a gas at room temperature. Sulfur dioxide is used to prevent mold in postharvest grapes and sanitize wine-storage equipment (EPA 2021). These products are sold as compressed liquids that turn into gas when applied. Formaldehyde is used as an antimicrobial fumigant, often to disinfect spaces, equipment, and commodities in poultry, swine, and citrus operations (EPA 2020a). Formaldehyde has a pungent odor and is a gas at room temperature (EPA 2008a).

Routes of Exposure

In general, people can be exposed to chemicals through dermal or ocular contact, inhalation, or ingestion. The most common route of exposure for fumigants is inhalation since they are applied as a gas in an enclosed space. This route of exposure may be particularly dangerous since fumigants can affect the lungs directly by inhibiting breathing, or they may be readily absorbed through the lungs and distributed throughout the body. Chemicals that may be toxic by one route of exposure may not be very toxic by other routes of exposure. For instance, fumigants generally have high toxicity from the inhalation route, but research shows that the risk from short-term dermal exposure is much lower (Gaskin et al. 2017) although some chemicals (e.g., methyl bromide, formaldehyde, and 1,3-D) may be absorbed through the skin.

Exposure may be considered acute or chronic. Acute exposure is generally a one-time short-term exposure to a pesticide and may require higher concentrations to elicit a toxic response. Chronic exposure involves repeated exposure over a longer period, which may cause health effects at a lower concentration of exposure due to the longer and more frequent contact with the chemical. For fumigation specifically, inhaling even small amounts can be dangerous due to the inherent nature of the chemicals; they are designed explicitly to harm living organisms that they contact.

Fumigant compounds will have exposure limits that are set at levels to prevent health effects. Exposure limits vary by chemical, and there are different exposure limits to prevent acute exposure-related effects and chronic exposure-related effects. Many occupational exposure limits can be found in the National Institute for Occupational Safety and Health (NIOSH) Pocket Guide to Chemical Hazards, which also includes information about first aid (NIOSH 2020).

Inhalation is the most common route of exposure to fumigant pesticides and can occur during and after fumigant application. Inhalation of fumigants may result in route-of-entry effects such as nasal irritation, coughing, and difficulty breathing, but most chemicals can also be absorbed through the lungs and distributed throughout the body, leading to the involvement of other organ systems and systemic effects. Exposure may occur if a person enters a treatment area before the labeled reentry period or if the space is improperly or poorly ventilated. Applicators may be exposed while setting up equipment or while monitoring fumigant levels. Care must be taken that all appropriate personal protective equipment is used. Fumigants often require the use of specific respirators, and workers should check the label to ensure that they are using the correct respirator. Respirators should be properly fitted for the worker prior to use, and the filters or canisters should be maintained and replaced regularly. Bystanders may be exposed to fumigants if the treatment area is not properly sealed, which allows gas to escape, or if the applicators did not maintain a proper buffer distance and applied fumigants too close to occupied spaces without notification and evacuation.

Dermal exposure is a common route of exposure for pesticide handlers and can often occur when proper personal protective equipment is not used. It is important for pesticide handlers to follow all precautions on the label, wash hands after handling pesticides or containers, and immediately wash any exposed body part after an accidental splash or spill. Dermal exposure may also occur from pesticide drifting onto other workers or bystanders or from entry into a treated area before chemical residues are dispersed or dry. The most common signs of dermal exposure include redness and irritation. Prolonged exposure or exposure to concentrated products may lead to more severe effects. Some chemicals (e.g., methyl bromide, formaldehyde, and 1,3-D) may also be absorbed through the skin, especially during prolonged contact or contact with broken skin, and can then be distributed throughout the body.

Ingestion of fumigant chemicals is less likely but can occur in different situations. For instance, a pesticide handler who does not wash their hands before eating, drinking, or smoking may ingest small amounts of chemicals. Some pesticides are stored illegally in old food or beverage containers and may then be mistakenly ingested. Pesticides may also be accidentally applied to types of food that they are not labeled for, which may leave a residue behind. In the event of deliberate ingestion with the intention of self-harm, there is a much higher exposure dose and more severe effects. Ingestion of fumigants may result in route-of-entry effects such as irritation and corrosion of the esophagus and stomach, but most chemicals can also be absorbed through the gastrointestinal tract and distributed throughout the body, which leads to the involvement of other organ systems and systemic effects.

Ocular exposure can occur if a chemical splashes or spills into the eyes, especially when a handler is not using proper personal protective equipment. Nearby workers and bystanders may also be susceptible to ocular exposure from drift from a pesticide sprayer. Applicators may also have ocular exposure if they touch or rub their eyes with contaminated gloves or hands, or if they handle dust or powder formulations without eye protection. Ocular exposure often results in local effects, such as itchy, irritated eyes, and in severe cases, corrosive damage that may be irreversible.

Toxicity

Most fumigants are highly toxic to humans and other living things. Some fumigants affect humans and pests by interfering with an organism's ability to breathe, while others disrupt other essential processes of the organism. The ability to cause toxic effects depends on several factors, including the amount of fumigant in the environment (concentration), the length of time the person is exposed (duration), how often the person is exposed (frequency), environmental factors (temperature and humidity), and other factors such as underlying health conditions and lifestyle.

Methyl Bromide

After exposure to methyl bromide, neurological and respiratory effects are the most common symptoms. Symptoms may be delayed by 2–48 h after exposure (ATSDR 2020a). Methyl bromide is well-absorbed through the respiratory and gastrointestinal tracts, where it can be widely distributed throughout the body including the central nervous system. Methyl bromide interacts with the sulfhydryl groups on enzymes, which ultimately leads to reduced glutathione levels. It is broken down quickly into several metabolites, including bromide ions and carbon dioxide.

Acute effects from methyl-bromide-inhalation exposure include involvement of the central nervous system and the respiratory system. Even though symptoms include convulsions, methyl bromide is a nervous system depressant. Initial symptoms include headache, dizziness, weakness, nausea, vomiting, and slurred speech. More severe effects may develop later, especially if the exposure was to a high concentration. More severe effects include ataxia, tremors, paralysis, and tonic–clonic seizures (Reigart and Roberts 2013). Many symptoms resolve after several days, but long-term effects may linger depending on the severity of the exposure. Acute respiratory effects include cough, edema, hemorrhagic lesions, and dyspnea. At higher exposure levels there may be effects on the cardiovascular, reproductive, hepatic, and renal systems. Acute exposure to the skin or eyes often leads to damage at the exposure point (i.e., erythema, edema, and blisters on the skin and eyelids) and conjunctivitis.

Health effects from chronic (long-term or repeated) exposure to methyl bromide have been studied less. Neurological symptoms may develop, such as headache, weakness, muscle aches, and fatigue. Peripheral neuropathies may occur, such as impaired gait and behavioral changes, and the liver and kidney may show mild dysfunction (Aribou and Ng 2022; ATSDR 2020b). EPA has classified methyl bromide as "not likely to be carcinogenic to humans" (Fehir 2022).

Chloropicrin

Chloropicrin exposure can result in the onset of symptoms shortly after exposure (15–30 min), including irritation of the eyes, airways, and exposed skin. Immediate ocular and respiratory effects are likely due to stimulation of the trigeminal nerve (Godshall and Perron 2018). Other modes of action for additional effects on the respiratory, neurological, and gastrointestinal systems are less well-known. Some experiments suggest that the parent compound is responsible for toxicity by inhibiting pyruvate dehydrogenase and succinate dehydrogenase activity and interacting with hemoglobin, interrupting oxygen transport (EPA 2008b).

In general, chloropicrin is an irritating agent, and eye irritation is regarded as the most sensitive health effect. NIOSH (2011) lists possible symptoms of inhalation exposure as irritation leading to coughing, choking, difficulty breathing, or shortness of breath; feeling of tightness in the chest; pulmonary edema; nausea, vomiting, and diarrhea; headache; dizziness, orthostatic hypotension, anxiety, lethargy, and fatigue; and cyanosis. Gastrointestinal effects may persist for weeks. Although less common, ingestion of chloropicrin can lead to irritation and damage to the gastrointestinal tract as well as typical gastrointestinal effects such as stomach pain, nausea, and vomiting. Ingestion may also lead to dyspnea, dizziness, headache, and cyanosis. Acute exposure to the skin or eyes often leads to damage at the exposure point, such as skin irritation and blisters due to dermal exposure and lacrimation and eye damage from acute ocular exposure. EPA has classified chloropicrin as "not likely to be carcinogenic to humans" (Fehir 2022).

Sulfuryl Fluoride

Sulfuryl fluoride may be absorbed through the lungs and distributed throughout the body (kidney, brain, spleen, and other tissues), but the highest levels of the chemical will be found in the respiratory tract after inhalation. Once in the body, most sulfuryl fluoride is eliminated through the urine. Sulfuryl fluoride breaks down quickly in the body into sulfate and fluoride ions. It has been proposed that fluoride is the metabolite responsible for most toxic effects from sulfuryl fluoride exposure (CalEPA 2006; Aribou and Ng 2022).

As with many fumigant chemicals, the primary effects of inhalation exposure are neurotoxicity and respiratory toxicity. Since chloropicrin is often used as a warning agent in structures fumigated with sulfuryl fluoride, some case-reported symptoms may be due to inhalation exposure to one or both compounds. In cases where workers or bystanders are exposed to sulfuryl fluoride, symptoms include irritated nose and throat, coughing, difficulty breathing, nausea, dizziness, numbness of hands, disorientation, headache, restlessness, and seizures (CalEPA 2006; Reigart and Roberts 2013). In severe cases, death has been reported. Acute exposure to the skin or eyes often leads to damage at the exposure point, such as damage to the eyes and skin.

Workers who are repeatedly exposed to sulfuryl fluoride over a long period may experience neurological effects (e.g., reduced performance on cognitive tests and pattern memory tests) and reduced olfactory function. Many of these workers are also co-exposed to other fumigants, such as methyl bromide and chloropicrin, so these may be confounding risk factors for chronic health effects (CalEPA 2006). Additionally, because sulfuryl fluoride metabolism can result in elevated levels of fluoride in the body, fluorosis may occur, which affects the bones and teeth of exposed individuals (Aribou and Ng 2022). EPA has classified sulfuryl fluoride as "not likely to be carcinogenic to humans" (Fehir 2022).

Phosphine

Phosphine is rapidly absorbed and distributed throughout the body after inhalation exposure. Ingestion of metal phosphides may also occur, either incidentally or from intentional poisonings. Once ingested, metal phosphides are rapidly metabolized to phosphine in the gastrointestinal tract. Metal phosphides can be absorbed by the skin, but phosphine gas generally does not affect the skin or eyes (ATSDR 2014b). Once in the body, phosphine can disrupt the sympathetic nervous system (possibly by inhibiting acetylcholinesterase activity), suppress energetic metabolic pathways, and cause oxidative damage on a cellular level (Karimani et al. 2018; Nath et al. 2011).

Acute phosphine exposure primarily affects the cardiovascular, respiratory, and neurological systems. Metabolic changes in cardiac muscle can lead to alterations in transmembrane potentials. These changes can lead to cardiac arrest, peripheral vascular collapse, and pulmonary edema, often within 12–24 h after exposure. Other cardiovascular symptoms include hypotension, reduced cardiac output, tachycardia, and arrhythmia. At high doses, the liver may also be damaged, which can be fatal. Neurological symptoms include headaches, restlessness, dizziness, impaired gait, trembling during movement, and double vision. In severe cases of phosphine poisoning, the exposed person may experience seizures. Respiratory symptoms include cough and shortness of breath, as well as fluid in the lungs (pulmonary edema), which may not appear until 3 or more days after exposure. Respiratory symptoms can result from both respiratory and oral exposure. Due to its high toxicity, phosphine exposure can also affect the gastrointestinal tract (nausea, vomiting, and diarrhea), liver (jaundice, enlarged liver, elevated serum transaminases, and bilirubin in the blood), and kidneys (ATSDR 2014b; Reigart and Roberts 2013).

There is less information available on the chronic effects of phosphine exposure. Exposure to phosphine for several days may lead to reactive airway dysfunction syndrome (RADS). Repeated, long-term exposure to phosphine may lead to anemia; bronchitis; and visual, speech, and motor disturbances (ATSDR 2014b; Aribou and Ng 2022).

1,3-Dichloropropene

1,3-Dichloropropene (1,3-D) is easily absorbed into the body due to its size and chemical properties, such as lipid solubility (ATSDR 2008). Once absorbed, 1,3-D is distributed throughout the body, but the highest levels are found at the portal-of-entry (e.g., nasal passages, larynx, trachea, and lung for inhalation exposure) as well as in organs associated with chemical metabolism and elimination (i.e., liver, kidney, and bladder). 1,3-D is metabolized and eliminated relatively quickly from the body. Metabolism may produce epoxide degradates and reactive intermediates that exert toxicity, such as by inducing lipid peroxidation (ATSDR 2008).

The most common symptoms from 1,3-D exposure are due to portal-of-entry effects. After acute inhalation exposure, irritation of the respiratory tract and bronchospasms may occur. High levels of exposure may eventually lead to cardiac effects, such as tachycardia and hypovolemia, as well as liver and kidney toxicity (ATSDR 2008; Reigart and Roberts 2013). Ocular exposure may lead to irritation and erythema of the eyes. Dermal exposure to 1,3-D can result in skin irritation, erythema, and edema, with necrosis following severe dermal exposure.

Repeated dermal exposure to 1,3-D can result in skin sensitization. Additionally, EPA has classified 1,3-D as having "suggestive evidence of carcinogenic potential" based on animal studies that have shown liver tumors in male rats after oral exposure (Godshall et al. 2019). Studies in rodents have shown hypertrophy/hyperplasia of the nasal respiratory mucosa after chronic inhalation exposure to 1,3-D (Godshall et al. 2019). Human epidemiology studies have not provided evidence of an association between repeated, long-term 1,3-D exposure and health effects although subclinical markers of renal damage were seen in one study of an occupationally exposed population (ATSDR 2008).

Metam-Sodium, Metampotassium, Dazomet, and Methyl Isothiocyanate

Metam-sodium, metam-potassium, and dazomet are rapidly converted to MITC both in the environment and in vivo (Lowit and Facey 2005). Another important degradate of metam-sodium, both in vivo and in the environment, is carbon disulfide

(CS_2). Toxic effects from application of and exposure to metam-sodium, metam-potassium, dazomet, and MITC may be due to MITC or CS_2 or from another MITC metabolite, methyl isocyanate (MIC). After exposure, MITC is readily absorbed and distributed throughout the body, with the highest uptake in the liver, kidneys, and lungs. Elimination from the body occurs within hours or days, mainly through urine, with MITC, CO_2, and CS_2 also being excreted through respiration via the lungs (Lowit and Facey 2005). The mode of action of MITC is unknown, but reactions with sulfhydryl groups of glutathione or proteins have been hypothesized (Shelat et al. 2018a).

Acute inhalation of MITC produces portal-of-entry and other respiratory effects, such as scratchy throat, salivation, coughing, and shortness of breath (Smith 2009). Severe exposure may result in pulmonary edema, which leads to respiratory distress and coughing bloody, frothy sputum (Reigart and Roberts 2013). Exposure to MITC vapor also leads to itchy and burning eyes and may irritate and burn the skin (Lowit and Facey 2005; Smith 2009). Eye irritation often occurs prior to more severe symptoms. Oral exposure in animals produced nonspecific effects.

There is limited information on the effects in humans from long-term repeated exposure to metam-sodium, metam-potassium, dazomet, and MITC. Animal studies in rodents and dogs have shown histological changes in the nasal passages and lungs, which is consistent with exposure to an irritating chemical. In long-term, repeat dose studies in animals that were exposed orally to metam-sodium and MITC, effects included liver effects such as fatty degeneration and clinical chemistry changes (Shelat et al. 2018b). Both chemicals are skin sensitizers with repeated dermal exposure. MITC and metam-sodium are classified by EPA as "likely to be carcinogenic to humans" based on animal studies (Fehir 2022).

Dimethyl Disulfide

Dimethyl disulfide (DMDS) is absorbed into the body after exposure due to its low molecular weight and lipophilicity, where it can be excreted as cysteine disulfide (EFSA et al. 2019). As an insecticide, DMDS disrupts the normal functioning of an insect's mitochondria, but the toxic mode of action in mammals is unknown (EPA 2010).

Acute inhalation exposure to DMDS generally results in portal-of-entry effects, specifically irritation and damage to the respiratory tract (EPA 2010; EFSA et al. 2019). Exposure to higher concentrations will lead to more severe effects in the respiratory tract, regardless of the length of exposure (EPA 2010). Studies in rodents indicate that inhalation exposure may lead to neurotoxicity at concentrations much higher than those that cause nasal irritation. Systemic effects in animal studies include decreases in body weight and food consumption. DMDS is irritating to the eyes (EFSA et al. 2019).

Chronic inhalation exposure to DMDS also results in nasal irritation at levels similar to acute exposure (EPA 2010). Repeat dermal exposure studies in rabbits have shown that DMDS is very irritating to the skin, leading to erythema, edema, and ischemic necrosis (EPA 2010). It is important to note that DMDS usually volatilizes from the skin, so the exposure duration in animal studies is much longer than would typically occur in humans. DMDS is a skin sensitizer (EFSA et al. 2019). EPA did not assess the carcinogenic potential due to its use profile (Fehir 2022), but its carcinogenic potential cannot be excluded considering the inflammatory and irritant changes in the nasal and respiratory tracts of exposed animals (EFSA et al. 2019).

Chlorine Dioxide

Chlorine dioxide is readily taken up into the body after exposure (ATSDR 2004). It quickly breaks down into chlorite ions and then into chloride ions. Chloride can be used for normal physiological processes and is eliminated through the urine. Chlorine dioxide and chlorite react to water, including the water contained in the moist body tissues. They are strongly oxidizing, resulting in irritation of the tissues to which they have contact (ATSDR 2004).

Inhalation of chlorine dioxide can lead to irritation of the respiratory tract, coughing, bronchitis, and pulmonary edema (NIOSH 2019). Ingestion can cause irritation of the mouth, esophagus, or stomach (ATSDR 2004). Chlorine dioxide may be irritating to the skin and eyes (EPA 2006). It is not classifiable as to its carcinogenicity. In animal studies, neurodevelopmental effects have been noted in animals orally exposed during critical periods, but the relevance to human neurodevelopment is unclear (ATSDR 2004).

Sulfur Dioxide

Sulfur dioxide is readily taken up into the body upon exposure. It is quickly hydrolyzed into sulfites, which can be taken up into the blood and distributed throughout the body. Sulfites are then metabolized to sulfate, primarily in the liver, and then eliminated via the urinary tract (EPA 2021). In the body, sulfites can interact with biomolecules mainly through three reactions: removing disulfide bonds in proteins, autooxidation which generates free radicals, and cytosine addition (Drew et al. 2020). Sulfur dioxide can also produce sulfurous acid upon contact with moist mucus membranes in the respiratory tract, and this acid acts as a direct irritant and prevents sinus drainage (Drew et al. 2020).

The respiratory tract is the main target of toxic effects from sulfur dioxide exposure. Sulfur dioxide reacts with moist mucus membranes to produce sulfurous acid, which irritates the respiratory passages leading to vagal stimulation and airway smooth-muscle contraction. Changes in specific airway resistance or forced expiratory volume may be seen within minutes of exposure (Drew et al. 2020). Effects from chronic exposure to sulfur dioxide are less studied, and EPA has determined that it is not currently classifiable as to its carcinogenicity to humans (Fehir 2022). Animal studies have not shown changes to lung function or histology after chronic exposure (Drew et al. 2020).

Formaldehyde

After exposure to formaldehyde, the chemical is taken up through the lungs, skin, or gastrointestinal tract although eating food may delay the latter. Formaldehyde is then rapidly metabolized to formic acid or formate, which can cause toxicity (Reigart and Roberts 2013). The toxic mode of action may include interaction with molecules on cell membranes and with proteins and DNA. Formic acid (which is ionized to formate) may lead to acid-base imbalance (ATSDR 2014a). Oxidative stress-induced cytotoxicity and changes in gene expression related to cell proliferation, metabolism, and cell cycle have been hypothesized as potential mechanisms of toxicity after formaldehyde exposure (ATSDR 2010).

Acute inhalation exposure to formaldehyde can result in neurological effects, such as headache; irritability; sleep disturbance; and impairment of dexterity, memory, and equilibrium. The most sensitive effects of formaldehyde inhalation are irritation of the respiratory tract, which causes symptoms such as nose and throat irritation, cough, chest pain, shortness of breath, and wheezing. More severe exposure can lead to impacts in the lower respiratory tract such as swelling of the throat, inflammation and narrowing of the bronchi and inflammation and accumulation of fluid in the lungs. These symptoms may continue to worsen even for more than 12 h after exposure and persist for several days (ATSDR 2014a). Some individuals are more sensitive to formaldehyde exposure and may show signs of asthma and dermatitis at low levels of exposure (ATSDR 2010, 2014a). Formaldehyde vapors can also irritate the eyes, which causes discomfort and lacrimation, with high levels leading to corneal opacification and vision loss. Formaldehyde ingestion can cause portal-of-entry effects such as corrosion of the gastrointestinal mucosa, particularly in the pharyngeal mucosa, epiglottis, and esophagus, as well as other gastrointestinal issues like nausea, vomiting, and diarrhea. Systemic toxicity may also occur after ingestion, including metabolic acidosis, central nervous system depression, respiratory distress, and renal failure (ATSDR 2014a). Dermal exposure leads to skin irritation and possible allergic dermatitis (Reigart and Roberts 2013).

Chronic formaldehyde exposure has been linked to effects on the central nervous system, namely an increased frequency of headaches; depression and mood changes; sleep disorders; and diminished dexterity, memory, and equilibrium (ATSDR 2014a). Chronic exposure may also result in allergy-type reactions, such as asthma-like symptoms and dermatitis. Formaldehyde is considered a carcinogen and is weakly linked to an increased risk of nasal cancer in exposed humans, which is consistent with findings from animal studies (ATSDR 2014a). Human studies have also noted an increased risk of leukemia in workers who have been occupationally exposed to formaldehyde (ACS 2022).

Treatment

Generally, treatment for fumigant exposure–related effects is supportive care and symptom management. The patient should be removed from the exposure area, after which contaminated clothing should be removed and any exposed skin or eyes should be flushed with water or saline for at least 15 min. This will prevent further absorption of the chemicals and allow for additional medical treatment to proceed. See Chap. 14 Toxic Gases for more detailed information on medical treatment.

Whenever possible, medical staff or first responders should identify the product used and obtain a copy of the product label and safety data sheet (SDS). The label and SDS both contain important information about the first aid required for exposed individuals. The label identifies the active ingredient and concentration, and the SDS provides more detailed information about the chemical properties, first aid, and toxic effects. The SDS may also list any inert ingredients that are in the product that responders should be aware of.

Airway protection is critical due to the toxic nature of fumigants and the primary exposure route of inhalation for fumigant poisonings. Oxygen administration may be needed to maintain perfusion. Suction of oral secretions may be necessary, and severe cases may require intubation and ventilation if the patient presents with respiratory distress (Reigart and Roberts 2013).

Depending on the fumigant, toxic effects may be seen immediately (e.g., chloropicrin or sulfur dioxide) or may take hours or days to begin or to worsen (e.g., methyl bromide, phosphine, or formaldehyde). Respiratory effects may be mild and clear without intervention after exposure ends, but patients should remain under observation to ensure that more severe effects do not develop. If more severe symptoms are present, then the patient should be treated in an intensive care unit. Chest X-rays and pulmonary function tests, especially forced expiratory volume (FEV1) and forced vital capacity (FVC), may be used to assess the extent of respiratory distress (Reigart and Roberts 2013; Murthy 2004). Inhalation of some fumigants may cause bronchospasms, which can be treated with aerosolized bronchodilators such as albuterol, with consideration of the health of the myocardium prior to choosing and administering the bronchodilator (ATSDR 2014b, c).

After exposure, urine and serum samples can be taken regularly to look for markers of kidney and liver damage. Typical markers include creatinine, blood urea nitrogen (BUN), glomerular filtration rate (GFR), urinalysis looking for cells and sediment, serum alkaline phosphatase (ALP), lactate dehydrogenase (LDH), alanine aminotransferase (ALT), aspartate aminotransferase (AST), and bilirubin levels (Reigart and Roberts 2013).

Most fumigants do not have specific biomarkers to test for exposure, and for those that do, the measurements are only useful within hours or days of exposure due to rapid metabolism and elimination from the body. For instance, the measurement of bromide ions in serum may be indicative of methyl bromide exposure, but other chemical exposures and endogenous metabolism may also produce bromide ions. The same holds true for sulfuryl fluoride exposure and serum fluoride levels (Reigart and Roberts 2013). Formaldehyde is an endogenous chemical that can be present even in nonexposed patients

(ATSDR 2015). Some studies of people exposed via inhalation to 1,3-D show that urinary levels of mercapturic acid correlated to 1,3-D exposure levels, but as elimination is rapid, the clinical usefulness is limited (ATSDR 2008).

Some fumigants, such as methyl bromide, phosphine, and sulfuryl fluoride, are neurotoxicants that can cause seizures. Benzodiazepines such as lorazepam may be used for seizure control. Some methyl bromide cases may be resistant to control from benzodiazepines and diphenylhydantoin, so thiopental anesthesia may be required (Reigart and Roberts 2013). Seizure-control medication may require ventilation assistance, and the patient should be monitored for hypotension, cardiac dysrhythmias, hypoglycemia, electrolyte disturbances, and hypoxia (Reigart and Roberts 2013). Patients with chronic exposure to neurotoxic agents such as methyl bromide, phosphine, and sulfuryl fluoride may be periodically assessed for neurologic function to detect long-term effects as early as possible for intervention (Reigart and Roberts 2013).

In the case of ingestion, gastric emptying within 60 min of ingestion followed by activated charcoal may be administered. For some chemicals, although ingestion is rare, emesis should not be induced due to aspiration risk. These include methyl bromide, phosphine, dimethyl disulfide, and MITC (ATSDR 2014a, 2020b; PubChem [Internet] 2004a, b). Activated carbon may help adsorb chemicals remaining in the stomach and reduce further chemical absorption into the body. Charcoal administration is most effective if given within 60 min of pesticide ingestion. Charcoal may be contraindicated in patients with any of the following: unprotected airway; decreased consciousness without intubation; neurological impairment without intubation; ingestion of corrosive substances; ingestion of a hydrocarbon with a high risk of aspiration; or risk of bleeding or perforation due to recent surgery or medical conditions like coagulopathy (Reigart and Roberts 2013).

Acute dermal exposure to high levels of some fumigants may result in blistering and chemical burns, which should be treated as such. Additionally, many fumigants, such as 1,3-D, MITC, DMDS, and formaldehyde, are skin sensitizers, so patients who are exposed repeatedly may experience dermatitis and other allergy-type skin effects.

Chemical-specific diagnosis and treatment include an electrocardiogram (ECG) after exposure to chloropicrin, phosphine, and sulfur dioxide (Murthy 2004). Ingestion of corrosive agents, such as chloropicrin and formaldehyde, may require an endoscopic examination of the esophagus and stomach (NIOSH 2011). Formaldehyde exposure may cause metabolic acidosis, and the excess formic acid in the blood may require dialysis for removal (ATSDR 2010). For fumigants that may rely on glutathione for detoxification, such as 1,3-D and phosphine, N-acetylcysteine administration may help increase tissue levels of glutathione (ATSDR 2008; Karimani et al. 2018). Phosphine-poisoned patients may also be treated with magnesium sulfate to protect against fatal cardiac effects such as arrhythmia (Reigart and Roberts 2013).

Some populations may be especially susceptible to the toxic effects of fumigant exposure. Patients with underlying respiratory diseases or risk factors may be at higher risk of adverse health effects after exposure since inhalation is the main route of exposure and target for toxic insult. This includes people with asthma, chronic obstructive pulmonary disease (COPD), and smokers (Reigart and Roberts 2013). Children who are inadvertently exposed may also be at greater risk because they breathe a higher volume of air compared to their total size and many fumigants are heavier than air and may settle closer to the ground (e.g., chloropicrin, sulfuryl fluoride, and phosphine), which is closer to the child's breathing zone than the breathing zone of an adult.

Workers who handle and apply fumigants regularly may be at risk of long-term health effects, especially on the respiratory and neurological systems, as well as certain forms of cancer. These workers can be screened routinely for long-term effects including testing for laboratory evidence of liver and kidney damage. Additionally, many patients who are occupationally exposed to fumigants may be exposed to several different chemicals, either together (such as chloropicrin used as a warning agent with other fumigants) or over a series of days and tasks. Providers should take a comprehensive approach to health history questionnaires to capture the full extent of their patients' chemical exposure.

References

ACS (American Cancer Society) [Internet]. [cited 2023 December 13]. Formaldehyde and Cancer Risk; [about 6 screens]. 2022. Available from: https://www.cancer.org/cancer/risk-prevention/chemicals/formaldehyde.html.

Aribou ZM, Ng WT. Targeted medical examinations for workers exposed to fumigants. J Occup Med Toxicol. 2022;17:20.

ATSDR (Agency for Toxic Substance and Disease Registry). Toxicological profile for chlorine dioxide and chlorite. Atlanta: Centers for Disease Control and Prevention; 2004. p. 191.

ATSDR (Agency for Toxic Substance and Disease Registry). Toxicological profile for dichloropropenes. Atlanta: Centers for Disease Control and Prevention; 2008. p. 361.

ATSDR (Agency for Toxic Substance and Disease Registry). Addendum to the toxicological profile for formaldehyde. Atlanta: Centers for Disease Control and Prevention; 2010. p. 149.

ATSDR (Agency for Toxic Substance and Disease Registry). Medical management guidelines for formaldehyde [Internet]. Atlanta: Centers for Disease Control and Prevention; 2014a. Oct 21 [cited 2023 Dec 1]. 24 p. Available from: https://www.atsdr.cdc.gov/MHMI/mmg111.pdf.

ATSDR (Agency for Toxic Substance and Disease Registry). Medical management guidelines for phosphine [Internet]. Atlanta: Centers for Disease Control and Prevention; 2014b. Oct 21 [cited 2023 Dec 1]. 18 p. Available from: https://www.atsdr.cdc.gov/MHMI/mmg177.pdf.

ATSDR (Agency for Toxic Substance and Disease Registry). Medical management guidelines for sulfur dioxide [Internet]. Atlanta: Centers for Disease Control and Prevention; 2014c. Oct 21 [cited 2023 Dec 1]. 18 p. Available from: https://www.atsdr.cdc.gov/MHMI/mmg116.pdf

ATSDR (Agency for Toxic Substance and Disease Registry). ToxFAQs for Formaldehyde [Internet]. Atlanta: Centers for Disease Control and Prevention; 2015. May 12 [cited 2023 Dec 1]. 2 p. Available from: https://www.atsdr.cdc.gov/toxfaqs/tfacts111.pdf

ATSDR (Agency for Toxic Substance and Disease Registry). Toxicological profile for bromomethane. Atlanta: Centers for Disease Control and Prevention; 2020a. p. 184.

ATSDR (Agency for Toxic Substance and Disease Registry). Medical management guidelines for methyl bromide (Bromomethane) [Internet]. Atlanta: Centers for Disease Control and Prevention; 2020b. Mar 12 [cited 2023 Dec 1]. 20 p. Available from: https://www.atsdr.cdc.gov/MHMI/mmg27.pdf

Becker J, Chism W, Kaul M. Overview of the use and usage of soil fumigants. Washington, DC: US Environmental Protection Agency, Biological and Economic Analysis Division; 2005.

CalDPR (California Department of Pesticide Regulation). Burrowing vertebrate pest fumigation: a study manual for private applicators. Sacramento: California Environmental Protection Agency; 2023. p. 71.

CalEPA (California Environmental Protection Agency). Sulfuryl fluoride (Vikane) risk characterization document volume I health risk assessment. Sacramento: California Environmental Protection Agency; 2006. p. 162.

Drew D, Donovan W, Liccione J, Lowe K. Inorganic sulfites. Draft human health risk assessment in support of registration review. Washington, DC: US Environmental Protection Agency, Health Effects Division; 2020. 40 p.

EFSA (European Food Safety Authority), Anastassiadou M, Arena M, Auteri D, Barmaz S, Brancato A, Bura L, Carrasco Cabrera L, Chaideftou E, Chiusolo A, Court Marques D, Crivellente F, De Lentdecker C, Egsmose M, Fait G, Ferreira L, Greco L, Ippolito A, Istace F, Jarrah S, Kardassi D, Leuschner R, Lostia A, Lythgo C, Mangas I, Miron I, Molnar T, Padovani L, Parra Morte JM, Pedersen R, Reich H, Santos M, Serafimova R, Sharp R, Stanek A, Streissl F, Sturma J, Szentes C, Terron A, Tiramani M, Vagenende B, Villamar-Bouza L. Peer review of the pesticide risk assessment of the active substance dimethyl disulfide. EFSA J. 2019;17(11):5905.

EPA (US Environmental Protection Agency). Office of Prevention, Pesticides and Toxic Substances. Reregistration Eligibility Decision (RED) for chlorine dioxide and sodium chlorite (Case 4023). Washington, DC: US Environmental Protection Agency; 2006. p. 124.

EPA (US Environmental Protection Agency). Office of Pesticide Programs. Reregistration eligibility decision for formaldehyde and paraformaldehyde. Washington, DC: US Environmental Protection Agency; 2008a. p. 89.

EPA (US Environmental Protection Agency). Acute exposure guideline levels (AEGLs) chloropicrin (CAS Reg. No, 76-06-2) interim. Washington, DC: US Environmental Protection Agency; 2008b. p. 52.

EPA (US Environmental Protection Agency). Office of Pesticide Programs. Amended Reregistration Eligibility Decision (RED) for chloropicrin. Washington, DC: US Environmental Protection Agency; 2009a. p. 197.

EPA (US Environmental Protection Agency). Office of Pesticide Programs. Amended Reregistration Eligibility Decision (RED) for Dazomet. Washington,

DC: US Environmental Protection Agency; 2009b. p. 178.

EPA (US Environmental Protection Agency). Office of Pesticide Programs. Amended Reregistration Eligibility Decision (RED) for the methyldithiocarbamate salts (metam-sodium, metam-potassium) and methyl isothiocyanate (MITC). Washington, DC: US Environmental Protection Agency; 2009c. p. 232.

EPA (US Environmental Protection Agency). Pesticide fact sheet dimethyl disulfide [Internet]. Virginia: US Environmental Protection Agency; 2010. Jul 9 [Cited 2023 Dec 1]. Available from: https://www3.epa.gov/pesticides/chem_search/reg_actions/pending/fs_PC-029088_09-Jul-10.pdf

EPA (US Environmental Protection Agency). Dimethyl Disulfide (DMDS) proposed interim registration review decision case number 7454. Washington, DC: US Environmental Protection Agency; 2019. p. 18.

EPA (US Environmental Protection Agency). Use report for formaldehyde (CAS RC 50-00-0). Washington, DC: US Environmental Protection Agency, Office of Pollution, Prevention, and Toxics; 2020a. p. 96.

EPA (US Environmental Protection Agency). Methyl bromide interim registration review decision case number 0335. Washington, DC: US Environmental Protection Agency; 2020b. p. 28.

EPA (US Environmental Protection Agency). Inorganic sulfites: sodium metabisulfite and sulfur dioxide interim registration review decision case numbers 7019 and 4056. Washington, DC: US Environmental Protection Agency; 2021. p. 38.

EPA (US Environmental Protection Agency). Aluminum phosphide, magnesium phosphide, and phosphine amended proposed interim registration review decision case numbers 0025, 0645, and 7608. Washington, DC: US Environmental Protection Agency; 2023. p. 95.

EPA (US Environmental Protection Agency) [Internet]. [cited 2023 Dec 1]. Sulfuryl Fluoride; [about 2 screens]. 2023 Jul. 5. Available from: https://www.epa.gov/ingredients-used-pesticide-products/sulfuryl-fluoride.

Fehir R. Chemical evaluated for carcinogenic potential by the Office of Pesticide Programs. Inorganic sulfites. Draft human health risk assessment in support of registration review. Washington, DC: US Environmental Protection Agency, Health Effects Division; 2022. 29 p

Gaskin S, Heath L, Pisaniello D, Edwards JW, Logan M, Baxter C. Dermal absorption of fumigant gases during HAZMAT incident exposure scenarios-methyl bromide, sulfuryl fluoride, and chloropicrin. Toxicol Ind Health. 2017;33(7):547–54. https://doi.org/10.1177/0748233716689651.

Godshall JG, Perron MM. Chloropicrin: draft human health risk assessment of conventional uses for registration review. U.S. Environmental Protection Agency, Health Effects Division; 2018. p. 36.

Godshall JG, Kramer GF, Phang W. 1,3-Dichloropropene (Telone): draft human health risk assessment for registration review. Washington, DC: US Environmental Protection Agency, Health Effects Division; 2019. p. 74.

Karimani A, Mohammadpour AH, Zirak MR, Rezaee R, Megarbane B, Tsatsakis A, Karimi G. Antidotes for aluminum phosphide poisoning—an update. Toxicol Rep. 2018;5:1053–9. https://doi.org/10.1016/j.toxrep.2018.10.009.

Lowit A, Facey J. 4th Revised toxicology disciplinary chapter for: metam sodium (PC Code 039003) and methyl isothiocyanate (MITC, PC Code 068103). Washington, DC: US Environmental Protection Agency, Health Effects Division; 2005.

Murthy LI. Specific medical tests or examinations published in the literature for OSHA-regulated substances. Washington, DC: National Institute for Occupational Safety and Health (NIOSH); 2004. 1 p

Nath NS, Bhattacharya I, Tuck AG, Schlipalius DI, Ebert PR. Mechanisms of phosphine toxicity. J Toxicol. 2011;2011:494168. https://doi.org/10.1155/2011/494168.

NIOSH (National Institute for Occupational Safety and Health) [Internet]. Chloropicrin emergency response card; [about 11 screens]. 2011. [cited 2023 Dec 1]. Available from: https://www.cdc.gov/niosh/ershdb/emergencyresponsecard_29750034.html.

NIOSH (National Institute for Occupational Safety and Health) [Internet]. Chlorine dioxide; [about 3 screens]. 2019. [cited 2024 Jan 4]. Available from: https://www.cdc.gov/niosh/npg/npgd0116.html.

NIOSH (National Institute for Occupational Safety and Health) [Internet]. NIOSH packet guide to chemical hazards; [about 2 screens]. 2020. [cited 2023 Dec 1]. Available from: https://www.cdc.gov/niosh/npg/default.html.

NPIC (National Pesticide Information Center) [Internet]. Structural fumigation; [about 2 screens]. 2019. [cited 2023 Dec 1]. Available from: http://npic.orst.edu/pest/fumigation.html.

Olinger C, Mendez E, Vogel D. 1,3-Dichloropropene: HED human health risk assessment for phase 5; DP Barcode: D337328, PC Code: 029001. Washington, DC: US Environmental Protection Agency, Health Effects Division; 2007.

PubChem [Internet]. PubChem compound summary for CID 12232, dimethyl disulfide. Bethesda, MD: National Library of Medicine (US), National Center for Biotechnology Information; 2004a. [cited 2023 Dec. 11]. Available from: https://pubchem.ncbi.nlm.nih.gov/compound/Dimethyl-Disulfide

PubChem [Internet]. Bethesda, MD: National Library of Medicine (US), National Center for Biotechnology Information; 2004b. PubChem compound summary for CID 3001858, Metam; [cited 2023 Dec. 8]. Available from: https://pubchem.ncbi.nlm.nih.gov/compound/Metam.

Reigart JR, Roberts JR. Fumigants. In: US Environmental Protection Agency, Office of Pesticide Programs. Recognition and management of pesticide poisonings.

6th ed. Washington, DC: US Government Printing Office; 2013. p. 161–72.

Shelat S, Schlosser C, Piper S. Dazomet and methyl isothiocyanate: draft human health risk assessment of conventional uses for registration review. Washington, DC: US Environmental Protection Agency, Health Effects Division; 2018a. p. 47.

Shelat S, Schlosser C, Piper S. Metam sodium; Metam potassium; and methyl Isothiocyanate: draft human health risk assessment of conventional uses for registration review. Washington, DC: US Environmental Protection Agency, Health Effects Division; 2018b. p. 61.

Smith C. Metam sodium: third revision of the HED human health risk assessment. Washington, DC: U.S. Environmental Protection Agency, Health Effects Division; 2009. p. 507.

Petroleum Products

13

William J. Meggs

Introduction

Farm vehicles, machinery, and structures are generally maintained and repaired on farms. Potential health hazards exist from toxicants used in these activities, including exposure to diesel fuels, gasoline, kerosene, hydraulic fluids, degreasers, lubricants, paints, paint thinners, and greases (Shaver and Tong 1991). Occupational routes of exposure are inhalation and skin contact. Ingestions can occur by curious small children playing around work sites. Intentional ingestions are usually in mentally disturbed older individuals. Siphoning of fuels from tanks by sucking on hoses to start the flow can lead to inadvertent ingestions and aspirations.

Fuels

Gasoline, kerosene, and diesel fuel are mixtures of hydrocarbons that can vary across products. Gasoline contains 4–12 carbon atoms per molecule. Diesel fuel has heavier molecules containing 9–25 carbon atoms per molecule. Kerosene is intermediate with 9–16 atoms per molecule. These products are extremely flammable and explosive, so they must be handled with great caution. Additives to fuels can have toxic effects. Benzene added to fuel can have hematological toxicity (Snyder 2012). Tetraethyl lead was used as an anti-knocking agent with the risk of lead toxicity. Volatility decreases as the number of carbon atoms increases, so gasoline is the most volatile fuel. Inhalation of fuel fumes can have irritant effects on the eyes and respiratory tract. Inhalation of vapors in confined spaces can have central nervous depressive effects, and fatalities have occurred from respiratory depression. In addition, myocardial sensitization to endogenous catecholamines can lead to cardiac dysrhythmias (Agency for Toxic Substances and Diseases Registry, ATSDR 1995a). Ingested fuels are poorly absorbed while aspiration of even small amounts can cause massive lung damage, so emesis should be avoided after ingestions. Massive ingestions can cause central nervous system depression. Treatment of inhalation is to move to fresh air while supporting respirations and protecting the airway. Skin exposure can cause dermatitis. Treatment of ingestions is supportive care with cardiac and respiratory monitoring. Leakage of fuel storage tanks contaminates groundwater and leads to chronic ingestion of fuels and additives for farm personnel who use well water.

Fuel storage tanks present on farms, in particular underground storage tanks, develop leaks and contaminate groundwater. Between 75,000 and 100,000 underground storage tanks leak mil-

W. J. Meggs (✉)
Brody School of Medicine, East Carolina University, Greenville, NC, USA
e-mail: meggsw@ecu.edu

W. J. Meggs, R. L. Langley (eds.), *Farm Toxicology*, https://doi.org/10.1007/978-3-031-80441-0_13

lions of gallons of gasoline into groundwater each year (ATSDR 1995b). Methyl tertiary butyl ether (MTBE), a flammable compound with a noxious odor, is added to gasoline as an anti-knocking agent in place of tetraethyl lead. Exposures can cause difficulty concentrating, headache, nausea, dizziness, weakness, and lightheadedness (New Jersey Department of Health 2006). Lead toxicity may be a problem in countries that still use lead as an anti-knocking agent. Prior to being banned as a gasoline additive in the United States, lead from vehicle exhaust contaminated air and soil and caused considerable toxicity in children.

Organic Solvents

Organic solvents are used as degreasers, to dissolve substances, and in cleaning. Solvents as a class can cause central nervous system depression with respiratory depression. Acute exposure such as by heavy use in unventilated space or intentional inhalational exposures to get high can cause euphoria followed by headache, dizziness, and in extreme cases, seizure, coma, and death (White and Proctor 1997). Sensitization of the myocardium to endogenous catecholamines can lead to cardiac dysrhythmias. Chronic exposures can lead to encephalopathy with neuropsychological disabilities including disabilities with memory, concentration, cognition, and mood (Dick 2006). Specific solvents can have unique toxicities. For example, carbon tetrachloride is toxic to the liver (Garner 1969). Benzene is toxic to the bone marrow and can cause leukemia and aplastic anemia (Snyder 2012). N-hexane is associated with peripheral neuropathies with chronic exposures (Guimarães-Costa et al. 2018). Methylene chloride, used as a paint stripper, is metabolized to carbon monoxide, resulting in cardiac and neurotoxicity (Hoang et al. 2021). Trichloroethylene, a widely used organic solvent that contaminates groundwater, has been identified as a cause of Parkinson's disease in human studies and animal models (Dorsey et al. 2023) (Table 13.1). Exposure to solvents during pregnancy increases the risk of miscarriage, stillbirth, preterm birth, a low birth weight, and birth defects (Centers for Disease Control (CDC) 2023). Inhalation of solvents for euphoric effects, known as huffing or glue-sniffing, can lead to encephalopathy with chronic use and malformations if inhaled by pregnant women.

Table 13.1 In addition to neurological and cardiac toxicity common to all solvents, some have specific toxicities

Carbon tetrachloride	Hepatotoxicity
Benzene	Aplastic anemia, leukemia
N-hexane	Peripheral neuropathy
Methylene chloride	Metabolized to carbon monoxide
Trichloroethylene	Parkinson's disease

Hydraulic Fluid

Hydraulic fluids are used to transmit energy in fluid-filled pressurized mechanical systems. Examples include vehicle transmissions, braking systems, and power steering. Hydraulic drive systems are used in agricultural equipment. Mineral oil distilled from petroleum is the basis for the majority of hydraulic fluids. Additives are used to prevent corrosion, foaming, wear, and oxidation. Products can vary widely in their chemical composition.

Organophosphate esters are added to hydraulic fluids as anti-wear agents. Acute exposures to hydraulic fluids can cause toxicity like exposure to organophosphate pesticides (see Chap. 5), with inhibition of acetylcholinesterase causing cholinesterase toxidrome, muscle weakness, and paralysis of respiratory muscles. Seizures and coma can occur from the inhibition of acetylcholinesterase in the central nervous system. Organophosphate-induced delayed neuropathy can also occur. Chronic effects include peripheral neuropathy from axonopathy with motor weakness. Neuropsychological disabilities have also been reported (ATSDR 1997). Treatment of acute poisoning is with atropine and pralidoxime (see Chap. 5).

High-Pressure Injection Injuries

Grease is used to lubricate joints in vehicles and is a complex mixture of compounds that can include petroleum distillates, trichloroethylene, acetone, and other materials. It is applied under pressure by grease guns. Pain sprayers also dispense complex mixtures under pressure. Inadvertent high-pressure injections into farm and other workers occur when the opening is directed into the skin. Hands and fingers are the most common sites of injection.

The site of injection often appears as a small puncture that can be painless, but the injected material can spread down tissues and cause inflammation and necrosis. Even injections of water or air can cause compartment syndrome. Emergent surgical intervention with the removal of foreign material and debridement is needed to minimize the devastating damage that can occur. Loss of function and amputations can result. Factors affecting prognosis are latency time to surgical intervention, the type of fluid mixture injected, pressure and volume of injection, and amount of direct tissue damage (Verhoeven and Hierner 2008).

Systemic toxicity can occur depending on the nature of the material (Lewis et al. 1998). Injection with paints containing lead should be monitored with serial lead measurements and evaluations for toxicity. Appropriate treatment can include surgical removal and chelation therapy. Renal failure, hemolysis, and allergic reactions have been reported in association with high-pressure injection injuries (Verhoeven and Hierner 2008).

The importance of early referral to a hand surgeon is critical, even for high-pressure injection injuries that initially appear minor and benign.

Dermal Exposures

Oil folliculitis, also known as oil acne, occurs from exposure to lubricating oils, degreasers, and other petroleum products (Finnie 1960). Physical findings of black comedones, pustules, furuncles, and carbuncles have been described (Maibach et al. 2021). The mainstay of treatment is avoidance, with protection of the skin from exposure.

Gasoline can cause a defatting or degreasing dermatitis from solubilizing dermal lipids. Skin-cracking and peeling can be seen. With prolonged or severe exposure, erythema and blistering occurs (AtSDr 2014).

Pulmonary Exposures

Toxicity to the pulmonary system varies with the volatility and viscosity of petroleum products. Volatile compounds pose inhalational risks as respiratory irritants, with results ranging from rhinosinusitis to bronchospasm and pulmonary edema. Inhalation exposures can have systemic effects involving the neurological system like sedation, dizziness, ataxia, and euphoria. The dominant cardiovascular effect of inhalation is sensitization of the myocardium to endogenous catecholamines, resulting in dysrhythmias that can be fatal.

Aspiration is more dangerous with hydrocarbons of low viscosity. Ingestions of hydrocarbons like mineral oil followed by emesis are associated with aspiration. Even small amounts can cause devastating pneumonitis and in severe cases, pulmonary necrosis (Curtis et al. 2024). Fatalities have occurred from aspiration of petroleum products.

Aspiration and inhalation of oils can lead to exogenous lipoid pneumonia that may be acute or chronic (Marchiori et al. 2011). Clinical manifestations are highly variable and can range from an incidental autopsy finding to acute reparatory failure requiring ventilatory support. Chest X-ray findings are also variable. Severity varies with the amount, duration, and nature of oil aspirated or inhaled. Host factors such as age and preexisting pulmonary disease can also impact severity. Intentional ingestion in adults and unintentional ingestion in small children of oils used for farm vehicles followed by aspiration can lead to acute exogenous lipoid pneumonia. In addition, oils in foods, laxatives such as mineral oil, oil-based medications, radiographic contrast media, and nasal application of oil-based treatments for upper-airway disease can be significant. Diagnosis is based on the history of exposure followed by respiratory signs and symptoms. Oil-based aspirate from bronchoalveolar lavage and lung biopsy can be definitive but is only performed in severe cases.

Treatment of inhalation exposures is primarily supportive care, with removal from the exposure to fresh air. Oxygen supplementation and bronchodilators are used as needed. Rarely, intubation and assisted ventilation are required. Bronchoalveolar lavage can be diagnostic with oil in the lavage fluid and possibly be of therapeutic benefit.

References

ATSDR. Toxicological profile for automobile gasoline. 1995a. https://wwwn.cdc.gov/TSP/ToxProfiles/ToxProfiles.aspx?id=468&tid=83.

ATSDR. Public health statement for automotive gasoline. 1995b. https://www.atsdr.cdc.gov/ToxProfiles/tp72-c1-b.pdf.

ATSDR. Toxicological profile for hydraulic fluid. 1997. https://wwwn.cdc.gov/TSP/ToxProfiles/ToxProfiles.aspx?id=757&tid=141.

ATSDR. Medical management guidelines for gasoline. 2014. https://wwwn.cdc.gov/TSP/MMG/MMGDetails.aspx?mmgid=465&toxid=83.

CDC. Solvents—reproductive health. 2023. https://www.cdc.gov/niosh/topics/repro/solvents.html.

Curtis J, Metheny E, Sergent SR. Hydrocarbon toxicity. 2024. https://www.ncbi.nlm.nih.gov/books/NBK499883/. Accessed 23 Jan 2024.

Dorsey ER, et al. Trichloroethylene: an invisible cause of Parkinson's disease? J Parkinsons Dis. 2023;13:203–18.

Finnie JS. Oil folliculitis. A study of 200 men employed in an engineering factory. Br J Ind Med. 1960;17:130–40. PMID: 13822949; PMCID: PMC1038037.

Garner RC. Toxicity of carbon tetrachloride. Br Med J. 1969;22:777. https://doi.org/10.1136/bmj.1.5646.777-b. PMID: 5769869; PMCID: PMC1982783.

Guimarães-Costa R, Schoindre Y, Metlaine A, Lefaucheur JP, Camdessanché JP, Maisonobe T, Léger JM. N-hexane exposure: a cause of small fiber neuropathy. J Peripher Nerv Syst. 2018;23:143–6.

Hoang A, Fagan K, Cannon DL, Rayasam SDG, Harrison R, Shusterman D, Singla V. Assessment of methylene chloride-related fatalities in the United States, 1980–2018. JAMA Intern Med. 2021;181(6):797–805. https://doi.org/10.1001/jamainternmed.2021.1063. PMID: 33871539; PMCID: PMC8056315

Lewis H, Clarke P, Kneafsey B, Brennen M. A 10–year review of high-pressure injection injuries to the hand. J Hand Surg (Br). 1998;23B:479–81.

Maibach HI, Li BS, Cary JH. Chapter 17. In: Ladou J, Harrison R, editors. Occupational and environmental medicine. 6th ed; 2021.

Marchiori E, Zanetti G, Mano CM, Hochhegger B. Exogenous lipoid pneumonia. Clinical and radiological manifestations. Respir Med. 2011;105:659–66.

New Jersey Department of Health 2006. Hazardous substances fact sheet. Methyl-tert-buyl-ether. https://nj.gov/health/eoh/rtkweb/documents/fs/1293.pdf. Accessed 19 Dec 2023.

Shaver CS, Tong T. Chemical hazards to agricultural workers. Occup Med. 1991;6:391–413. PMID: 1948526.

Snyder R. Leukemia and benzene. Int J Environ Res Public Health. 2012;9:2875–93. https://doi.org/10.3390/ijerph9082875. Epub 2012 Aug 14. PMID: 23066403; PMCID: PMC3447593.

Verhoeven N, Hierner R. High-pressure injection injury of the hand: an often underestimated trauma: case report with study of the literature. Strategies Trauma Limb Reconstr. 2008;3:27–33. https://doi.org/10.1007/s11751-008-0029-9. Epub 2008 Feb 2.

White RF, Proctor SP. Solvents and neurotoxicity. Lancet 1997;26:1239–43.

14 Toxic Gases

Jennifer Parker-Cote

See Chart 14.1.

Chart 14.1 Toxic gases

Toxic gas	Common application	Mode of toxicity
Anhydrous ammonia	Agricultural fertilizer	Caustic, liquefactive necrosis
Carbon monoxide	Internal combustion engines, fires, gasoline-powered equipment	Tissue hypoxia from carboxyhemoglobin, inhibition of cellular respiration
Hydrogen sulfide	Manure storage tanks, pulp–paper mills, roofing-asphalt tanks, oil and gas production, chemical suicide, leather industry, slaughterhouse-waste lagoons	Inhibition of cellular respiration by inhibition of cytochrome a_3 oxidase, which interrupts oxidative phosphorylation, leading to cellular hypoxia and anaerobic metabolism
Fumigants		
Aluminum phosphide/ phosphine gas	Pest control for grain storage and transport	Noncompetitive inhibition of cytochrome c oxidase, leading to blockage of the electron transport chain and oxidative phosphorylation
1,3-Dichloropropene	Pest control (nematodes) for crops (sweet potatoes, almonds, strawberries, grapes, and carrots)	Unclear mechanism of toxicity
Chloropicrin	Crowd control, soil fumigant in orchards and greenhouses	Lacrimator, respiratory irritant
Methyl isothiocyanate	Fungicidal, herbicidal, and nematocidal. Used on golf greens, nonbearing crops, turf sites, ornamental sites, compost piles, field nurseries, potting soils, strawberries, tomatoes, and timber	Not well-known, stimulates chemesthesis
Nitrogen dioxide	Silage, silos (grain, grass, corn)	Simple asphyxiant, pulmonary epithelial injury, corrosive injury

J. Parker-Cote (✉)
Division of Medical Toxicology, Department of Emergency Medicine, East Carolina University-Brody School of Medicine, Greenville, NC, USA
e-mail: parkercotej16@ecu.edu

W. J. Meggs, R. L. Langley (eds.), *Farm Toxicology*, https://doi.org/10.1007/978-3-031-80441-0_14

Anhydrous Ammonia

Anhydrous ammonia is an agricultural fertilizer that is stored as a liquid at subzero temperatures and high pressures (Amshel et al. 2000; Baker 1993). Agricultural workers are most likely to be exposed during distribution. Typically, when injected into soil, the ammonia gas is rapidly absorbed (Baker 1993). Exposed individuals should seek care immediately to avoid irreversible damage.

Anhydrous ammonia is not only used as an agricultural fertilizer but is also applied to animal feeds to control mold growth, added to corn silage, and used in the manufacture of synthetic fibers and methamphetamine production, refrigeration, petroleum industry, explosives industry, and cleaning products (White et al. 2007).

When combined with water, anhydrous ammonia is very caustic and results in chemical burns when exposed. Tissues with high moisture content such as the eyes, skin, and respiratory track are extremely vulnerable to cell destruction by liquefactive necrosis. Liquefactive necrosis involves the destruction of cells by hydrolytic enzymes that can lead from superficial to full-thickness tissue loss and perforation (Baker 1993). Cold-induced thermal injuries occur from the storage of anhydrous ammonia as a liquid at subzero temperatures (Baker 1993).

The acute effects of toxicity increase as the concentration of anhydrous ammonia increases. Nose irritation occurs at concentrations of 5 ppm (Baker 1993). At concentrations of 1700 parts per million (ppm), serious lung damage can occur with irreversible scarring, leading to chronic lung disease and pulmonary edema. At acutely high levels, symptoms such as coughing, laryngospasm, bronchoconstriction, and glottic edema can be seen (Baker 1993; White et al. 2007). Acute respiratory distress syndrome (ARDS) and acute lung injury can be seen after acute exposure. Rapid respiratory arrest can occur at concentrations of 5000 ppm (Baker 1993).

Chronic effects such as persistent damage to the cornea from ulceration result in partial or complete visual loss (White et al. 2007). Bacterial or fungal infections can occur after lung injury, which predisposes patients to infection. Resultant scarring of lung tissue can lead to decreased oxygen perfusion. Chronic exposure to mild or moderate levels of anhydrous ammonia can lead to obstructive lung disease (Padappayil and Borger 2021).

In the agricultural setting, if a patient is having respiratory distress or depressed mental status, clinicians should include other differential diagnoses such as exposures to hydrogen sulfide or carbon monoxide. In addition, irritative gases, such as acrolein, ethylene oxide, formaldehyde, hydrogen chloride, and sulfur dioxide, may cause a similar respiratory presentation (Padappayil and Borger 2021). Other caustics should be considered with ingestion. Sodium hydroxide, potassium hydroxide, and calcium hydroxide can cause similar chemical skin burns (Padappayil and Borger 2021). Other causes of acute respiratory distress must be considered when the history is not clear such as anaphylaxis, aspiration, and status asthmaticus.

Initial workup depends on the severity of the exposure. Minor exposures may not require any laboratory evaluation, while severe exposures may require extensive workup. General laboratory evaluation may consist of complete blood count (CBC), electrolytes, blood urea nitrogen, creatinine, lactic acid, coagulation studies, type and screen, and monitoring of urinary output (Padappayil and Borger 2021). Asymptomatic patients may be monitored in the emergency department for 6 hours of observation and tolerance of food (Padappayil and Borger 2021). Patients with respiratory exposure may require stabilization of the airway, arterial blood gas, and chest radiograph. Further pulmonary assessment may be warranted with the assessment of pulmonary function, bronchoscopy, and ventilation and perfusion scans. Inhaled steroids are not beneficial (White et al. 2007).

Carbon Monoxide

Carbon monoxide (CO) is the product of incomplete combustion of carbon-containing compounds. It is an odorless, colorless, tasteless gas that makes it hard to detect. It is a leading cause of poisoning morbidity and mortality in the United States and accounts for approximately 450 unintentional non-fire-related deaths annually (Hampson 2016). Excluding fire-related deaths, accidental carbon monoxide poisoning deaths outnumbered intentional deaths in 2021 (543 vs. 524) (Hampson 2023). In 2021, approximately 28,900 deaths worldwide were attributed to unintentional carbon monoxide poisoning (Moberg et al. 2023) More than half of all cases occur in homes during fall or winter, secondary to faulty furnaces (Hampson 2023; Tomaszewski 2019).

There are many associated carbon monoxide exposures due to the use of gasoline-powered equipment during storms, blizzards, hurricanes, and other natural disasters. Generators are associated with carbon monoxide outbreaks. Internal combustion engines such as trucks, cars, boats, and other gasoline-powered equipment also potentially place agricultural workers at risk. 50% of unintentional CO deaths are caused by motor vehicle exhaust (Cobb and Etzel 1991; Tomaszewski 2019; Mott et al. 2002). Other potential exposures can be from wood pellet storage, coffee roasting, formic acid decomposition mixed with sulfuric acid, underground mining explosions, methylene chloride (paint strippers), and methylene bromide (solvent for chemical manufacture, gauge fluid, and in fire-extinguishing fluids) (Tomaszewski 2019; National Center for Biotechnology Information 2023).

Carbon monoxide inhibits cellular respiration by binding to mitochondrial cytochrome oxidase, leading to oxidative stress and causing mitochondrial damage. It is rapidly absorbed and binds to hemoglobin, leading to tissue hypoxia. Hemoglobin has approximately 200–250 times greater affinity for CO than oxygen (Tomaszewski 2019). This leads to a leftward shift of the oxyhemoglobin dissociation curve, resulting in a decrease of the offloading of oxygen to tissues (Coburn 1970). Approximately 15% of carbon monoxide is bound to myoglobin and contributes to myocardial impairment from decreased oxygen extraction (Coburn 1970).

The earliest symptoms of CO poisoning are nonspecific and can present with viral-like symptoms characterized by headache, nausea, vomiting, and dizziness. Viral-like symptoms can lead to a missed diagnosis by a clinician, especially during the winter months when viral illnesses occur and indoor heating equipment is used (Dolan et al. 1987). Headache is the most common symptom and is often described as a constant, dull, frontal headache. Carbon monoxide exposure should be considered if multiple family members from the same household or multiple people from the same building present with similar symptoms, particularly if the time of onset is the same. Viral illness among a group is more likely to have a staggering time of onset. Headache has been associated with carboxyhemoglobin levels of 15–20% (Stewart et al. 1973).

Acute mortality from carbon monoxide is usually a result of ventricular dysrhythmias (Allred et al. 1991). Agricultural workers with a prior history of coronary artery disease may experience angina even with low levels of exposure to carbon monoxide. Myocardial ischemia and myonecrosis are seen in significant exposures (Cha et al. 2014). Neurologic involvement from minor symptoms like headache to major symptoms such as coma can occur. Cherry-red skin is not a common presentation (2 to 3%), but it does represent the failure to extract oxygen from arterial blood, vasodilatation, and tissue ischemia (Risser et al. 1995). An uncommon but classic skin finding for carbon monoxide poisoning is the presence of cutaneous bullae secondary to pressure necrosis versus the direct effect of CO on the epidermis (Tomaszewski 2019).

Approximately 50% of patients who sustain severe symptoms from CO poisoning develop persistent or delayed neurocognitive symptoms (Gorman et al. 1992; Raphael et al. 1989; Weaver et al. 2002). Patients with persistent neurological symptoms suffer various behavioral, neurologic, memory, and learning difficulties. Most cases are associated with a loss of consciousness in the acute phase of CO poisoning (Copel et al. 1982). The majority of cases present within 2–40 days of the initial event (Choi 1983). Some studies report that persistent cognitive sequelae resolve in one-third to one-fourth of cases over the course of a year (Choi 1983; Weaver et al. 2002).

Agricultural workers can be potentially exposed to a wide range of toxic agents but may also suffer from non-toxicological pathology. Clinicians need to be vigilant to rule out other causes for altered mental status, loss of consciousness, headache, nausea, and vomiting such as simple asphyxiants, hydrogen sulfide exposure, cerebrovascular accident or intracranial hemorrhage, endocrine abnormalities, or trauma.

Initial treatment for carbon monoxide exposure should involve scene safety and personal protective equipment (PPE). It is always a concern that rescuers can become second victims. After removing the victim from the source of carbon monoxide, apply 100% oxygen by a non-rebreather mask or endotracheal intubation, along with cardiac monitoring. The mean half-life of carboxyhemoglobin at room air is 249–320 minutes (min); with 100% oxygen, that decreases to approximately 74–80 min (Rose et al. 2017). Hyperbaric oxygen (HBO) can reduce carboxyhemoglobin half-life to 20 min (range 4–86 min) (Weaver et al. 2000).

Proponents of hyperbaric oxygen suggest that its use can prevent ischemic reperfusion injury and the development of delayed neurologic sequelae. There is debate over its utility in victims without loss of consciousness, altered mental status, coma, or seizure (Tomaszewski 2019). A more recent Cochrane Collaboration review and the American College of Emergency Physician guidelines report conflicting data and insufficient evidence to support HBO for CO poisoning (Buckley et al. 2011; Wolf et al. 2017). It is reasonable to discuss with a regional poison center or hyperbaric facility if a patient is a candidate for hyperbaric oxygen therapy. Patients presenting with altered mental status, loss of consciousness, carboxyhemoglobin levels >25%, cerebellar dysfunction, pregnancy (carboxyhemoglobin level > 15%), fetal distress, equivocal cases with age > 35 and prolonged exposure (>24 h), arrhythmias, cardiac dysfunction, seizures, and coma may be candidates for hyperbaric oxygen therapy (Tomaszewski 2019). There are barriers to HBO treatment due to cost and transport time to facilities with a chamber.

CO-oximetry is used to measure the percentage of hemoglobin saturated with carbon monoxide. Blood samples for the measurement of carboxyhemoglobin levels can be drawn from an arterial or venous source. The normal level for a nonsmoker is 0–2% and for a smoker, 4–10% (Radford and Drizd 1982). Carboxyhemoglobin levels may not correlate with the severity of the disease, prediction of outcomes, or development of delayed neurologic sequelae. Also, the administration of hydroxocobalamin, after concerns for cyanide toxicity from a structure fire, can provide a falsely reassuring reading (Livshits et al. 2012; Pace et al. 2012). Carboxyhemoglobin can be misinterpreted as oxyhemoglobin and misread by pulse oximetry as normal. Some prehospital providers (fire departments) may have newer pulse oximeters (pulse CO-oximetry) that read carboxyhemoglobin noninvasively and are used as screening tools in the field but may overestimate carboxyhemoglobin levels (Barker and Badal 2008). It is recommended that pulse CO-oximetry be not used independently to diagnose carbon monoxide toxicity and cannot substitute for carboxyhemoglobin measurement as per the most recent American College of Emergency Physician guidelines (Wolf et al. 2017).

Laboratory analysis with significant metabolic acidosis and elevated lactate levels occurs in severe CO poisoning (Sokal and Kralkowska 1985). Initial laboratory evaluation may consist of basic metabolic panel (BMP), lactate, arterial blood gas (ABG), creatine phosphokinase (CPK), troponin, brain natureitic peptide (BNP), 12-lead electrocardiogram (EKG), toxicology testing depending on the severity of symptoms, and past medical history (Sokal and Kralkowska 1985; Chamberland et al. 2004). Symptomatic patients should have continuous cardiac monitoring, and clinicians should obtain a 12-lead EKG to evaluate for any ischemia or dysrhythmias. The patient may have mild elevations of creatine phosphokinase (CPK) secondary to rhabdomyolysis rather than cardiac ischemia. Elevations in troponin levels are seen even in patients without coronary artery disease after significant CO exposure

(Chamberland et al. 2004). Patients with altered mental status, loss of consciousness, or other neurological deficits may require head computer tomography (CT) or brain magnetic resonance imaging (MRI). Changes can be seen on head CT within 12 hours of exposure. After severe CO exposure, globus pallidus lesions are a common radiologic finding and are generally bilateral and symmetric (Weaver 2009). MRI is more sensitive but may not be readily available at certain facilities, or the patient may not be stable enough to undergo MRI.

Disposition depends on initial presentation, initial carboxyhemoglobin levels, and persistence of symptoms. Persistent neurologic sequelae may initially be present and develop later in the disease course. Some patients have symptoms for months, years, or permanently.

Hydrogen Sulfide

Hydrogen sulfide forms from the bacterial decomposition of proteins of sulfur-containing products such as fish, eggs, sewage, and manure (Gerasimon et al. 2007; Strickland et al. 2003). Hydrogen sulfide is an irritating colorless gas with the odor of "rotten eggs" (Holstege 2019).

Farm laborers may encounter hydrogen sulfide while working near livestock due to presence of manure storage tanks. There are other agricultural and industrial sources: pulp–paper mills, the leather industry, roofing-asphalt tanks, and oil and gas production (Chou and Selene 2006). Multiple victims can present with "knockdown," and rescuers can succumb to the gas as they attempt to retrieve victims using inadequate personal protective equipment (Ng et al. 2019). Workers can be exposed to hydrogen sulfide through suicide attempts by mixing common household detergents with sulfuric acid to create hydrogen sulfide gas (Ng et al. 2019; Kamijo et al. 2013; Reedy et al. 2011).

Hydrogen sulfide is lipid-soluble and is rapidly distributed to tissues. Its primary mechanism of toxicity is interference with cellular respiration by inhibition of cytochrome a_3 oxidase, which interrupts oxidative phosphorylation leading to cellular hypoxia and anaerobic metabolism (Ng et al. 2019; Chou and Selene 2006). Other mechanisms of toxicity involve alteration of neurotransmitter release and inhibitory neuronal transmission, cytotoxicity, and free radical injury (Olson 2012; Truong et al. 2006).

Acute hydrogen sulfide produces an immediate profound central nervous system (CNS) impairment, causing coma, rapid loss of consciousness, and cardiopulmonary arrest at levels of 500 ppm. Apnea occurs suddenly at 1000 ppm (Reiffenstein et al. 1992). Neurologic symptoms can include headache, weakness, ataxia, syncope and convulsions, olfactory nerve paralysis, and hearing difficulties. Along with systemic symptoms, mucous-membrane irritation and corrosive injury can occur to the eyes, nasal passages, and respiratory tissues. "Gas eye" can occur due to keratoconjunctivitis from eye involvement and lead to corneal abrasions and ulcers (Lambert et al. 2006). There is little dermal absorption, but irritation can occur.

Perception of gas odor extinguishes, and olfactory nerve dysfunction occurs at 100–150 ppm (Holstege 2019).

In those who survive to reach an emergency department, metabolic and lactic acidosis is seen on initial laboratory evaluation. Clinicians should consider secondary traumatic injuries from falls after sudden loss of consciousness.

Low-level exposures to hydrogen sulfide can produce chronic effects and can be seen in sewer, gas, and oil workers. Irritation of the mucus membranes, nasal and pharyngeal area, and eyes can occur. Other symptoms reported from chronic low-level exposures are fatigue, ataxia, headache, dizziness, and memory difficulties. Long-term pulmonary effects such as decreased lung volumes can be seen in sewer workers with chronic exposures (Richardson 1995).

Clinicians should consider other possible causes for sudden rapid unresponsiveness in their workup and differential diagnosis such as carbon monoxide poisoning, hydrogen cyanide (fires), organophosphates and carbamates, trauma, other causes of cardiopulmonary arrest such as arrhythmias, other simple asphyxiants, stroke, or overdose.

First responders must ensure scene safety and wear appropriate PPE as first responders can become victims in the agricultural setting where hydrogen sulfide is a potential source. Remove the patient from the source and apply oxygen. It is essential to consider potential secondary trauma from a fall. The application of supplemental oxygen is key as it competitively reactivates oxidative phosphorylation by inhibiting hydrogen sulfide from binding to cytochrome oxidase. It is suggested to decontaminate clothes, eyes, and skin (Jiang et al. 2016). The odor of "rotten eggs" may be present on the patient's clothes, even blood and bodily secretions, or exhaled air. Silver jewelry can darken secondary to exposure (Chou and Selene 2006). Clinical suspicion is based on history and physical examination. If exposure is a concern, workers can complete safety measures such as atmospheric testing prior to entering an area, but gas can dissipate prior to assessment. Currently, there is no method to measure hydrogen sulfide or its metabolites rapidly and directly. The presence of an elevated thiosulfate level (urine or blood sources) indicates exposure but does not determine the severity of exposure (Holstege 2019). In the emergency department, reassessing airway status and managing appropriately should be the primary concern upon initial evaluation. An arterial blood gas (ABG) may reveal acidemia with an elevated lactate. Oxygen saturation will most likely be normal on the ABG. An elevated oxygen on mixed venous oxygen measurement may be present due to decreased oxygen consumption. Sulfhemoglobin is generally not present with hydrogen sulfide poisoning and is not useful for diagnosis. CBC, BMP, troponin, EKG, carboxyhemoglobin, and chest X-ray may help differentiate the presentation. Supportive care for hypotension with intravenous fluids and vasopressors may be indicated. Any arrhythmias should be managed as per advanced cardial life support (ACLS) protocols. MRI and CT of the brain may show globus pallidus and subcortical white-matter demyelination. Abnormalities may be present for weeks or months with serious exposures (Callender et al. 1993).

If the patient survives the initial insult, disposition depends on the initial presentation and stabilization of the patient.

Fumigants

Metal Phosphides and Phosphine Gas

In the agricultural industry, metal phosphides (aluminum phosphide, zinc phosphide, magnesium phosphide, and calcium phosphide) are distributed as pellets, sometimes called "rice tablets," to protect grain from rodents in silos and ships' holds and during transportation. When metal phosphides encounter moisture, phosphine gas is released (Sciuto et al. 2016; Proudfoot 2009; Gurjar et al. 2011).

Phosphine gas is odorless, colorless, and highly explosive. Secondary to impurities during the pellet manufacturing process, there is a presence of the odor of garlic or fish (Sciuto et al. 2016; CDC 2011). Fatality rates range from 70–100% (Meena et al. 2015). Death typically occurs within 12–24 hours (Sciuto et al. 2016). Phosphine gas can be absorbed through the gastrointestinal (GI) tract and respiratory tract and, minimally, transdermally (CDC 2011). Cellular damage occurs through noncompetitive inhibition of cytochrome c oxidase, leading to blockage of the electron transport chain and oxidative phosphorylation. This leads to widespread cellular damage and ion dysfunction (Shadnia and Soltaninejad 2019).

Clinical manifestations depend on the duration, route, and time since exposure (Gurjar et al. 2011). Acutely, patients present with primarily pulmonary manifestations such as airway irritation, breathlessness, chest tightness, and cough with green fluorescent sputum. Other signs and symptoms that can be present are tachycardia, headache, nausea, vomiting, electrolyte disturbance, hypoglycemia, diarrhea, numbness, impaired gait, paresthesias, muscle weakness, and diplopia. After ingestion or inhalation, the odor of garlic or fish may be noted on the patient's breath. Cardiopulmonary arrest or collapse, hypotension, ventricular dysrhythmias, and seizures may occur in severe exposures (CDC 2011; Shadnia and

Soltaninejad 2019). In rare cases, liver failure, kidney failure, pulmonary edema, myocardial infarction, disseminated intravascular hemolysis, and methemoglobinemia have been reported (Sciuto et al. 2016; Shadnia and Soltaninejad 2019).

Exposure to chronic low levels of phosphine gas has resulted in anemia; bronchitis; gastrointestinal symptoms; kidney failure; and visual, speech, and motor disturbances (CDC 2011).

Considerations of other sources such as toxic gases like hydrogen sulfide and carbon monoxide, trauma, stroke, overdose, and cardiac dysrhythmias should be considered in those presenting with altered mental status, unresponsiveness, and seizures.

Victims of phosphine-gas exposure should immediately be removed from the source and oxygen applied. Phosphine is very volatile, and exposure from off-gassing can occur. First responders and medical personnel should be aware of the concern for ignition. Appropriate PPE and respirators are required, particularly for exposures from ingestions (Mital et al. 1992). After exposure from ingestion, decontamination with potassium permanganate (1:10,000) by gastric lavage has been used, as well as activated charcoal and coconut oil (Gurjar et al. 2011). After cutaneous exposure, thorough irrigation with water is important if absorption is a concern (Mehrpour et al. 2012). Treatment is supportive with ventilatory support; monitoring; intravenous fluids; sodium bicarbonate; vasopressors; and the management of electrolyte disturbances, acidemia, and hypoglycemia as needed (Hashemi-Domeneh et al. 2016). Multiple studies and case reports site a mortality reduction up to 50% with the use of magnesium sulfate, potentially from cell-membrane stabilization and prevention of fatal arrhythmias. Magnesium sulfate has an antiperoxident effect and limits free radical damage. Variable dosages and frequency have been reported: 3 grams (g) given over 3 hours, followed by 6 g over 24 hours for 3–5 days; 1 g as a bolus, then 1 g every hour for the next 2 hours, and then 1–1.5 g every 6 hours for 5–7 days; 4 g bolus, 2 g after 1 hour, and then 1 g every three-hourly; and 3 g bolus, followed by 6 g infusion over the next 12 hours for 5–7 days (Gurjar et al. 2011; Chugh et al. 1994a, b, 1997; Gupta and Ahlawat 1995). N-acetylcysteine has been shown to improve mortality rates in human clinical trials and is recommended (Agarwal et al. 2014; Tehrani et al. 2013). Intramuscular vitamin E injections may decrease mortality as per some studies (Halvaei et al. 2017). Veno-arterial extracorporeal membrane oxygenation has shown benefit in short-term survival in refractory cardiogenic shock and severe acidemia. Hemodialysis does not effectively remove hydrogen phosphide but is recommended in refractory acidosis and fluid overload (Gurjar et al. 2011).

Acutely, specific blood or urine levels are not recommended and not helpful as analysis for phosphine in blood or urine is ineffective because phosphine is rapidly oxidized to phosphite and hypophosphite (Proudfoot 2009; Yadav et al. 2007). If a clinician has doubts about exposure, then a diagnosis can be made by the use of a silver nitrate paper test. Gastric contents that contain phosphine will turn the paper black due to silver phosphate (Gurjar et al. 2011; Goel and Aggarwal 2007; Chugh et al. 1989; Mital et al. 1992). Hydrogen sulfide may also change the color of silver nitrate, so lead acetate paper can be used to differentiate the two (hydrogen sulfide will turn the lead acetate paper to a black color) (Gurjar et al. 2011). Phosphine exposure can be confirmed by the application of ammonium molybdate solution to the silver nitrate paper that has turned black as the paper should turn blue if phosphine is present (Curry 1976). Arrhythmias are common and an EKG along with cardiac monitoring should be obtained (Sciuto et al. 2016; Siwach et al. 1998). As pulmonary symptoms are the primary concern after exposure, chest X-ray is useful to assess for pulmonary edema or acute respiratory distress syndrome (Sciuto et al. 2016). Metabolic acidosis with elevated lactic acid indicates significant toxicity and mortality (Shadnia and Soltaninejad 2019; Erfantalab et al. 2017). Along with evaluation for metabolic acidosis, clinicians should obtain a complete blood count, measurement of electrolytes and magnesium, and liver and kidney function tests. An echocardiogram to evaluate cardiac function may benefit as global hypokinesis and decreased ejection fraction are reported in some exposures (Sciuto et al. 2016; Akkaoui et al. 2007).

Other Fumigants (Also see Chap. 12)

1,3-Dichloropropene

1,3-Dichloropropene is a soil fumigant that is solubilized in soybean oil and used for the control of nematodes for crops such as sweet potatoes, almonds, strawberries, grapes, and carrots (EPA 2020; Gharibi et al. 2020). Agricultural workers are primarily exposed via inhalation. It is rapidly absorbed by the lungs, GI tract, and dermal routes. It has an odor similar to chloroform. Hydrogen chloride and phosgene are formed after thermal breakdown of 1,3-dichloropropene (Blanc 2012). The exact mechanism of toxicity is not clear (Shadnia and Soltaninejad 2019). Clinical effects seen after oral and inhalational exposures are extensive including systemic symptoms, gastrointestinal symptoms, pulmonary symptoms, CNS depression, and acute kidney injury (Hernandez et al. 1994). Dermal exposures report hypersensitivity, erythema, and diaphoresis (Hayes 2010). Chronic long-term effects include asthma, lymphoma, and histiocytic lymphoma (Gharibi et al. 2020). Liver and kidney function tests should be monitored, but there is no specific antidote for 1, 3-dichloropropene. Changes on chest X-ray may lag behind clinical symptoms by 8 hours (Hernandez et al. 1994). Treatment is supportive with ventilatory support, decontamination, and protection of personnel with appropriate personal protective equipment. With ingestion, activated charcoal is reasonable but of no proven value. With ingestions, orogastric lavage is reasonable if presenting shortly after ingestion. Monitor for 24 hours after exposure (Shadnia and Soltaninejad 2019).

Chloropicrin

Chloropicrin is a highly volatile soil fumigant and is also used in crowd control due to its ability to cause lacrimation. It is used as a soil fumigant in orchards and greenhouses and added to other fumigants as a warning agent. Inhalational exposure typically causes eye, nose, throat, and upper-respiratory-tract irritation (EPA 2018). Breakdown products include oxides of nitrogen (Durrani et al. 2018). Exposure can occur through ingestion and dermally, causing GI symptoms and blisters, respectively. Treatment involves irrigation of eyes and skin, and symptoms typically resolve after 15–30 min following decontamination. Respiratory irritation can result in bronchospasm and pulmonary edema. Bronchospasm can be treated with beta-2 agonists (CDC 2011).

Methyl Isothiocyanate

Methyl isothiocyanate (MITC) is the breakdown product of dazomet, metam-sodium, and metam-potassium. It is a highly volatile fumigant that is fungicidal, herbicidal, and nematocidal. It is used on golf courses, nonbearing crops, turf sites, ornamental sites, field nurseries, compost piles, potting soils, strawberries, and tomatoes. It is also used to prevent wood rot on pilings, utility poles, and timber. Its mechanism of toxicity is not well-known, but MITC is thought to stimulate chemesthesis, which is the activation of receptors associated with sensations of pain, touch, or thermal perception (Gadagbui et al. 2014). Metam-sodium is associated with acute and persistent irritant-induced asthma (National Research Council 2013). It has been noted to have a horseradish-like odor. Clinical effects include eye irritation, lacrimation, systemic symptoms (headache, nausea, and vomiting), and respiratory effects and is a known dermal sensitizer (EPA 2008). Treatment consists of removal from the area and supportive measures with oxygen and corticosteroids that can be helpful with persistent reactive airway symptoms. It is recommended after unintentional ingestion to dilute with water but not induce emesis. Also, in significant ingestions, activated charcoal and gastric lavage can be considered. With dermal exposures, decontamination with soap and water is recommended.

Nitrogen Dioxide

Nitrogen dioxide forms after the decomposition of silage from recently filled silos. It is recommended that silos should be avoided for 3 weeks after filling. There may be an odor of bleach and yellow-to-brown gas observed near the silos. Silo-gas is a combination of nitrogen dioxide and carbon dioxide. Silo-filler's disease is the chronic effect of delayed-onset pulmonary toxicity from exposure. The primary mechanism of toxicity of Silo-filler's disease is asphyxiation from the rapid depletion of oxygen, pulmonary epithelial injury from reactive nitrogen intermediates, and corrosive injury to pulmonary tissue from nitric acid that is formed when nitrogen dioxide dissolves in the aqueous environment of the lower respiratory tract (Groves and Ellwood 1989; Skjolaas et al. 2010; Nelson and Odujebe 2019). Acute effects involve acute asphyxiation. Chronic effects due to inadequate ventilation can be fatal. Chronic effects from delayed-onset pulmonary toxicity can lead to bronchiolitis obliterans. Treatment is primarily supportive with removal to fresh air, application of oxygen, and decontamination of skin and clothing. A relapse can occur 2–6 weeks after the original exposure and can be equal in severity. Airway support may involve mechanical ventilation, or noninvasive positive pressure ventilation. Delayed-onset pulmonary toxicity may have to be treated in the long term with corticosteroids (Sherwood 2020).

Conclusion

In summary, scene safety is essential on farms after exposure to a toxic gas as first responders and medical personnel can easily become second victims if not using appropriate personal protective equipment. Consider if decontamination is needed. Initial treatment should be supportive, focusing on the airway, breathing, and circulation. Call your regional poison control center for further guidance and care.

References

Agarwal A, Robo R, Jain N, Gutch M, Consil S, Kumar S. Oxidative stress determined through the levels of antioxidant enzymes and the effect of N-acetylcysteine in aluminum phosphide poisoning. Indian J Crit Care Med. 2014;18(10):666–71. https://www.ncbi.nlm.nih.gov/pubmed/25316977. https://doi.org/10.4103/0972-5229.142176.

Akkaoui M, Achour S, Abidi K, Himdi B, Madani A, Zeggwagh AA, Abouqal R. Reversible myocardial injury associated with aluminum phosphide poisoning. Clin Toxicol. 2007;45(6):728–31.

Allred EN, Bleecker ER, Chaitman BR, Dahms TE, Gottlieb SO, Hackney JD, et al. Effects of carbon monoxide on myocardial ischemia. Environ Health Perspect. 1991;91:89–132. https://doi.org/10.2307/3430988.

Amshel CE, Fealk MH, Phillips BJ, Caruso DM. Anhydrous ammonia burns case report and review of the literature. Burns. 2000;26(5):493–7. https://doi.org/10.1016/S0305-4179(99)00176-X.

Baker DE. Using agricultural anhydrous ammonia safely. University Extension, University of Missouri. 1993. https://nasdonline.org/1085/d000875/using-agricultural-anhydrous-ammonia-safely.html.

Barker SJ, Badal JJ. The measurement of dyshemoglobins and total hemoglobin by pulse oximetry. Curr Opin Anaesthesiol. 2008;21(6):805–10. https://www.ncbi.nlm.nih.gov/pubmed/18997533. https://doi.org/10.1097/ACO.0b013e328316bb6f.

Blanc PD. Evaluation of the patient with occupational chemical exposure. In: Olson KR, Anderson IB, Benowitz NL, Blanc PD, Clark RF, Kearney TE, Kim-Katz SY, Wu AHB, editors. Section IV environmental and occupational toxicology. Poisoning & drug overdose. 6th ed. New York: McGraw Hill Lange; 2012. p. 617.

Buckley NA, Juurlink DN, Isbister G, Bennett MH, Lavonas EJ. Hyperbaric oxygen for carbon monoxide poisoning. Cochrane Database Syst Rev. 2011;4:CD002041. https://doi.org/10.1002/14651858.CD002041.pub3.

Callender TJ, Morrow L, Subramanian K, Duhon D, Ristovv M. Three-dimensional brain metabolic imaging in patients with toxic encephalopathy. Environ Res. 1993;60(2):295–319. https://doi.org/10.1006/enrs.1993.1039.

Centers for Disease Control. The National Institute for Occupational Safety and Health, (NIOSH). Phosphine: lung damaging agent; 2011. https://www.cdc.gov/niosh/ershdb/emergencyresponsecard_29750035.html. Accessed 1 Jan 2024.

Cha YS, Cha KC, Kim OH, Lee KH, Hwang SO, Kim H. Features and predictors of myocardial injury in carbon monoxide poisoned patients. Emerg Med J. 2014;31(3):210–5. https://doi.org/10.1136/emermed-2012-202152.

Chamberland DL, Wilson BD, Weaver LK. Transient cardiac dysfunction in acute carbon monoxide poisoning. Am J Med. 2004;117(8):623–5. https://doi.org/10.1016/j.amjmed.2004.04.025.

Choi S. Delayed neurologic sequelae in carbon monoxide intoxication. Arch Neurol. 1983;40(7):433–5. https://doi.org/10.1001/archneur.1983.04050070063016.

Chou CH, Selene J. Syracuse Research Corporation, United States. Agency for Toxic Substances and Disease Registry. Toxicological profile for hydrogen sulfide. U.S. Dept. of Health and Human Services, Public Health Service, Agency for Toxic Substances and Disease Registry; 2006.

Chugh SN, Ram S, Chugh K, Malhotra KC. Spot diagnosis of aluminium phosphide ingestion-an application of simple test. J Assoc Physicians India. 1989;37:219–20.

Chugh SN, Kumar P, Aggarwal HK, Sharma A, Mahajan SK, Malhotra KC. Efficacy of magnesium sulphate in aluminium phosphide poisoning-comparison of two different dose schedules. J Assoc Physicians India. 1994a;42:373–5.

Chugh SN, Kamar P, Sharma A, Chugh K, Mittal A, Arora B. Magnesium status and parenteral magnesium sulphate therapy in acute aluminum phosphide intoxication. Magnes Res. 1994b;7:289–94.

Chugh SN, Kolley T, Kakkar R, Chugh K, Sharma A. A critical evaluation of anti-peroxidant effect of intravenous magnesium in acute aluminium phosphide poisoning. Magnes Res. 1997;10:225–30.

Cobb N, Etzel RA. Unintentional carbon monoxide-related deaths in the united states, 1979 through 1988. JAMA. 1991;266(5):659–63. https://www.ncbi.nlm.nih.gov/pubmed/1712865. https://doi.org/10.1001/jama.266.5.659.

Coburn RF. The carbon monoxide body stores. Ann N Y Acad Sci. 1970;174(1):11–22. https://www.ncbi.nlm.nih.gov/pubmed/4943970. https://doi.org/10.1111/j.1749-6632.1970.tb49768.x.

Copel JA, Bowen F, Bolognese RJ. Carbon monoxide intoxication in early pregnancy. Obstet Gynecol. 1982;59(6 Suppl):26S–8S. https://pubmed.ncbi.nlm.nih.gov/7088422/.

Curry A. Poison detection in human organs. 3rd ed. Springfield, IL: Charles C Thomas; 1976. p. 128–9.

Dolan MC, Haltom TL, Barrows GH, Short CS, Ferriell KM. Carboxyhemoglobin levels in patients with flu-like symptoms. Ann Emerg Med. 1987;16(7):782–6. https://doi.org/10.1016/S0196-0644(87)80575-9.

Durrani TS, Blanc PD, Hiatt P, Olson KR, Timur S. The toxic hazards of industrial and occupational chemicals. In: Olson KR, Anderson IB, Benowitz NL, Blanc PD, Clark RF, Kearney TE, Kim-Katz SY, Wu AB, editors. Poisoning & drug overdose. 7th ed. New York: McGraw Hill; 2018. https://accessmedicine.mhmedical.com/content.aspx?bookid=2284&sectionid=248386031. Accessed 15 Dec 2023.

Environmental Protection Agency. US environmental protection agency office of pesticide programs. Red fact sheet: Dazomet. 2008. https://archive.epa.gov/pesticides/reregistration/web/pdf/dazomet-fs.pdf. Accessed 1 Jan 2024.

Environmental Protection Agency. U.S. environmental protection agency office of pesticide programs. Red fact sheet: Chloropicrin. 2018. https://www3.epa.gov/pesticides/chem_search/reg_actions/reregistration/fs_PC-081501_10-Jul-08.pdf. Accessed 28 Dec 2023.

Environmental Protective Agency. Trans-1,3-dichloropropene. 2020. https://sor.epa.gov/sor_internet/registry/substreg/searchandretrieve/advancedsearch/externalSearch.do?p_type=CASNO&p_value=10061-02-6#top. Accessed 28 Dec 2023.

Erfantalab P, Soltaninejad K, Shadnia S, Zamani N, Hassanian-Moghaddam H, Mahdavinejad A, et al. Trend of blood lactate level in acute aluminum phosphide poisoning. World J Emerg Med. 2017;8(2):116–20. https://doi.org/10.5847/wjem.j.1920-8642.2017.02.006.

Gadagbui B, Vincent M, Willis A. In: Wexler P, editor. Methyl isothiocyanate. Encyclopedia of toxicology. 3rd ed. Amsterdam: Elsevier Science & Technology; 2014. p. 310–3.

Gerasimon G, Bennett S, Musser J, Rinard J. Acute hydrogen sulfide poisoning in a dairy farmer. Clin Toxicol. 2007;45(4):420–3. https://doi.org/10.1080/15563650601118010.

Gharibi H, Entwistle MR, Schweizer D, Tavallali P, Cisneros R. The association between 1,3-dichloropropene and Asthma Emergency Department visits in California, USA from 2005 to 2011: a bidirectional-symmetric case crossover study. J Asthma. 2020;57(6):601–9. https://doi.org/10.1080/02770903.2019.1590596.

Goel A, Aggarwal P. Pesticide poisoning. Natl Med J India. 2007;20:182–91.

Gorman DF, Clayton D, Gilligan JE, Webb RK. A longitudinal study of 100 consecutive admissions for carbon monoxide poisoning to the Royal Adelaide Hospital. Anaesth Intensive Care. 1992;20(3):311–6. https://doi.org/10.1177/0310057X9202000306.

Groves JA, Ellwood PA. Gases in forage tower silos. Ann Occup Hyg. 1989;33:519–35.

Gupta S, Ahlawat SK. Aluminum phosphide poisoning—a review. J Toxicol Clin Toxicol. 1995;33:19–24.

Gurjar M, Baronia AK, Azim A, Sharma K. Managing aluminum phosphide poisonings. J Emerg Trauma Shock. 2011;4(3):378–84. https://www.ncbi.nlm.nih.gov/pubmed/21887030. https://doi.org/10.4103/0974-2700.83868.

Halvaei Z, Tehrani H, Soltaninejad K, Abdollahi M, Shadnia S. Vitamin E as a novel therapy in the treatment of acute aluminum phosphide poisoning. Turk J Med Sci. 2017;47(3):795–800. https://www.ncbi.nlm.nih.gov/pubmed/28618724. https://doi.org/10.3906/sag-1512-6.

Hampson NB. U.S. mortality due to carbon monoxide poisoning, 1999–2014. Accidental and intentional deaths. Ann Am Thorac Soc. 2016;13(10):1768–74. https://www.ncbi.nlm.nih.gov/pubmed/27466698. https://doi.org/10.1513/AnnalsATS.201604-318OC.

Hampson NB. Carbon monoxide poisoning mortality in the United States from 2015-2021. Clin Toxicol. 2023;61(7):483–91. https://doi.org/10.1080/15563650.2023.2237667.

Hashemi-Domeneh B, Zamani N, Hassanian-Moghaddam H, Rahimi M, Shadnia S, Erfantalab

P, Ostadi A. A review of aluminium phosphide poisoning and a flowchart to treat it. Arh Hig Rada Toksikol. 2016;67(3):183–93. https://doi.org/10.1515/aiht-2016-67-2784.

Hayes WJ. Handbook of pesticide toxicology. 3rd ed. New York: Academic Press, Elsevier Science & Technology; 2010. p. 764–5.

Hernandez AF, Martin-Rubi JC, Ballesteros JL, Oliver M, Pla A, Villanueva E. Clinical and pathological findings in fatal 1,3-dichloropropene intoxication. Hum Exp Toxicol. 1994;13(5):303–6. https://doi.org/10.1177/096032719401300502.

Holstege CP. Chapter 123: Cyanide and hydrogen sulfide. In: Nelson LS, Howland MA, Lewin NA, Smith SW, Goldfrank LR, Hoffman RS, editors. Goldfrank's toxicologic emergencies. 11th ed. New York: McGraw-Hill Education; 2019.

Jiang J, Chan A, Ali S, Saha A, Haushalter KJ, Lam WL, et al. Hydrogen sulfide—mechanisms of toxicity and development of an antidote. Sci Rep. 2016;6:20831. PMID: 26877209; PMCID: PMC4753484. https://doi.org/10.1038/srep20831.

Kamijo Y, Takai M, Fujita Y, Hirose Y, Iwasaki Y, Ishihara S. A multicenter retrospective survey on a suicide trend using hydrogen sulfide in Japan. Clin Toxicol. 2013;51(5):425–8. https://doi.org/10.3109/15563650.2013.799676.

Lambert TW, Goodwin VM, Stefani D, Strosher L. Hydrogen sulfide (H 2S) and sour gas effects on the eye. A historical perspective. Sci Total Environ. 2006;367(1):1–22. https://doi.org/10.1016/j.scitotenv.2006.01.034.

Livshits Z, Lugassy DM, Shawn LK, Hoffman RS. Falsely low carboxyhemoglobin level after hydroxocobalamin therapy. N Engl J Med. 2012;367(13):1270–1. https://doi.org/10.1056/NEJMc1114820.

Meena MC, Mittal S, Rani Y. Fatal aluminum phosphide poisoning. Interdiscip Toxicol. 2015;8(2):65–7. https://pubmed.ncbi.nlm.nih.gov/27486362 https://www.ncbi.nlm.nih.gov/pmc/articles/PMC4961899/. https://doi.org/10.1515/intox-2015-0010.

Mehrpour O, Jafarzadeh M, Abdollahi M. A systematic review of aluminum phosphide poisoning. Arch Ind Hyg Toxicol. 2012;63:1.

Mital HS, Mehrotra TN, Dwivedi KK, Gera M. A study of aluminum phosphide poisoning with special reference to its spot diagnosis by silver nitrate test. J Assoc Physicians India. 1992;40(7):473–4. https://www.ncbi.nlm.nih.gov/pubmed/1282918.

Moberg ME, Hamilton EB, Zeng SM, Bryazka D, Zhao JT, Feldman R, et al. Global, regional, and national mortality due to unintentional carbon monoxide poisoning, 2000–2021: results from the Global Burden of Disease Study 2021. Lancet Public Health. 2023;8(11):E839–49. https://doi.org/10.1016/S2468-2667(23)00185-8.

Mott JA, Wolfe MI, Alverson CJ, Macdonald SC, Bailey CR, Ball LB, et al. National vehicle emissions policies and practices and declining US carbon monoxide–related mortality. JAMA. 2002;288(8):988–95. https://doi.org/10.1001/jama.288.8.988.

National Center for Biotechnology Information. PubChem Compound Summary for CID 3024, Dibromethane. 2023. https://pubchem.ncbi.nlm.nih.gov/compound/Dibromomethane. Accessed 30 Dec 2023.

National Research Council. Acute exposure guideline levels for selected airborne chemicals, vol. 15. 2013. https://www.ncbi.nlm.nih.gov/books/NBK201333/.

Nelson LS, Odujebe OA. Chapter 121. Simple asphyxiants and pulmonary irritants. In: Nelson LS, Howland MA, Lewsin NA, Smith SW, Goldfrank LR, editors. Goldfrank's Toxicologic emergencies. New York: McGraw-Hill Education; 2019.

Ng PC, Hendry-Hofer TB, Witeof AE, Brenner M, Mahon SB, Boss GR, et al. Hydrogen sulfide toxicity: mechanism of action, clinical presentation, and countermeasure development. J Med Toxicol. 2019;15(4):287–94. https://doi.org/10.1007/s13181-019-00710-5.

Olson KR. A practical look at the chemistry and biology of hydrogen sulfide. Antioxid Redox Signal. 2012;17(1):32–44. https://doi.org/10.1089/ars.2011.4401.

Pace R, Bon Homme M, Hoffman RS, Lugassy D. Effects of hydroxocobalamin on carboxyhemoglobin measured under physiologic and pathologic conditions. Clin Toxicol (Phila). 2012;52(7):647–50. https://doi.org/10.3109/15563650.2014.939659.

Padappayil RP, Borger J. Ammonia toxicity. StatPearls; 2021. https://www.ncbi.nlm.nih.gov/books/NBK546677/.

Proudfoot AT. Aluminum and zinc phosphide poisoning. Clin Toxicol (Phila). 2009;47(2):89–100. https://doi.org/10.1080/15563650802520675.

Radford EP, Drizd TA. Blood carbon monoxide levels in persons 3–74 years of age: United States, 1976–80. Adv Data. 1982;1982(76):1–24. https://www.ncbi.nlm.nih.gov/pubmed/10257767.

Raphael JC, Elkharrat D, Jars-Guincestre MC, Chastang C, Chasles V, Vercken JB, Gajdos P. Trial of normobaric and hyperbaric oxygen for acute carbon monoxide intoxication. Lancet. 1989;2(8660):414–9. https://doi.org/10.1016/s0140-6736(89)90592-8.

Reedy SJD, Schwartz MD, Morgan BW. Suicide fads: frequency and characteristics of hydrogen sulfide suicides in the United States. West J Emerg Med. 2011;12(3):300–4. https://www.ncbi.nlm.nih.gov/pubmed/21731786.

Reiffenstein RJ, Hulbert WC, Roth SH. Toxicology of hydrogen sulfide. Annu Rev Pharmacol Toxicol. 1992;32(1):109–34. https://www.ncbi.nlm.nih.gov/pubmed/1605565. https://doi.org/10.1146/annurev.pharmtox.32.1.109.

Richardson DB. Respiratory effects of chronic hydrogen sulfide exposure. Am J Ind Med. 1995;28(1):99–108. https://doi.org/10.1002/ajim.4700280109.

Risser D, Bönsch A, Schneider B. Should coroners be able to recognize unintentional carbon monoxide-related deaths immediately at the death scene? J Forensic

Sci. 1995;40(4):596–8. https://doi.org/10.1520/JFS13832J.

Rose JJ, Wang L, Xu Q, McTiernan CF, Shiva S, Tejero J, Gladwin MT. Carbon monoxide poisoning: pathogenesis, management, and future directions of therapy. Am J Respir Crit Care Med. 2017;195(5):596–606. https://doi.org/10.1164/rccm.201606-1275CI.

Sciuto AM, Wong BJ, Martens ME, Hoard-Fruchey H, Perkins MW. Phosphine toxicity: a story of disrupted mitochondrial metabolism. Ann N Y Acad Sci. 2016;1374(1):41–51. https://doi.org/10.1111/nyas.1308.

Shadnia S, Soltaninejad K. Chapter 108. Fumigants. In: Nelson LS, Howland MA, Lewin NA, Smith SW, Goldfrank LR, Hoffman RS, editors. Goldfrank's toxicologic emergencies. 11th ed. New York: McGraw-Hill Education; 2019.

Sherwood B. Acute inhalation injury. In: Occupational and environmental lung disease; 2020. p. 70–85.

Siwach SB, Singh H, Jagdish KVK, Bhardwaj G. Cardiac arrhythmias in aluminium phosphide poisoning studied by on continuous holter and cardioscopic monitoring. J Assoc Physicians India. 1998;46(7):598–601. https://www.ncbi.nlm.nih.gov/pubmed/12152839.

Skjolaas CA, Muck R, Holmes B. Silo gas and Silo-Filler's disease: safety notes. 2010. https://fyi.extension.wisc.edu/forage/silo-gas-and-silo-fillers-disease/. https://fyi.extension.wisc.edu/forage/silo-gas-and-silo-fillers-diseas.

Sokal JA, Kralkowska E. The relationship between exposure duration, carboxyhemoglobin, blood glucose, pyruvate and lactate and the severity of intoxication in 39 cases of acute carbon monoxide poisoning in man. Arch Toxicol. 1985;57(3):196–9. https://www.ncbi.nlm.nih.gov/pubmed/4062554. https://doi.org/10.1007/BF00290887.

Stewart RD, Peterson JE, Fisher TN, Hosko MJ, Baretta ED, Dodd HC, et al. Experimental human exposure to high concentrations of carbon monoxide. Arch Environ Health. 1973;26(1):1–7. https://doi.org/10.1080/00039896.1973.10666210.

Strickland J, Cummings A, Spinnato JA, Liccione JJ, Foureman GL. Toxicological review of hydrogen sulfide. Washington, DC: U.S. Environmental Protection Agency; 2003. https://cfpub.epa.gov/ncea/iris/iris_documents/documents/toxreviews/0061tr.pdf.

Tehrani H, Halvaie Z, Shadnia S, Soltaninejad K, Abdollahi M. Protective effects of N-acetylcysteine on aluminum phosphide-induced oxidative stress in acute human poisoning. Clin Toxicol (Phila). 2013;51(1):23–8. https://doi.org/10.3109/15563650.2012.743029.

Tomaszewski C. Chapter 122. Carbon monoxide. In: Nelson LS, Howland MA, Lewin NA, Smith SW, Goldfrank LR, Hoffman RS, editors. Goldfrank's toxicologic emergencies. 11th ed. New York: McGraw-Hill Education; 2019.

Truong DH, Eghbal MA, Hindmarsh W, Roth SH, O'Brien PJ. Molecular mechanisms of hydrogen sulfide toxicity. Drug Metab Rev. 2006;38(4):733–44. https://doi.org/10.1080/03602530600959607.

Weaver LK. Carbon monoxide poisoning. N Engl J Med. 2009;360:1217.

Weaver LK, Howe S, Hopkins R, Chan KJ. Carboxyhemoglobin half-life in carbon monoxide-poisoned patients treated with 100% oxygen at atmospheric pressure. Chest. 2000;117(3):801–8. https://doi.org/10.1378/chest.117.3.801.

Weaver LK, Hopkins RO, Chan KJ, Churchill S, Elliott CG, Clemmer TP, Orme JF, Thomas FO, Morris AH. Hyperbaric oxygen for acute carbon monoxide poisoning. N Engl J Med. 2002;347(14):1057–67. https://doi.org/10.1056/NEJMoa013121.

White CE, Park MS, Renz EM, Kim SH, Ritenour AE, Wolf SE, Cancio LC. Burn center treatment of patients with severe anhydrous ammonia injury: case reports and literature review. J Burn Care Res. 2007;28(6):922–8. https://www.ncbi.nlm.nih.gov/pubmed/17925646. https://doi.org/10.1097/BCR.0b013e318159a44e.

Wolf SJ, Maloney GE, Shih RD, Shy BD, Brown MD, American College of Emergency Physicians. Correction: Correction to 'clinical policy: critical issues in the evaluation and management of adult patients presenting to the emergency department with acute carbon monoxide poisoning' [annals of emergency medicine 69 (2017) 98–107.e6]. Ann Emerg Med. 2017;70(5):758. https://doi.org/10.1016/j.annemergmed.2017.03.036.

Yadav J, Athawal BK, Dubey BP, Yadav VK. Spontaneous ignition in case of celphos poisoning. Am J Forensic Med Pathol. 2007;28:353–5.

15 Welding Hazards

David Lipton

Introduction

Welding is an important part of farm operations to maintain, repair, and modify equipment, machinery, and facilities. On and off the farm, the welding process can be varied and complex. The National Institute for Occupational Safety and Health (NIOSH), lists over 80 different welding and allied processes (NIOSH 1988). On farms, the types of welding processes can be highly varied (Roehl 2007).

Welding fuses metals together under intense heat and is the strongest way to bond metals. Other allied processes include brazing and soldering. Brazing joins metal pieces with fillers to bond parts together. The melting point of the filler materials is lower than that of the base metals. Brazed joints have less strength than welded joints. Soldering uses filler materials at lower temperature than brazing. Soldered joints have less strength that brazed joints. The most common uses for soldering include the assembly of electronic components, plumbing, and assembly of jewelry and decorative items (NIOSH 1988).

On farms, welding in confined spaces can be an especially hazardous activity. Confined spaces are places not intended for human occupancy but are large enough for a worker to enter. They have limited or restricted means of entry or exit and limited air flow. Farming operations must identify confined spaces and develop safe entry procedures for these spaces before working inside them (OSHA 2018). Welding may occur on equipment or in locations that do not meet the strict criteria of a confined space but may still have limited airflow for ventilation.

Welding Processes

Welding fuses metal parts together under heat by electrical arcs or high-temperature flames. Arc welding uses intense heat (at least 6500 °F) to melt the metal at the joint between the workpieces (TWI 2024a). Gas welding uses intense heat created by the combustion of oxygen and fuel gases to create the high temperature needed to fuse the base metal parts (TWI 2021).

In arc welding, an electric arc is applied between consumable or nonconsumable electrodes and the workpieces to be joined. Consumable electrodes are manually or mechanically fed into the arc and melt into or on the pool of molten metal. Consumable electrodes often contain fluxes, inert agents added to the electrode for better conduction of electric current, to prevent oxidation and contamination. The American Welding Society classifies electrodes using an alphanu-

D. Lipton (✉)
North Carolina Department of Health and Human Services, Occupational and Environmental Epidemiology Branch, Raleigh, NC, USA
e-mail: david.lipton@dhhs.nc.gov

W. J. Meggs, R. L. Langley (eds.), *Farm Toxicology*, https://doi.org/10.1007/978-3-031-80441-0_15

meric system that identifies whether the product is a stick electrode, solid wire, or tubular wire and the chemistry, composition (fillers and fluxes), and type of shielding gas if required (Hobart Brothers 2023). Safety data sheets and manufacturer specification sheets can supply users with information to select appropriate electrodes for the task and understand associated hazards.

In all welding processes, the base metals and filler materials react under intense heat with oxygen, nitrogen, and other air contaminants. Welds are protected by shielding gases, either supplied from compressed gas cylinders or generated by consumable electrodes. The fluxes in consumable electrodes are nonmetal ingredients that form slag under the intense heat of welding. Slag is a glass-like (vitreous) material that solidifies before the weld, protecting the joint from contamination. After the weld has cooled, the slag is removed by chipping and grinding (TWI 2021).

Consumable Electrode Methods

Metal Inert Gas (MIG) Welding

Metal inert gas welding (MIG) is a common type of consumable electrode arc welding. Sometimes, MIG welding is called gas metal arc welding (GMAW). A welding gun supplies the consumable electrode, typically a wire fed from a spool along with a shielding gas to protect the weld. Shielding gases are either argon or helium, supplied from compressed gas cylinders.

Shielded Metal Arc Welding (SMAW)

Also known as manual metal arc welding (MMAW) or flux shield arc welding (FSAW), SMAW (commonly called stick welding) uses consumable electrodes, which when consumed, produce shielding gases, filler metal, and slag. It is versatile and can be used to join ferrous and nonferrous materials in a wide range of thicknesses. No compressed gas cylinders are required.

Hardfacing

Hardfacing is a form of manual metal arc welding used to protect and extend the service life or minimize wear by adding a metal layer to the wear surfaces to protect them from damage. Hardfacing can be used for buildup or rebuilding, overlays, or a combination. Consumable electrodes can be low-alloy iron-base alloys that contain chromium, molybdenum, and manganese. High-alloy hardfacing electrodes contain 12–50% alloy content with the addition of nickel (Ni) and cobalt or cobalt–chromium–tungsten alloys and tungsten carbide materials (Pradeep et al. 2010). Little research is available about how consumable electrodes used for hardfacing contribute to welder exposure to air contaminants.

Flux-Cored Arc Welding (FCAW)

An alternative to SMAW, FCAW uses a continuously fed consumable flux-cored electrode. Shielding gases and fluxes are produced as the electrode is consumed to protect the weld from contamination.

Submerged Arc Welding (SAW)

Another variant of shield metal arc welding uses consumable electrodes, which create a conductive blanket of flux that involves the formation of an electric arc path between the part to be welded and the electrode. The flux also helps prevent spatter and sparks while suppressing fumes and ultraviolet (UV) radiation.

Nonconsumable Electrode Methods

Tungsten Inert Gas (TIG) Welding

Also known as gas tungsten arc welding (GTAW), TIG welding uses a nonconsumable tungsten electrode to create the arc and an inert shielding gas to protect the weld against atmospheric contamination. Simultaneously, filler materials may be added via a filler rod in the welder's other hand.

Steel, stainless steel, chromoly steel, aluminum, nickel alloys, magnesium, copper, brass, bronze, and even gold can be TIG-welded. TIG welding allows for precise control of the weld puddle when appearances are important for the final weld. Fewer sparks and spatter are produced in TIG welding, with no flux or slag to chip away compared to the consumable arc weldiing process.

Plasma Arc Welding (PAW)

Like TIG welding, PAW uses an electric arc between a nonconsumable electrode and an anode, which are placed within the body of the torch. The electric arc is used to ionize the gas in the torch and create plasma, which is then pushed through a fine borehole (TWI 2024a).

Oxyacetylene Welding

Oxyacetylene welding, commonly referred to as gas welding, is a process that relies on the combustion of oxygen and acetylene or other fuel gases. When mixed in correct proportions in a hand handheld torch or blowpipe, the flame can reach about 6000 °F. Fuel gases, supplied from compressed gas cylinders, are most often acetylene and occasionally methylacetylene-propadiene stabilized gas (MAPP™), propylene, natural gas, and propane. Oxygen is also supplied from a compressed gas cylinder. The fuel gases and oxygen are regulated to the proper mixture for complete combustion and high temperature. Oxyacetylene welding is most often used to weld or cut thin metal pieces. Since the temperature can be controlled, it can also be used for heating tasks, heating heavy stock for bending, brazing, and soldering (TWI 2024b).

Hazards of Welding

Hazards are conditions that may cause harm. Welders, helpers, and nearby persons are exposed to multiple chemical and physical hazards. Chemical hazards include exposure to components of welding fume, a complex mixture of metals, metallic oxides, silicates, and fluorides and their condensation/oxidation products, other particulate matter, and a variety of gases. Physical hazards include electric shock; intense ultraviolet, visible, and infrared (IR) radiation; noise; injuries from handling materials (workpieces and compressed gas cylinders); and heat-related injuries and illnesses.

Risks of Welding

Risks are the probability and severity of harm from a hazard. Farmers and farmworkers are exposed daily to chemical agents, physical agents, and biological agents. Previous and/or concurrent occupational exposures, among other factors, can influence the overall health of the farming population. Epidemiological studies on health effects from welding in agricultural settings, especially for chronic and long-term exposures, cannot be isolated and studied without considering these variables. For these reasons, there are few high-quality studies on the health risks of welders in farming.

Several challenges are present when evaluating the potential risks of welding on farms. There are a variety of welding processes, electrodes, and base metals. There is a lack of high-quality data on the composition of metal fumes and gases in the welder's breathing zones. There is also little data on the extent, use, and effectiveness of engineering controls, administrative controls, work practices, and personal protective equipment to control exposures in farmers (AWS-1 1979).

Occupational Illnesses Associated with Welding

Metal Fume Fever

A common acute illness associated with welding is metal fume fever. Metal fume fever is a flu-like illness with symptoms including headache, fever, chills, muscle aches, thirst, nausea, vomiting, chest soreness, fatigue, gastrointestinal pain, weakness, and tiredness. The symptoms usually start several hours after exposure; the attack may last 6–24 h. Complete recovery occurs without intervention within 24–48 h. Metal fume fever is more likely to occur after a period away from the job, on Mondays, or after vacations. Zinc from welding on galvanized metals is the most common cause of metal fume fever although other metals including aluminum, cadmium, and copper are also associated with this disorder (Ahsan et al. 2009).

Chemical Pneumonitis

Very high levels of fumes from cadmium, chromium, or nickel can cause chemical pneumonitis, but this is uncommon (Jenkins and Pechter 2017). Other inhalational chemical hazards in the work environment may include ozone and nitrogen oxides from arc processes, exhausts from generators and vehicles, solvents, oils, and thermal byproducts of organics that can include phosgene.

Pneumonia

There is an increase in the incidence and severity of pulmonary infections in welders with an excess in mortality from pneumonia (Jenkins and Pechter 2017). This is thought to be due to chronic chemical irritation of the airway epithelium or perhaps from a subtle immunosuppression caused by the inhalation of metal oxide fume particles or halide salts used as welding fluxes. Some research has suggested that welders are at greater risk than the general public for developing lower-airway infections due to *Streptococcus pneumonia* (Suri et al. 2016).

Occupational Asthma

There are case reports (Vandenplas et al. 1995; Hannu et al. 2007; MSU 2010) of occupational asthma in welders. Asthma is an obstructive respiratory disease that includes both airway hypersensitivity and irritation of the linings of the airways. The agents causing or aggravating asthma from welding cannot be definitively identified since welding fumes are a complex mixture of metal oxide particulates and irritant gases. Vandenplas et al. (1995) postulate that chromium and nickel are part of the underlying cause of hypersensitivity reactions characteristic of asthma due to the fact that trivalent (Cr +3), hexavalent (Cr +6) (Bregnbak et al. 2015), and nickel (Ahlström et al. 2019) are known to cause allergic contact dermatitis. The Association of Occupational and Environmental Clinics labels stainless steel welding and gas metal arc welding of mild steel as capable of causing asthma (AOEC 2009–2012).

Pneumoconiosis

Siderosis is a pneumoconiosis resulting from significant iron accumulation in the lungs; it is common in steel welders and is usually benign without significant changes in pulmonary function. Rarely, it may lead to pulmonary fibrosis. Chronic tin inhalation can present similarly to siderosis. Welders may work in shipyards or other environments with potential asbestos exposure, putting them at risk of asbestosis and other asbestos-related lung diseases. In addition, welders often use grinding and machining tools; abrasives may release crystalline silica and machining may release hard metal carbides of tungsten, cobalt, titanium, or tantalum, creating the risk of silicosis or interstitial lung disease, respectively (Jenkins and Pechter 2017). An interstitial lung disease known as hard metal lung disease has been observed in welders who used powdered tungsten carbide (WC) and cobalt while welding to produce a welded material, a process called sintering, hence the term “sintered carbides” or cemented carbides (Mizutani et al. 2016).

Bronchitis and Chronic Obstructive Pulmonary Disease (COPD)

Welders and others exposed to dust, gases, and fumes have an increased rate of noninfectious chronic bronchitis (cough on most days for 3 or more months for two consecutive years) (Jenkins and Pechter 2017). Meldrum et al. (2005) found that welding was an occupation associated with an increased prevalence of COPD.

Cancer

The International Agency for Research on Cancer (IARC) has classified arsenic, beryllium, cadmium, and hexavalent chromium as group 1 carcinogens, agents with sufficient evidence of causing cancer in humans and animals. Ultraviolet light is also a group 1 carcinogen with sufficient evidence to cause cancer in humans and animals (IARC 2012).

The National Toxicology Program has classified hexavalent chromium (Cr +6) and nickel and nickel compounds from welding on stainless steel as human carcinogens (NTP 2021a, b).

A study of cancer risk among Canadian welders found elevated risks for lung cancer, mesothelioma, bladder cancer, and kidney cancer. When restricted to blue-collar workers, lung cancer and mesothelioma risks were attenuated, while bladder and kidney cancer risks increased. A confounder is that the excess risk of lung cancer and mesothelioma may be partly attributable to factors including smoking and asbestos. Welding-specific exposures may increase bladder and kidney cancer risks, and particular sources of exposure should be investigated (MacLeod et al. 2017).

Specific Contaminants Generated During Welding

Metal Fume

Metal fume is formed as metals vaporize when in contact with an intense electric arc or hot flames. Vaporization is a change of state from a solid to a vapor. Metals often oxidize when vaporized. Vaporized metals typically start as particles less than 1 μm in diameter. Metal vapors quickly cool, condense, and agglomerate into particles with a size range of 1–7 μm (Cena et al. 2014).

The hazards associated with metal fumes are dependent on the particle size in the fumes. Particle size is a major determinant of where the particles may deposit in the respiratory tract and the level of bioavailability. As the particle size decreases, their ability to penetrate deeper into the respiratory system increases. In addition, as particle size decreases, diffusion has a stronger effect and further increases deposition rates in all regions of the respiratory system.

Particles greater than 10 μm in diameter tend to settle quickly from air and if inhaled, deposit in the oral–pharyngeal region (nose and mouth). Particles with a diameter between 2 and 10 μm tend to penetrate deeper into the lungs and deposit in the tracheobronchial region of the respiratory tract. Particles between 0.2 and 5 μm in diameter can penetrate deep into the respiratory bronchioles and alveoli (air exchange regions).

Particle size of about 0.3 μm diameter is known as the most penetrating particle size (MPSS). Deposition of particles larger than MPSS tends to be driven by impaction and interception. Particles less than 0.3 μm are in the diffusion regime. The effects of diffusion tend to increase as particles become smaller than the MPSS. Particles less than 0.1 μm tend to behave like gases. At the size of 0.3 μm, all the filtration methods, interception, impaction, and diffusion are the least effective. Because of this phenomenon, high efficiency particulate air (HEPA) filters are tested against 0.3-μm aerosol (Lee and Liu 1980).

Particle size also plays a role in interaction with the systems, organs, and cells. As particle size decreases, the surface area to volume area of a particle increases, which increases the potential for irritation, inflammation, and uptake of toxic substances. Other factors that influence the extent and location of particle deposition include density and shape, airway geometry, and the individual's breathing pattern (Cena et al. 2014).

When consumable electrode methods are used, sources of vaporized metals include base metals, metals in fillers, and components of fluxes. The base metals are the primary sources of metal fumes in nonconsumable electrodes and oxyacetylene welding or cutting. Metal vaporization from alloys depends on alloys, the temperature at which the metals vaporize, and the voltage and amperage of the arc. Aluminum, cadmium, cobalt, chromium, copper, iron, lead, manganese, magnesium, molybdenum, nickel, titanium, and zinc as metal oxides can be present in welding fumes. Metal fumes generated from welding on stainless steel usually contain chromium, iron, manganese, and nickel (Fe, Cr, Mn, and Ni) compared to mild steel, which may contain mostly iron.

Hazards of Specific Metals

Aluminum

Vandenplas et al. (1995) report a case of occupational asthma thought to be related to flux-cored manual metal arc welding on aluminum. Aluminum has also been associated with metal fume fever.

Cadmium

Small amounts of cadmium are found in several types of flux-cored electrodes (AWS-V 1985). Occasionally, cadmium can be found in anti-rust paint and, occasionally, electroplated onto steel, nuts, bolts, and rivets. Short-term inhalational exposure to cadmium is associated with metal fume fever. Chronic and long-term exposure to cadmium oxide fume is associated with kidney damage because cadmium causes chronic renal tubular damage. Long-term exposure to cadmium is also associated with pulmonary emphysema and bone diseases such as osteomalacia and osteoporosis. Cadmium exposure may also cause anemia, teeth discoloration, and loss of smell (MIOSHA 2020).

Copper

The highest copper concentrations are found when copper and its alloys are welded. Another minor source is copper-coated gas metal arc electrodes. Inhalation of copper oxide fumes may cause irritation of the upper respiratory tract and may result in a form of metal fume fever, characterized by flu-like symptoms such as chills, fever, nausea, and vomiting.

Chromium

Chromium fume is generated when welding stainless steel and steel alloys containing chromium. Chromium exists in various oxidation states from 0 to +6. Of these oxidation states, the best known are 0, +2, +3, and +6. Chromium in its +3-oxidation state (trivalent) is the most stable, including chromic oxide and chromic chloride. Hexavalent chromium (Cr +6) compounds are important industrially; examples include chromium oxide (CrO_3), chromates, and dichromates.

Chromium (III) trivalent is known to be a respiratory irritant and asthma trigger. Chromium VI is classified as a known human carcinogen.

Lead

Lead vaporizes at about 800 °F. Welding on metals containing lead alloys or painted with lead-based paint causes massive release of lead fumes, which are known health hazards. Lead-based paint was commonly used on agricultural machinery and structures due to its durability and corrosion resistance.

Manganese

Manganese oxide is used as a flux agent in the coatings of shielded metal arc electrodes, in the core of flux-cored arc electrodes, and as an alloying element in the steel used in electrodes. Some special steels containing high manganese may produce high concentrations of manganese oxide in the fume.

A longitudinal cohort study among welders examined the relationship between exposure to manganese in welding fumes and movement disorders, called parkinsonism. The study found that the progression of parkinsonism increased with cumulative manganese exposure. The association between welding exposure and parkinsonism progression appeared particularly marked in welders who did flux-cored arc welding in a confined space or workers whose baseline examination was within 5 years of the first welding exposure (Racette et al. 2017).

Nickel

Nickel is present in stainless steel (typically 8–15%) and nickel alloys. Some nickel compounds have been identified as carcinogens, and some research indicates that welding fumes containing nickel, chromium, and other metals may be potentially mutagenic (IARC 2012).

Zinc

Metal fume fever is the name for an illness that is caused primarily by exposure to zinc oxide fumes (ZnO) in the workplace. The main cause of this exposure is usually breathing in the fumes from welding, cutting, or brazing on galvanized metal. Iron and steel are protected against rusting by submerging them in a bath of hot molten zinc (i.e., galvanizing). Studies indicate that the most common cause of metal fume fever is overexposure to zinc fumes from welding, burning, or brazing galvanized steel. Other elements, such as copper and magnesium, may cause similar effects.

Hazards of Specific Gases

Toxic gases, including ozone (O_3), nitrogen oxides (NO_x), carbon dioxide, and carbon monoxide, are generated during common arc welding processes. The types and amounts of gases depend on the welding process. Inert shielding gases that reduce oxidation in SAW, GMAW, and TIG welding reduce the generation of gases produced compared to MMAW. In contrast, intense ultraviolet light in GMAW and TIG welding can intensify the photochemical formation of gases such as O_3 and NO_x (Riccelli et al. 2020).

Ozone

Ozone is a strong oxidant produced by the photochemical reactions of oxygen in the air in the presence of ultraviolet light. It produces reactive oxygen species in tissues and alters pulmonary function and bronchial responsiveness. Ozone is produced when oxygen reacts with ultraviolet light in the wavelength range of 185 nm. It is a severe respiratory irritant; exposure to levels above 0.3 parts per million parts of air (ppm) can cause extreme discomfort while exposure to 10 ppm for several hours can cause pulmonary edema. Ozone is unstable in the air and its decomposition may be accelerated by metal oxide fumes. The amounts of ozone produced by welding vary depending on the base metal, the type of welding activity, and the composition of electrodes. Plasma arc cutting appears to produce the greatest amount of ozone (Liu et al. 2007).

Oxides of Nitrogen

Oxides of nitrogen are products of oxidation reactions between nitrogen and oxygen in the air and reactions between oxygen and nitrogen in the presence of intense ultraviolet light. At low levels, oxides of nitrogen are irritants to mucus membranes of the respiratory tract. Longer-term and higher exposures can exacerbate preexisting lung disease, irritate alveoli and bronchioles, and cause pulmonary edema. In extreme cases, exposure to oxides of nitrogen is associated with bronchiolitis obliterans and an increase in methemoglobin in the blood (Jones et al. 1973; ATSDR 2014a).

Carbon Monoxide

Carbon monoxide (CO) is a byproduct of the incomplete combustion of carbonaceous materials present in electrodes and is present during oxyfuel gas welding. Welding for maintenance and repairs often occurs in the field. Portable generators or portable welding machines using gasoline as a fuel source may be used and generate CO. Carbon monoxide from these combustion sources may accumulate in poorly ventilated areas (CPSC 2022), resulting in CO poisoning (asphyxiation may occur with high exposure levels).

Carbon Dioxide

Carbon dioxide (CO_2) is also a product of combustion during oxyfuel welding from incomplete combustion of carbonates or organic materials in electrodes. It can also be a byproduct of Metal

Active Gas welding (MAG) welding. At low concentrations, gaseous carbon dioxide appears to have little toxicological effect. At higher concentrations, it leads to an increased respiratory rate, tachycardia, cardiac arrhythmias, and impaired consciousness. Concentrations >10% may cause convulsions, coma, and death (Langford 2005).

Phosphine

Phosphine (PH_3) is a colorless gas with a garlic-like or decaying fish–like odor. It can be generated as a byproduct when welding metals coated with phosphate-based corrosion inhibitors (Work safe Alberta 2009). Most phosphine exposures occur by inhalation of the gas or ingestion of metallic phosphides (usually of a pesticide), but dermal exposure to phosphides can also cause systemic effects. Phosphine is a respiratory-tract irritant that attacks primarily the cardiovascular and respiratory systems, causing peripheral vascular collapse, cardiac arrest and failure, and pulmonary edema (ATSDR 2014b).

Phosgene

Phosgene, having the chemical formula $COCl_2$, is a colorless gas with an odor like musty hay. It is formed by the decomposition of chlorinated hydrocarbon solvents exposed to ultraviolet light. It reacts with moisture in the lungs to produce hydrogen chloride, which in turn destroys lung tissues. For this reason, any use of chlorinated solvents should be far away from welding operations or any operation in which ultraviolet radiation or intense heat is generated (Nieuwenhuizen and Groeneveld. 2000).

Other Particulate Matter

Other particulate matter can be generated based on the composition of the electrodes used for arc welding including silica, silicates, and fluorides. Silica is often a component in shielded metal arc electrodes and from the flux composition of flux-cored arc electrodes. Fluoride compounds may also be present on the coverings of shielded metal arc electrodes or the flux and slag compositions of flux-cored arc electrodes or submerged arc welding.

Other Hazards

Light: Ultraviolet, Visible, and Infrared Radiation

All welding processes emit intense ultraviolet, visible, and infrared light. However, the spectrum and intensity will differ based on the welding process, electrode size, applied current, base metal, and composition of the electrodes. Damage to the skin or eyes can be caused by physical injury or photochemical reactions.

Ultraviolet light is subdivided into UV-A (wavelengths in the range of 315–400 nm), UV-B (280–315 nm), and UV-C (100–280 nm). Visible light has a wavelength between approximately 380 nm and approximately 760 nm. Of special concern is blue light with a wavelength between 380 and 550 nm. Infrared light is subdivided into near-infrared (760–1400 nm), mid-infrared (1400–3000 nm), and far-infrared (3000 nm–1 mm). The type of effect, injury thresholds, and damage mechanisms vary significantly with wavelength and may overlap (Flores 2018).

Ultraviolet Light

Ultraviolet (UV) radiation interacts strongly with living organisms. The short wavelength and relatively high photon energy can excite electrons and photochemical reactions. Ultraviolet radiation is part of the spectrum of ionizing radiation (high UV frequencies) while visible and infrared are not. Intense ultraviolet light is absorbed by the cornea. Short-term high-intensity exposure to ultraviolet light causes irritant and inflammatory responses called keratoconjunctivitis, also known as flash burn, welders' flash, or arc eye.

Like sunburn, effects from prolonged and repeated exposure to ultraviolet light can be cumulative including an increased risk for cataracts and epidermoid carcinoma of the bulbar conjunctiva (Takahashi et al. 2020).

Exposure to UV light may occur when face shields are not in place before striking an arc. Helpers and others adjacent to welding activities may be exposed to UV light if they are not wearing appropriate personal protective equipment. Welding is just one of the many ways that agricultural workers are exposed to ultraviolet light.

Visible Light

When exposed suddenly to a highly intense visible light source, most people exhibit an aversion response that includes blinking and turning their heads. The aversion response is quick, often less than 0.25 s. Short bursts of high-intensity visible light (<0.25 s) may cause "flash blindness," a temporary and reversible condition (US Navy 1963).

Blue-light retinal injury can result from viewing either an extremely bright light for a short duration or a less bright light for a longer duration. Measurement of the spectral radiance of the sun has shown that the exposure limits for blue light can easily be exceeded when viewing the sun. Directly viewing the sun is very hazardous and should be avoided. Even typical or "normal" outdoor exposure to sunlight can result in damage to the retina over a period of many years. Lifelong exposure to the blue-light portion or possibly the entire visible spectrum of ambient sunlight can increase the risk of age-related macular degeneration, a leading cause of blindness in older persons.

Longer-term exposure to intensive visible light can suppress the aversion response, and staring directly at a high-intensity light source, such as the sun during an eclipse or arc welding activities can cause photo retinopathy, which is thought to be more related to photochemical damage than thermal injury (Magnavitia 2002).

Infrared Light

Infrared (IR) light is absorbed by tissues and converted to heat. The eyes and skin are the organs most susceptible to damage by infrared radiation. Thermal injury is strongly dependent upon heat conduction from the irradiated tissue. When exposure is less intense, surrounding tissue conducts heat away from the exposed site. In general, shorter exposures require higher temperatures to produce the same degree of damage. The injury from accidental exposure to arc lamps or the sun, for example, is both thermal and photochemical.

IR radiation below 3000 nm will penetrate different depths of the cornea to varying degrees, depending on the specific wavelength. The iris can absorb energy only at wavelengths below approximately 1300 nm. IR thermal injury may have significant biological effects on the human skin. The IR rays induce free radicals in the dermis and diminish the skin's antioxidant capacity, the main cause of premature skin aging. Both the skin and the cornea are opaque to wavelengths >1400 nm. Exposure to IR radiation in this region causes injury through thermal mechanisms, with absorbed radiation being converted to heat.

The most common eye disease associated with near-infrared radiation is cataracts. Prolonged exposure to IR radiation causes a gradual but irreversible opacity of the lens. Other forms of damage to the eye from IR exposure include formation of scotoma, which is a loss of vision due to the damage to the retina. Even low-level IR absorption can cause symptoms such as redness of the eye, swelling, or hemorrhaging.

Cataracts caused by near-infrared radiation have been noted historically in glassblowers and furnace workers. Radiation between 800 and 1200 nm is most likely responsible for temperature increases in the lens itself because of its spectral absorption characteristics. Visible wavelengths may also contribute to the problem since the heat absorbed by the iris could result in heat transfer to the lens. The US Department of Labor has guidance on selecting appropriately shaded lenses in welding helmets and goggles (OSHA 2012).

Noise

Welding activities are loud. MMAW, MIG welding, flame-cutting, grinding, and chipping to remove slag create high noise levels between 95 and 105 Decibels on the A-Weighted Scale adjusted to reflect the sensitivity of the human ear (dBA), depending on the diameter of consumable electrodes, the current, the type and thickness of metals being welded, and other factors. Noise is the sound pressure level measured in decibels. The dBA scale measures the sound pressure level weighted to the sensitivity of the human ear to frequencies in the 3000–5000-hertz spectrum. The frequency and duration of exposure to noise are essential to assess exposure.

Noise exposure is assessed based on the sound pressure level and exchange rate (dose). The exchange rate defines the increase or decrease in the sound level for a corresponding halving or doubling of the exposure time. For example, the OSHA–permissible exposure limit is 90 dBA with a 5-dB exchange rate. This means that a worker can be exposed to 90 dBA for 8 h, 95 dBA for 4 h, 100 dBA for 2 h, and 105 dBA for 1 h. Other recommendations include an 8 h limit of 85 dBA with a 3-dB exchange rate (ACGIH 2016).

OSHA requires a hearing conservation program when workers are exposed to 85 dBA for 8 h (50% dose). Although the actual time that high noise levels are generated during welding may be quite short, they can contribute to the daily dose of other hazardous sounds on a farm from equipment and operations. Even without measuring sound pressure levels, it is important to reduce noise from equipment through maintenance and isolation. Exposures can also be reduced by scheduling and rotating workers away from extended noise exposure areas. When these controls fail to reduce noise levels or are not feasible and administrative actions fail to decrease noise levels to acceptable levels, personal protective equipment (PPE) such as ear muffs or ear plugs are required. Plugs and muffs are ranked by their noise reduction rating (NRR), an estimate of the noise level reduced by the hearing protector. For example, in a 105-dBA work area, a device with an NRR of 25 dB would suggest an exposure level of 80 dBA. This assumes a perfect fit and that the worker is wearing the hearing protector the entire time that he or she is exposed to the 105-dBA noise level. Numerous field studies suggest that perfect wearing and use of hearing protection is rarely achieved. Most safety and health professionals discount the NRR on ear plugs and muffs by up to 50% (PSU 2022).

Electric Shock

Arc welding is generally a safe activity when the electric current path to the ground has less resistance through the welding equipment and workpieces compared to the path to the ground through the worker. Electric shock hazards are controlled by proper grounding; keeping equipment and cables in good condition; and avoiding standing in water, working on wet surfaces, working with wet hands, or wearing sweaty garments. Insulating gloves and boots and the use of insulating mats can reduce the potential for electric shock (CCOSH 2024).

Compressed Gases

Any compressed gas cylinders used in welding processes must be properly stored, handled, maintained, and used. Gas cylinders must be stored in an upright position and secured against falling or being knocked over, preferably in a gas cylinder cart or stand. Never move gas cylinders by rolling them on the ground. Always keep the protective safety cap on compressed gas cylinders when not in use (Oregon OSHA 2015).

Ergonomic and Traumatic Injuries

Welding activities can present several physical hazards to workers and helpers. Work materials may have sharp edges capable of causing cuts to exposed skin and penetrating eye injuries.

Sparks and flying slag are hot and may burn the worker if they contact his/her body. In addition, work areas must be free of combustible or flammable materials. Occasionally, welding activities (especially in confined spaces) can cause fires or explosions when the atmosphere is oxygen-enriched.

Large workpieces may be bulky or heavy and require lifting and placement in awkward positions. Holding pieces to be welded together, proper positioning of welding equipment, and positioning the body to observe the weld can place the welder in awkward positions and increase the risk of musculoskeletal injuries.

Shoulder pain and, more specifically, supraspinatus tendonitis appear to be associated with welding. The working theory is that a welder's shoulder may be in an awkward position with a high static load for lengthy periods of time (AWS-VI 1989). Body, posture, muscle force, repetition, duration, and frequency of activities influence the risk of injury.

Conclusion

The knowledge skills and ability to perform welding on a farm for maintenance, repair, or alteration of equipment, machinery, and facilities are essential to keep farms operational and productive. Unlike many activities on a farm, welding may be periodic and occur under expedient conditions. Nevertheless, hazard and risk assessments are required before welding, along with planning, preparation, and practice to ensure safe and successful work practices.

References

ACGIH (American Conference of Governmental Industrial Hygienists). TLVs® and BEIs® based on the documentation of the threshold limit values for chemical substances & biological exposure indices. 2016.

Ahlström MG, Thyssen JP, Wennervaldt M, Menné T, Johansen JD. Nickel allergy and allergic contact dermatitis: a clinical review of immunology, epidemiology, exposure, and treatment. Contact Dermatitis. 2019;81:227–41. https://doi.org/10.1111/cod.13327.

Ahsan SA, Lackovic M, Katner A, Palermo C. Metal fume fever: a review of the literature and cases reported to the Louisiana poison control center. J La State Med Soc. 2009;161(6):348–51.

AOEC (Association of Occupational and Environmental Clinics). Search welding in the look-up list. 2009–2012. http://www.aoecdata.org/ExpCodeLookup.aspx.

ATSDR (Agency for Toxic Substances and Disease Registry). Medical management guidelines for nitrogen oxides. 2014a. https://wwwn.cdc.gov/TSP/MMG/MMGDetails.aspx?mmgid=394&toxid=69.

ATSDR (Agency for Toxic Substances and Disease Registry). Medical management guidelines for phosphine. 2014b. https://wwwn.cdc.gov/TSP/MMG/MMGDetails.aspx?mmgid=1013&toxid=214.

AWS (American Welding Society). Effects of welding on health, I. 1979. https://aws-p-001-delivery.sitecorecontenthub.cloud/api/public/content/Effects-of-Welding-on-Health.

AWS (American Welding Society). Effects of welding on health, V. 1985.

AWS (American Welding Society). Effects of welding on health, VI. 1989.

Bregnbak D, Johansen JD, Jellesen MS, Zachariae C, Menné T, Thyssen JP. Chromium allergy and dermatitis: prevalence and main findings. Contact Dermatitis. 2015;73(5):261–80. https://doi.org/10.1111/cod.12436.

CCOSH (Canadian Center For Occupational Safety and Health). Welding electrical safety. 2024. https://www.ccohs.ca/oshanswers/safety_haz/welding/electric.html.

Cena LG, Chisholm WP, Keane MJ, Cumpston A, Chen BT. Size distribution and estimated respiratory deposition of total chromium, hexavalent chromium, manganese, and nickel in gas metal arc welding fume aerosols. Aerosol Sci Tech. 2014;48(12):1254–63.

CPSC (Consumer Product Safety Commission). Fatal incidents associated with non-fire carbon monoxide poisoning from engine-driven generators and other engine driven tools, 2011–2021. 2022. https://www.cpsc.gov/s3fs-public/Fatal-Incidents-Associated-with-Non-Fire-Carbon-Monoxide-Poisioning-from-Engine-Driven-Generators-and-Other-Engine-Driven-Tools-2011-2021.pdf?VersionId=w1it1Z8oqRDGpO9AzW5Bft.gdXClrCh.

Flores CL. Light and infrared radiation, Lawrence Berkley National Laboratories. 2018. https://ehs.lbl.gov/resource/documents/radiation-protection/non-ionizing-radiation/light-and-infrared-radiation/.

Hannu T, Piipari R, Tuppurainen M, Nordman H, Tuomi T. Occupational asthma caused by stainless steel welding fumes: a clinical study. Eur Respir J. 2007;29:85–90. https://doi.org/10.1183/09031936.0005810.

Hobart Brothers. Basics of AWS filler metal and electrode classification. 2023. https://www.hobartbrothers.com/resources/technical-articles/electrode-classification/.

IARC (International Agency for Research on Cancer). Arsenic, metals, fibres, and dusts. In: A review of human carcinogens, vol. 100C. Lyon: IARC; 2012.

Jenkins N, Pechter E. Welding—impact on occupational health. Occupational lung disease bulletin. Massachusetts Department of Public Health; 2017. https://www.mass.gov/doc/winter-2017-2018-welding-impact-on-occupational-health/download.

Jones GR, Proudfoot AT, Hall JI. Pulmonary effects of acute exposure to nitrous fumes. Thorax. 1973;28(1):61–5.

Langford NJ. Carbon dioxide poisoning. Toxicol Rev. 2005;24(4):229–35. https://doi.org/10.2165/00139709-200524040-00003.

Lee KW, Liu BYH. On the minimum efficiency and the Most penetrating particle size for fibrous filters K. J Air Pollut Control Assoc. 1980;30(4):377–81. https://doi.org/10.1080/00022470.1980.10464592.

Liu HH, Wu YC, Chen HL. Production of ozone and reactive oxygen species after welding. Arch Environ Contam Toxicol. 2007;53:513–8.

MacLeod JS, Harris MA, Tjepkema M, Peters PA, Demers PA. Cancer risks among welders and occasional welders in a National Population-Based Cohort Study: Canadian Census Health and Environmental Cohort. Saf Health Work. 2017;8(3):258–66. https://doi.org/10.1016/j.shaw.2016.12.001.

Magnavitia N. Photoretinitis: an underestimated occupational injury? Occup Med (Lond). 2002;52(4):223–5. https://doi.org/10.1093/occmed/52.4.223.

Meldrum M, Rawbone R, Curran AD, Fishwick D. The role of occupation in the development of chronic obstructive pulmonary disease (COPD). Occup Environ Med. 2005;62(4):212–4. https://doi.org/10.1136/oem.2004.015511.

MIOSHA (Michigan Occupational safety and Health Administration). MIOSHA Fact Sheet Cadmium Exposure in Construction. 2020. https://www.michigan.gov/leo/-/media/Project/Websites/leo/Documents/MIOSHA/Fact-Sheets/CSHD/Fact_C004.pdf.

Mizutani RF, Terra-Filho M, Lima E, Freitas CS, Chate RC, Kairalla RA, Carvalho-Oliveira R, Santos UP. Hard metal lung disease: a case series. J Bras Pneumol. 2016;42(6):447–52. https://doi.org/10.1590/S1806-37562016000000260.

MSU (Michigan State University College of Human Medicine). Asthma and welding Project Sensor News. Fall. 2010;21(4). https://oem.msu.edu/images/newsletter/ProjectSensor/v21n4.pdf.

Nieuwenhuizen MS, Groeneveld FR. Formation of phosgene during welding activities in an atmosphere containing chlorinated hydrocarbons. AIHAJ. 2000;61(4):539–43. https://doi.org/10.1080/15298660008984566.

NIOSH (National Institute for Occupational Safety and Health). Criteria for a Recommended Standard, Welding Brazing and Thermal Cutting, NIOSH Publication Number Publication 88-11. 1988. https://www.cdc.gov/niosh/docs/88-110/default.html.

NTP (National Toxicology Program Report on Carcinogens). Profile on chromium hexavalent compounds. 2021a. https://ntp.niehs.nih.gov/sites/default/files/ntp/roc/content/profiles/chromiumhexavalentcompounds.pdf.

NTP (National Toxicology Program Report on Carcinogens). Profile on nickel and nickel compounds. 2021b. https://ntp.niehs.nih.gov/sites/default/files/ntp/roc/content/profiles/nickel.pdf.

Oregon OSHA. Compressed gas safety. OR-OSHA (5/15) FS-09. 2015. https://osha.oregon.gov/OSHAPubs/factsheets/fs09.pdf.

OSHA (US Department of Labor, Occupational Safety and Health Administration). OSHA fact sheet protection against radiant energy during welding and cutting in shipyard employment. 2012. https://www.osha.gov/sites/default/files/publications/OSHAfactsheet-eyeprotection-during-welding.pdf.

OSHA (US Department of Labor, Occupational Safety and Health Administration). Fatal Facts Confined Space Entry on Farm No 16–2018. 2018. https://www.osha.gov/sites/default/files/publications/OSHA3939.pdf.

Pradeep GRC, Ramesh A, Prasad BD. A review paper on hard facing processes and materials. Int J Eng Sci Technol. 2010;2(11):6507–10.

PSU (Pennsylvania State University Cooperative Extension Service). Noise induced hearing loss in agriculture. 2022. https://extension.psu.edu/noise-induced-hearing-loss-in-agriculture.

Racette BA, Searles Nielsen S, Criswell SR, Sheppard L, Seixas N, Warden MN, Checkoway H. Dose-dependent progression of parkinsonism in manganese-exposed welders. Neurology. 2017;88(4):344–51. https://doi.org/10.1212/WNL.0000000000003533.

Riccelli MG, Goldoni M, Poli D, Mozzoni P, Cavallo D, Corradi M. Welding fumes, a risk factor for lung diseases. Int J Environ Res Public Health. 2020;17(7):2552. https://doi.org/10.3390/ijerph17072552.

Roehl C. Welding on the farm, selecting a welding unit for the farm or ranch. Miller Welding LLC; 2007. https://www.millerwelds.com/resources/article-library/welding-on-the-farm-selecting-a-welding-unit-for-the-farm-or-ranch#Portability.

Suri R, Periselneris J, Lanone S, Zeidler-Erdely PC, Melton G, Palmer KT, Andujar P, Antonini JM, Cohignac V, Erdely A, Jose RJ, Mudway I, Brown J, Grigg J. Exposure to welding fumes and lower airway infection with Streptococcus pneumoniae. J Allergy Clin Immunol. 2016;137(2):527–534.e7. https://doi.org/10.1016/j.jaci.2015.06.033.

Takahashi J, Nakashima H, Fujii N, Okuno T. Comprehensive analysis of hazard of ultraviolet radiation emitted during arc welding of cast iron. J Occup Health. 2020;62(1):e12091. https://doi.org/10.1002/1348-9585.12091.

TWI (The Welding Institute). What is oxy-acetylene welding? All you need to know. 2021. https://www.uti.edu/blog/welding/oxy-acetylene-welding.

TWI (The Welding Institute). What is arc welding—definition and process types. 2024a. https://www.twi-global.com/technical-knowledge/faqs/what-is-arc-welding.

TWI (The Welding Institute). What is the difference between welding, brazing and soldering. 2024b. https://www.twi-global.com/technical-knowledge/faqs/welding-brazing-and-soldering.

United States Navy. Visual impairment from exposure to high intensity light sources. 1963. https://apps.dtic.mil/sti/tr/pdf/AD0412960.pdfSOURCES.

Vandenplas O, Dargent F, Auverdin JJ, Boulanger J, Bossiroy JM, Roosels D, Vande WR. Occupational asthma due to gas metal arc welding on mild steel. Thorax. 1995;50(5):587–8.

Work Safe Alberta. Welder's guide to the hazards of welding fumes and gases. 2009. https://open.alberta.ca/dataset/b15f90d9-a316-41af-954b-ef45ddc3b833/resource/92687979-5230-442b-a49b-1860ceb63caa/download/whs-pub-ch032.pdf.

Freshwater Algal Toxins

16

Mina W. Shehee

Background

Cyanobacteria are prokaryotic photosynthetic bacteria (Madigan et al. 2022). They are part of natural aquatic ecosystems. Under certain environmental conditions (nutrient-rich, warm, calm waters), cyanobacteria can rapidly increase to large numbers (Rastogi et al. 2015). This explosive growth of one or more cyanobacterial species to large numbers is called an algal bloom (Nienaber and Steinitz-Kannan 2018). A harmful algal bloom (HAB) is an algal bloom that adversely affects the environment; human health; and/or pets, livestock, and wildlife (Huisman et al. 2018). Because of this nexus among humans, animals, and the environment, HABs are considered a One Health issue (CDC 2023b).

Cyanobacterial blooms occur mainly in freshwater (rivers, lakes, farm ponds, fisheries, and reservoirs) but may be present in estuarine and marine waters (Preece et al. 2017). In affected waters, cyanobacterial bloom may degrade water quality (discolor water and produce water tastes and odors), impair water-related recreational activities, and adversely impact aquatic life (CDC 2023a; Chapman 2010; Yunes 2019; Zurawell 2017). Toxins produced by cyanobacteria (also known as cyanotoxins) can be detected in animals and plants. However, these toxins can be eliminated, diluted, or detoxified (Codd et al. 2017; Ferrao-Filho and Kozlowsky-Suzuki 2011). Cyanotoxins have also been detected in dietary supplements (Roy-Lachapelle et al. 2017).

Cyanobacterial blooms are expected to increase in frequency, intensity, and distribution. This is mainly due to the increasing eutrophication of natural waters (nutrient pollution such as runoff after applying fertilizers to farmlands) along with the increasing temperatures of climate change (Chapra et al. 2017; Huisman et al. 2018). Humans are exposed to algal toxins through ingestion, inhalation, and dermal contact. Activities that can lead to exposure to cyanobacteria and their toxins include drinking inadequately treated water, eating contaminated fish, and recreational activities (swimming, skiing, jet skiing, and wading) in bloom waters. Occupations (e.g., aquaculture) that have contact with bloom waters may also be a source of exposure (Humpage and Cunliffe 2021; Chorus and Testai 2021). The presence–absence and concentration of toxins can vary by bloom. Approximately 25–75% of cyanobacterial blooms contain a toxin (Huisman et al. 2018; Blaha et al. 2009). The associated symptoms can vary by the type of toxin, concentration of toxin, and exposure length and type (CDC 2023b). See Table 16.1 for a summary of cyanotoxins. See Table 16.2 for a summary of World

M. W. Shehee (✉)
Biology Department, Indian River State College, Fort Pierce, FL, USA

W. J. Meggs, R. L. Langley (eds.), *Farm Toxicology*, https://doi.org/10.1007/978-3-031-80441-0_16

Table 16.1 Freshwater cyanotoxin summary[a,b]

Toxin	Chemical type	Mode of action	Target organs	Health effects	Carcinogenic[c]	Symptoms
Microcystins (MCY)	Cyclic heptapeptide	Protein phosphate inhibition	Liver	Hepatotoxic	IARC Group 2B possibly carcinogenic	Abdominal pain, nausea vomiting, headache, sore throat, blistering around mouth, and pneumonia[d]
Nodularins (NOD)	Cyclic pentapeptide	Protein phosphate inhibition	Liver	Hepatotoxic	IARC Group 3 not classifiable as a carcinogen	Symptoms similar to microcystins[e]
Cylindrospermopsin (CYN)	Guanidine alkaloid	Protein synthesis inhibition	Liver and kidneys	Hepatotoxic Nephrotoxic	Not listed	Gastrointestinal (vomiting and bloody diarrhea), fever, headache; kidneys: loss of electrolytes, water, and protein[d,f]
Anatoxin-a	Bicyclic amine alkaloid	Nicotinic agonist	Nerves	Neurotoxic	Not listed	Neurologic including numbness, tingling, or burning sensation, dizziness, blurred or double vision, drowsiness, ataxia including speech disturbances; salivation (Anatoxin-a(S)[d,g]
Saxitoxin	Alkaloid	Nerve cell sodium channel blocker; heart muscle calcium and potassium channel blocker	Nerves and muscles	Neurotoxic	Not listed	Initial: numbs or tingling in lips, mouth, face, and neck, prickling in fingers and toes; followed by: headache, dizziness, gastrointestinal (nausea, vomiting and diarrhea); severe symptoms: stumbling, twitching, convulsions, muscle and respiratory paralysis[h]

[a]Buratti et al. (2017)
[b]Codd et al. (2017)
[c]IARC (2010)
[d]CDC (2022b)
[e]Du et al. (2019)
[f]EPA (2015a)
[g]Bire et al. (2020)
[h]WHO (2017)

Health Organization guidelines and reference values for drinking and recreational waters. See Table 16.3 for a summary of the United States Environmental Protection Agency's (EPA's) 10-day health advisory (HA) levels for cyanotoxins in drinking water and swimming advisory levels in recreational waters.

Occupations that take place in or around bloom waters may be at risk of exposure to cyanobacterial intoxication. Examples of those involved in possible occupations include aquaculture or spray irrigation workers, livestock farmers, scientists, environmental or natural resource personnel, and environmental health

Table 16.2 Available World Health Organization (WHO) cyanotoxin recommended guideline (GV)/reference (RV) values[a]

Cyanotoxin	Water use	Value (μg/L)[b]	Value[c,d,e]
Microcystin-LR	Drinking	1	Provisional GV/lifetime
Microcystin-LR	Drinking	12	Provisional GV/short-term
Microcystin-LR	Recreational	24	Provisional GV
Cylindrospermopsin	Drinking	0.7	Provisional GV/lifetime
Cylindrospermopsin	Drinking	3	Provisional GV/short-term
Cylindrospermopsin	Recreational	6	Provisional GV
Anatoxin	Drinking	30	Health-based RV/acute
Antatoxin	Recreational	60	Health-based RV
Saxitoxin	Drinking	3	GV/acute
Saxitoxin	Recreational	30	GV

[a]References: Chorus and Welker 2021; WHO 2017
[b]Micrograms per liter, μg/L
[c]Provisional, value has a high level of uncertainty due to database limitations
[d]Reference Value (RV), the level where no adverse health effects are expected
[e]Guideline Value (GV), the concentration of a toxin does not exceed a tolerable risk

Table 16.3 Available United States Environmental Protection Agency (EPA) Cyanotoxin recommended 10-day advisory levels[a]

Cyanotoxin	Water use	Level (μg/L)[b]	Advisory[c,d,e]
Microcystins	Drinking	0.3	<6 years old[f] (health)
Microcystins	Drinking	1.6	≥6 years old (health)
Microcystins	Recreational	8	Swimming[g]
Cylindrospermopsin	Drinking	0.7	<6 years old[f] (health)
Cylindrospermopsin	Drinking	3.0	≥6 years old (health)
Cylindrospermopsin	Recreational	15	Swimming[g]

[a]References: EPA 2016a, 2019
[b]Micrograms per liter, mg/L
[c]If the cyanotoxin level exceeds the recommended drinking water health advisory on any day during the 10-day period, then adverse health effects may occur
[d]If the cyanotoxin level exceeds the recommended recreational swimming advisory on any day during the 10-day period, then adverse health effects may occur
[e]These advisory levels are recommendations, not regulations
[f]Includes vulnerable populations: pregnant women, nursing mothers, patients with pre-existing liver conditions, dialysis treatment patients, and the elderly
[g]Swimming advisory levels are based on children

professionals. Types of exposures include dermal contact, inhalation, and incidental ingestion (Chorus and Testai 2021; Stewart et al. 2009).

Epidemiological surveillance in the United States has been ongoing for decades through several consecutive programs including the Centers for Disease Control and Prevention's (CDC's) Waterborne Disease and Outbreak Surveillance System (WBDOSS), Harmful Algal Bloom-related Illness Surveillance System (HABISS), and One Health Harmful Algal Bloom System (OHHABS). These surveillance systems have demonstrated that adverse health effects may occur after exposure to cyanobacteria and their toxins (Hilborn et al. 2014; Backer et al. 2015).

For example, in 2021, 368 HAB events (311 confirmed and 57 suspected) were reported through the CDC's One Health Harmful Algal Bloom System (OHHABS), resulting in 117 human and 2715 animal illnesses (2018 confirmed cases, 669 probable cases, and 28 suspected cases). This program is made up of 16 reporting states. Most HAB events were reported during the summer months (peaking in August) and occurred in freshwaters (90% in lakes and reservoirs). Most human cases occurred in June while most animal cases occurred in August. Reported human cases were predominantly classified as probable (89%) with 46% of the cases occurring in people less than 18 years of age. The cyanobacterial toxin microcystin was the leading toxin identified during environmental testing. For humans, diarrhea, nausea, vomiting, headache, and rashes were the most reported signs or symptoms. Most animal illnesses occurred in wildlife (97%) and included many bat deaths (2018 cases). Dogs, cattle, and bats were affected the most. Vomiting and lethargy were the common symptoms in domestic pets (CDC 2023b).

Categories of Algal Toxins

Microcystin (MCY)

Microcystins are cyclic heptapeptides. There are over 275 microcystin congeners (Bouaicha et al. 2019). A congener is a variant of the toxin. Congeners are based on the type of amino acids and the specific site of methylation or demethylation. Microcystin-LR is the most common congener detected worldwide, in the northern temperate and boreal lakes in Canada, and in the United States (EPA 2015b; MacKeigan et al. 2023). An example of a microcystin-producing cyanobacteria is *Microcystis aeruginosa* (EPA 2015b). See Fig. 16.1 for examples of cyanobacterial blooms with associated microorganisms.

Microcystins are water-soluble and stable (Massey and Yang 2020; EPA 2015d). They may persist in the environment from weeks to months. The half-life of the toxin in the environment is approximately 2 weeks but depends upon bacteria degradation and sunlight exposure, among other environmental factors (EPA 2015b). They may persist in dried scum and sediments for 6 months.

Humans are exposed to microcystins through drinking water, recreational activities, consuming algal dietary supplements, eating finfish or shellfish, and possibly inhalation of aerosolized toxins all via contaminated bloom waters (CDC 2022a; Massey and Yang 2020; Backer 2012). Bloom waters used for irrigation can contaminate vegetable plants and microcystins have been detected in groundwaters (Melaram et al. 2022). After oral exposure, microcystins are absorbed by the gastrointestinal tract (ileum and jejunum). Microcystins that are not absorbed are eliminated in feces. Microcystins are distributed to the liver (the primary target organ) (Arman and Clarke 2021).

The mechanism of toxicity is protein phosphatase inhibition by unique amino acid components of microcystin. This inhibition process results in a buildup of phosphorylated proteins and is responsible for its hepatotoxicity. Oxidative stress, changes in cell morphology, and cell mortality are associated with the inhibition of protein phosphatases (Arman and Clarke 2021). Microcystin may be actively transported into other organ system cells (cardiovascular, renal, and respiratory) (Massey and Yang 2020). In general, microcystins are metabolized and detoxified by glutathione and cysteinyl conjugation. Excretion is through feces and urine (Arman and Clarke 2021).

The toxic effects of microcystins may include liver and kidney damage, gastroenteritis, reproductive effects, reduced ability to repair DNA, and tumor promotion (Arman and Clarke 2021). This is due to the amount of toxin, the length of exposure to the toxin, exposure type, and toxin type (there are various microcystin variants) (CDC 2022a). Inhalation of microcystins has been demonstrated to affect human bronchial epithelial cells (Li et al. 2016). Although aerosolized microcystins have been detected in the air, the serum levels of exposed persons were below the detection limit (Backer et al. 2010; Lim et al. 2023). Microcystins have met most but not all criteria to classify them as a possible endocrine disruptor (Zhang et al. 2022). The International Agency for Research on Cancer (IARC) classifies microcystin-LR as "possibly carcinogenic in humans" (IARC Group 2B) (IARC 2010). However, the United States Environmental Protection Agency (EPA) does not classify microcystin-LR as a carcinogen due to the lack of data (EPA 2015b).

Exposed patients may exhibit signs and symptoms of "abdominal pain, nausea, vomiting,

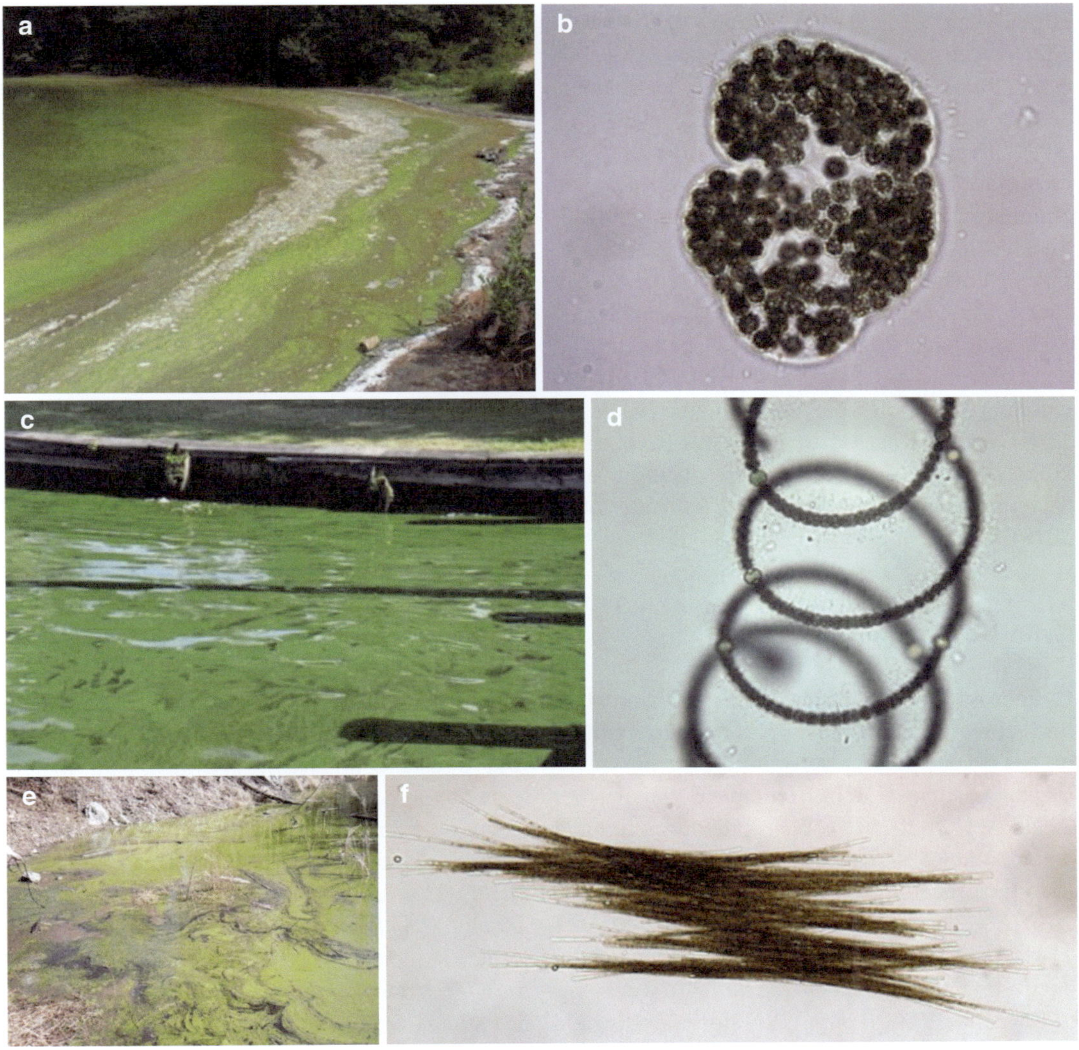

Fig. 16.1 Examples (genera) of cyanobacterial blooms with associated microorganisms. (Photos courtesy of North Carolina Department of Environmental Quality). (**a**) *Microcystis* bloom; (**b**) *Microcystis* Microscopic; (**c**) *Dilichospermum* (formerly (*Anabaena*) bloom; (**d**) *Dilichospermum* microscopic; (**e**) *Aphanizomenon* bloom; (**f**) *Aphanizomenon* microscopic

headache, diarrhea, sore throat, blistering around the mouth and pneumonia" (CDC 2022b). Liver biomarkers of alanine aminotransferase (ALT) and alkaline phosphatase (ALP) may not be reliable (Su et al. 2020). Microcystins can exacerbate underlying conditions such as type 2 diabetes, heart disease, and liver disease. Moreover, other pathogens may be present in the same waters as an algal bloom (*Vibrio species*) (Chatterjee and More 2023).

Nodularin (NOD)

Nodularins (NODs) are often co-detected with microcystins using congener-independent enzyme-linked immunoassays enzyme-linked immunosorbant assays (ELISA) tests (EPA 2016b). NODs are cyclic pentapeptides possessing many characteristics of microcystins (MCYs) (Du et al. 2019). NODs are hepatotoxic and cell-bound and inhibit protein phosphatases (Chen et al. 2013,

2021). There are at least ten variants of NOD with NOD-R being the most common variant (Huisman et al. 2018). They are stable in the environment and are water-soluble (Chen et al. 2021). However, NODs are found in brackish waters where they can bioaccumulate in finfish and shellfish (Fastner and Humpage 2021). Exposures to NODs are by swallowing bloom waters while swimming and consuming contaminated seafood (Chen et al. 2013). Like MCYs, NODs target the liver (Nienaber and Steinitz-Kannan 2018). NODs are listed as class 3 ("not classified as carcinogenic") (IARC 2010). A recommended tolerable daily intake value of 1 μg/L is extrapolated from MCY-LR (Chen et al. 2021). An example of a NOD-producing cyanobacterium is *Nodularia spumigena* (Huisman et al. 2018).

Cylindrospermopsin (CYN)

Cylindrospermopsin (CYN) is a guanidine alkaloid (Huisman et al. 2018). It is toxic to multiple organs (liver and kidney), inhibits protein synthesis, and damages DNA (Humpage and Fastner 2021; WHO 2020). CYN is hydrophilic and water-soluble (WHO 2017). The toxin is mainly found extracellularly (Du et al. 2019; WHO 2017). CYN is stable with a half-life of 11–15 days in surface waters. Depending on the environmental conditions, the half-life can be up to 8 weeks (EPA 2015a). CYN does not degrade with boiling (WHO 2020). CYNs are found primarily in tropical, subtropical, and warm temperate, fresh, or marine waters (EPA 2015a). An example of a CYN-producing cyanobacteria is *Raphidiopsis* (*Cylindrospermopsis*) *raciborskii* (Huisman et al. 2018).

Drinking water is the primary route of exposure. Exposures from drinking water are expected to be acute rather than chronic due to the seasonality of blooms (EPA 2015a). The risk of exposure may also be through recreational activities, mainly incidental ingestion of water during swimming (EPA 2019). Food ingestion may be another route of exposure. However, the data are limited. CYN is absorbed by the intestinal tract and excreted mainly in the urine and lesser amounts in feces. The target organ is the liver, but it can affect the kidneys and the spleen (EPA 2015a). CYN primarily inhibits protein synthesis (Humpage and Fastner 2021).

Adverse health effects may present as a "hepatoenteritis-like illness" (EPA 2015a). Signs and symptoms include "gastrointestinal symptoms, including vomiting and bloody diarrhea, as well as fever and headache" (CDC 2022b). There may be liver enlargement. Kidneys can be damaged with "loss of water, electrolytes, and protein" (EPA 2015a).

Anatoxin (ATX)

Anatoxin-a (ATX-a) is a neurotoxic bicyclic amine alkaloid (Buratti et al. 2017). It is found worldwide and is soluble in water (EPA 2015c). ATX-a rapidly degrades in water under light and high pH (Du et al. 2019). ATX-a occurs in benthic mats (underwater surfaces) and surface waters with varying concentrations (Buratti et al. 2017; Testai et al. 2016). Livestock, wildlife, and pets (dogs) deaths have been reported. Exposure is possible through ingesting contaminated water (drinking and recreational), food, algal supplements, skin contact (showering or bathing), or inhalation (EPA 2015c). Exposures are normally acute. Dogs and small children are at the most risk. The toxin is readily absorbed by the gastrointestinal tract into the bloodstream. ATX-a binds to acetylcholine receptors as a nicotinic agonist (EPA 2015c). ATX-a is not degraded by acetylcholinesterase (Christensen and Khan 2020). A variety of cyanobacteria can produce ATX-a including *Dolichospermum* (*Anabaena*) *species* (EPA 2015c).

Case reports and epidemiological data are lacking regarding ATX-a's health effects in humans (EPA 2015c). However, Bire et al. (2020) reported that ATX-a was a cause of food poisoning events (18 events from 2011 to 2018) involving 26 patients. None of the cases involved children. All patients had similar symptoms after consuming sea figs (*Microcosmus*). The most common symptoms included "ataxia, dizziness and accommodation disturbances (blurred vision, diplopia). Digestive disorders (nausea, vomiting and diarrhea) were also reported but were less frequent; so were asthenia, headaches, muscle cramps and paresthesia" (Bire et al. 2020). Leftovers from three events were analyzed for the presence of biotoxins. Marine biotoxins, including saxitoxin, tetrodotoxin, and domoic acid, among others, were ruled out. Concentrations of ATX-a were greater in the leftover sea figs compared to the control (concentrations193.7–1240.2 μg/kg in the leftovers and 22.5 μg/kg in the control) (Bire et al. 2020). It is hypothesized that a benthic marine ATX-a-producing cyanobacterium (*Hydrocleum* or *Trichodesium*) was involved (Bire et al. 2020). In animals, domestic pets, livestock (cattle), and wildlife, poisonings and deaths have been documented. Dogs are extremely susceptible to the effects of ATX-a. Death can happen rapidly (min) after symptoms occur (EPA 2015c; Colas et al. 2021).

Two other anatoxins have been described. However, data are limited. Anatoxin-a(S) (ATX-a(S)) is a natural organophosphate (Testai 2021). A new name for ATX-a(S) is guanitoxin (CDC 2022a). ATX-a(S) is a neurotoxin and causes salivation (Huisman et al. 2018; Nienaber and Steinitz-Kannan 2018). It can inhibit acetylcholinesterase. Symptoms include convulsions and respiratory failure, among others, in animal studies (Christensen and Khan 2020; Mahmood and Carmichael 1986). Homo-anatoxin (HTX) is an analog of ATX-a and its toxicity properties are like ATX-a (EPA 2015c). Currently, there are no EPA health advisory levels for anatoxin-a.

Saxitoxin (STX)

Saxitoxins (STXs) are neurotoxic alkaloids (Nienaber and Steinitz-Kannan 2018). The most familiar disease associated with STX is paralytic shellfish poisoning (PSP) from consuming contaminated marine shellfish. PSP is caused by eukaryotic microorganisms called dinoflagellates (Testai 2021). In freshwaters, prokaryotic microorganisms called cyanobacteria can produce STX (Ballot et al. 2017).Examples of STX-producing cyanobacteria genera are *Aphanizomenon*, *Dolichospermum*, and *Raphidiopsis* (Testai 2021). STX produced by marine dinoflagellates and freshwater cyanobacteria is the same (Testai 2021). STX is mainly hydrophilic (Christensen and Khan 2020; Testai 2021). Hence, STX is water-soluble and has the potential to bioaccumulate in freshwater shellfish (Testai 2021).

STX occurs worldwide in freshwater lakes, reservoirs, streams, and rivers (Christensen and Khan 2020). STX has been detected in benthic (bottom surfaces) and planktonic (water column) samples (Ballot et al. 2017). Toxin is cell-bound unless released from the cell by lysis or damage (WHO 2017). STX may persist in the environment for 1 or 2 months (Testai 2021). The most likely exposure risk would be incidental swallowing of contaminated recreational waters and consuming inadequately treated drinking water (WHO 2017).

STX is quickly absorbed in the gastrointestinal tract and distributed into body tissues. Its main target is the central nervous system (Testai 2021). Cyanobacterial STX is a potent neurotoxin that blocks sodium channels in neuronal cells. It can also affect heart-muscle calcium and potassium channels (Buratti et al. 2017). The initial symptoms of STX are numbness or tingling (lips, mouth, face, and neck) and prickling (fingers and toes). This is followed by headache, dizziness, gastrointestinal symptoms (nausea, vomiting, and diarrhea), and muscle weakness (limbs). Severe symptoms include neurologic symptoms (stumbling, twitching, and convulsions) and muscle and respiratory paralysis (WHO 2017). Death may occur within 2–24 h (Testai 2021). STX breaks down rapidly and is excreted in the urine (Christensen and Khan 2020; Testai 2021).

There is no antidote or detoxification treatment for STX poisoning (Ballot et al. 2017). STX does not degrade by cooking (Nienaber and Steinitz-Kannan 2018). There is no definitive information regarding repeat exposure to the toxin, reproductive and developmental toxicity, genotoxicity, or carcinogenicity (Testai 2021). Currently, there are no EPA health advisory levels for cyanobacterial saxitoxin.

Lipopolysaccharides (LPS)

Cell walls of cyanobacteria are thought to be gram-negative. Like other gram-negative bacteria, cyanobacteria possess an outer membrane containing lipopolysaccharides (LPS). In general, LPS can cause gastrointestinal symptoms, various skin reactions (e.g., allergic reactions or rashes), respiratory symptoms, fever, and headache. However, cyanobacterial LPS is not as toxic as other gram-negative bacteria (e.g., *Enterobacteriaceae*) LPS (Stewart et al. 2006). The concentration of cyanobacterial LPS is not expected to increase during drinking water treatent and represents a very low health risk by ingestion or inhalation (showering). In recreational waters, health effects that are assumed to be caused by exposure to cyanobacterial LPS may be due to other constituents in the water (Welker 2021). Further research is needed to delineate the role of LPS in cyanobacterial illnesses.

Beta-N-Methylamino-L-Alanine (BMAA)

BMAA is produced by most cyanobacteria. Its involvement with neurogenerative diseases (amyotrophic lateral sclerosis (ALS) and Parkinson's and Alzheimer's diseases) has been hypothesized (Chernoff et al. 2021). However, BMAA's role has been controversial as a cause of these diseases due to conflicting reports (Chernoff et al. 2021). Nugumanova et al. (2023) indicated that there is an increasing amount of experimental data that confirms BMAA's role in neurodegenerative diseases. Continued research is needed to clarify the role BMAA may have in these diseases.

Cyanobacterial Diagnosis, Treatment, and Prevention

The diagnosis of cyanobacterial intoxication is one of exclusion (ASTHO 2022). Seasonality, patient history, and routine diagnostic tests are keys to this process. Knowing when HABs occur can help with the diagnosis. In temperate regions, HABs occur mainly during late spring to early fall (May–October) and peak in August (EPA 2015b). Because of this seasonality, the risk of exposure to cyanotoxins would most likely be acute. However, sub-chronic or chronic exposures to cyanotoxins may occur in areas that have rainy/dry seasons, continuous year-long blooms, or repetitive exposures.

Asking the patient about potential exposures can help with the diagnosis. During the HAB season, patients with gastrointestinal, liver, nervous system, and skin symptoms should be asked exposure-activity questions. Questions to ask may include: "Have you visited any lake, river, or other natural body of water?"; "Did you (or your pet) swim or wade in, walk near, or have any contact with water?"; and "Did your symptoms begin after exposure to the water (min/h/days)?" (ASTHO 2022). In general, cyanobacterial illnesses mainly occur by exposure to freshwater bloom waters through recreational activities (CDC 2023b).

Because other contaminants such as organophosphates can have similar signs and symptoms as some cyanotoxins, routine diagnostic tests will aid with an exclusionary process. Currently, there are no definitive tests for diagnosing cyanotoxins. Cyanotoxin illnesses are underdiagnosed due to a lack of tests (ASTHO 2022). There are no antidotes for cyanotoxins (CDC 2022a). For most cyanobacterial illnesses, stop the exposure and provide supportive and symptomatic care (CDC 2022b). Poison control centers can be consulted for questions about possible cyanotoxin poisonings. Suspected cases of cyanotoxin should be reported, although not required, to the local health department. There are International Classification of Diseases, Tenth Revision, Clinical Modification (ICD-10-CM) codes available for contact with (Z77.121) or toxic effects from harmful algae or their toxins (T65.82) (ASTHO 2022).

The best personal prevention methods are recognition and avoidance of bloom waters (CDC 2023a). A cyanobacterial bloom may discolor the water and produce scums or mats. Recreational water should not be used if it has dead fish and dead animals in the water or on the shore (CDC 2023a). You cannot tell by looking at bloom waters whether they contain a toxin or not (CDC 2022a). The water needs to be tested for toxins.

Before going to a beach or lake, check for any swimming advisories that may have been issued in the area (CDC 2022c). Notify the state or local wildlife agencies and/or environmental health agencies if you notice dead animals and several dead fish in the water body.

Follow any health advisories (drinking water or recreational) given by the local health department as the source of drinking water may be a lake that has an ongoing algal bloom. Many of the cyanotoxins cannot be destroyed by boiling (EPA 2016a). Alternative sources of drinking water may be advised. Preschool children are especially vulnerable to cyanotoxins. This is due to their higher water intake rate by weight compared to adults (EPA 2015b). Other vulnerable populations include breastfeeding mothers, pregnant women, immunocompromised people, dialysis patients, and the elderly (EPA 2016a).

Occupations that take place in or around bloom waters may be at risk of exposure to cyanobacterial intoxication. The use of practical personal protective equipment, such as waterproof gloves and boots while sampling bloom waters, may help reduce the risk of exposure to cyanotoxins (Stewart et al. 2009). Because blooms may have respiratory effects (Backer 2012), the appropriate level of respiratory protection should be chosen judiciously. Safety plans about the adverse health effects of cyanotoxins and accidental immersion protocols help inform workers how to best avoid these exposures (Stewart et al. 2009).

Domestic pets (dogs) can be exposed to cyanotoxins by swimming in and drinking from bloom waters, eating mats or scum, and licking their wet fur (Backer and Miller 2016). Symptoms of cyanotoxin poisoning in dogs may include vomiting, excessive drooling, twitching, staggering, impaired balance, and a change in behavior. For a sick dog after exposure to bloom waters, time is of the essence. Symptoms may happen fast, sometimes within minutes (CDC 2021, 2022c). Rinse to get any of the bloom scum and mats or the bloom waters off the fur and seek veterinarian care as soon as possible (CDC 2022c). Often, animal (dog) illnesses and deaths after exposure to bloom waters are harbingers (epidemiological sentinel surveillance) of increased human health risks (Hilborn and Beasley 2015; Backer and Miller 2016).

Tools to help with cyanotoxin identification and health surveillance are available online. The CDC and U.S. EPA have flyers and handouts that can be downloaded. CDC has information of poison center professionals, veterinarians, and healthcare providers. The Association of State and Territorial Health Officials (ASTHO) has a "Clinician Toolbox for Physicians and Healthcare Providers" (ASTHO 2022). The Association of Public Health Laboratories has published a guidance that outlines algal toxin methodologies (APHL 2021). State and local health and environmental departments may have resources with state-specific recommended cyanotoxin action levels, procedures to report a bloom, and public education materials. The World Health Organization (WHO) has publications about cyanotoxins and recommended guideline values.

Conclusion

Freshwater cyanobacteria are often unrecognized and underreported. The lack of definitive tests for cyanotoxins and recognition of cyanobacterial illnesses contributes to underreporting and unrecognizing them. Research in the types of cyanobacteria that produce toxins, toxicology of exposure to these toxins in animals, the structure/chemistry of various cyanotoxins, and environmental or ecological characteristics of blooms and toxin production have all advanced understanding of the nature and extent of freshwater cyanobacteria and their toxins. However, the science of cyanotoxins is still developing. Research is needed to clarify the questions of cause and effect in humans and the discovery and development of diagnostic tests.

References

Arman T, Clarke JD. Microcystin toxicokinetics, molecular toxicology, and pathophysiology in preclinical rodent models and humans. Toxins (Basel). 2021;13(8):537.

Association for State and Territorial Health Officials (ASTHO). Cyanobacterial blooms and associated illnesses: a clinician toolbox for physicians and healthcare providers; 2022. https://www.astho.org/globalassets/pdf/cyanobacterial-blooms-and-associated-illnesses-presentation.pdf. Accessed 25 Sep 2023.

Association of Public Health Laboratories (APHL). Cyamotoxins: a guidance Document for Public Health Laboratories; 2021. https://www.aphl.org/aboutAPHL/publications/Documents/EH_2021_Cyanotoxin_Guide.pdf. Accessed 27 Nov 2023.

Backer LC. Freshwater algal blooms & public health. Lake Line. 2012;32(3):7–9. PMID: 26412937.

Backer LC, Miller M. Sentinel animals in a one health approach to harmful cyanobacterial and algal blooms. Vet Sci. 2016;3(2):8.

Backer LC, McNeel SV, Barber T, Kirkpatrick B, Williams C, Irvin M, et al. Recreational exposure to microcystins during algal blooms in two California Lakes. Toxicon (Basel). 2010;55(5):909–21.

Backer LC, Manassararam-Baptiste D, LePrell R, Bolton B. Cyanobacteria and algal blooms: review of health and environmental data from the harmful algal bloom-related illness surveillance system (HABISS) 2007–2011. Toxins (Basel). 2015;7(4):1048–64.

Ballot A, Bernard C, Fastner J. Saxitoxin and analogues. In: Meriluoto J, Spoff L, Codd GA, editors. Handbook of cyanobacterial monitoring and cyanotoxin analysis. Chichester: Wiley; 2017. p. 148–54.

Bire R, Bertin T, Dom I, Hort V, Scmitt C, Diogene J, Memee R, De Haro L, Nicholas M. First evidence of the presence of Anatoxin-A in sea figs associated with human food poisonings in France. Mar Drugs. 2020;18:285.

Blaha L, Babica P, Marsalek B. Toxins produced in cyanobacterial water blooms—toxicity and risks. Interdiscip Toxicol. 2009;2(2):36–41.

Bouaicha N, Miles CO, Beach DG, Labodi Z, Djabri A, Benayache NY, Nguyen-Quang T. Structural diversity, characterization, and toxicology of microcystins. Toxins (Basel). 2019;11:714.

Buratti FM, Manganelli M, Vichi S, Stafanelli M, Scardala S, Testai E, Funari E. Cyanotoxins: producing organisms, occurrence, toxicity, mechanism of action and human health toxicological risk evaluation. Arch Toxicol. 2017;91(3):1049–130.

Centers for Disease Control and Prevention (CDC). Veterinarian reference for cyanobacterial blooms; 2021. https://www.cdc.gov/habs/specific-groups/veterinarians-cyanobacteria.html. Accessed 3 Sep 2023.

Centers for Disease Control and Prevention (CDC). Cyanobacterial blooms: information for health care providers; 2022a. https://www.cdc.gov/habs/specific-groups/healthcare_providers.html. Accessed 25 Sep 2023.

Centers for Disease Control and Prevention (CDC). Facts about Cyanobacterial Harmful Algal Blooms for Poison Center Professionals; 2022b. https://www.cdc.gov/habs/materials/factsheet-cyanobacterial-habs.html. Accessed 25 Sep 2023.

Centers for Disease Control and Prevention (CDC). Protect yourself and your pets; 2022c. https://www.cdc.gov/habs/prevention-control.html. Accessed 25 Sep 2023.

Centers for Disease Control and Prevention (CDC). Harmful algal bloom (HAB)-associated illness: general information; 2023a. https://www.cdc.gov/habs/general.html. Accessed 14 Jun 2023.

Centers for Disease Control and Prevention (CDC). Summary report—One Health Harmful Algal Bloom System (OHHABS), United States, 2021; 2023b. https://www.cdc.gov/habs/data/2021-ohhabs-data-summary.html. Accessed 23 Jun 2023.

Chapman AD. Cyanobacteria. In: Algae source to treatment—manual of water supply practices M57. Denver, CO: American Water Works Association; 2010. p. 131.

Chapra SC, Boehlert B, Fant C, Bierman VJ, Henderson J, Mills D, Mas DML, Rennels L, Jantarasami L, Martinich J, Strzepek KM, Paerl HW. Climate change impacts on harmful algal blooms in U.S. freshwaters: a screening-level assessment. Environ Sci Technol. 2017;51:8933–43.

Chatterjee S, More M. Cyanobacterial harmful algal bloom toxin microcystin and increased vibrio occurrence as climate-change-induced biological co-stressors: exposure and disease outcomes via their interaction with gut-liver-brain axis. Toxins (Basel). 2023;15(4):289.

Chen Y, Shen D, Fang D. Nodularin in poisoning. Clin Chim Acta. 2013;425:18–29.

Chen G, Wang L, Wang M, Hu T. Comprehensive insights into the occurrence and toxicological issues of Nodularins. Mar Pollut Bull. 2021;162:111884.

Chernoff N, Faassen EJ, Hill DJ. B-Methylamino-L-alanine (BMAA). In: Chorus I, Welker M, editors. Toxic cyanobacteria in water. Abington: CRC Press; 2021. p. 123–36.

Chorus I, Testai E. Recreation and occupational activities. In: Chorus I, Welker M, editors. Toxic cyanobacteria in water. Abington: CRC Press; 2021. p. 333–67.

Chorus I, Welker M. Exposure to cyanotoxins: understanding it and short-term interventions to prevent it. In: Chorus I, Welker M, editors. Toxic cyanobacteria in water. Abington: CRC Press; 2021. p. 299.

Christensen VG, Khan E. Freshwater neurotoxins and concerns for human, animal, and ecosystem health: a review of Anatoxin-a and Saxitoxin. Sci Total Environ. 2020;20(736):139515.

Codd GA, Metcalf MJ, JS. Introduction: Cyanobacteria, Cyanotoxins. Their human impact, and risk management. In: Meriluoto J, Spoff L, Codd GA, editors. Handbook of cyanobacterial monitoring and cyanotoxin analysis. Chichester: Wiley; 2017. p. 6–7.

Colas S, Marie B, Lance E, Quiblier C, Tricoire-Leignel H. Anatoxin-a: overview on a harmful cyanobacterial neurotoxin from the environmental scale to the molecular target. Environ Res. 2021;193:110590.

Du X, Liu H, Yuan L, Wang Y, Ma Y, Wang R, Chen X, Losiewicz MD, Guo H, Zhang H. The diversity of bacterial toxins on structural characterization, distribution and identification: a systematic review. Toxins (Basel). 2019;11(9):530.

Fastner J, Humpage A. Hepatotoxic cyclic peptides—microcystins and nodularins. In: Chorus I, Welker M, editors. Toxic cyanobacteria in water. Abington: CRC; 2021. p. 21–52.

Ferrao-Filho ADS, Kozlowsky-Suzuki B. Cyanotoxins: bioaccumulations and effects on aquatic animals. Mar Drugs. 2011;9(12):2729–72.

Hilborn ED, Beasley VR. One health and cyanocateria in freshwater systems: animal illnesses and deaths are sentinel events for human health risks. Toxins (Basel). 2015;7(4):1374–95.

Hilborn ED, Roberts VA, Backer L, DeConno E, Egan JS, Hyde JB, Nicholas DC, Wiegert EJ, Billing LM, DiOrio M, Mohr MC, Hardy FJ, Wade TJ, Yoder JS, Hlavsa MC. Algal bloom-associated disease outbrreaks among users of freshwater lake—United States 2009–2010. MMWR Morb Mortal Wkly Rep. 2014;63(1):11–5.

Huisman J, Codd GA, Paerl HW, Ibelings BW, Verspagen JMH, Visser PM. Cyanobacterial blooms. Nat Rev Microbiol. 2018;16(8):471–83.

Humpage A, Cunliffe D. Drinking water. In: Chorus I, Welker M, editors. Toxic cyanobacteria in water. Abington: CRC Press; 2021. p. 305–32.

Humpage A, Fastner J. Cylindrospermopsin. In: Chorus I, Welker M, editors. Toxic cyanobacteria in water. Abington: CRC Press; 2021. p. 53–71.

International Agency for Research on Cancer (IARC). IARC Monographs on the evaluation of carcinogenic risks to humans. Ingested nitrate and nitrite and cyanobacterial peptide toxins, vol. 94. Lyon: IARC; 2010. p. 412. https://www.iarc.who.int/news-events/iarc-publications-iarc-monographs-volume-94/. Accessed 11 Nov 2023.

Li Y, Li J, Huang H, Yang M, Zhuang D, Cheng X, Zhang H, Fu X. Microcystin-LR induces mitochondria-mediated apoptosis in human bronchial epithelial cells. Exp Ther Med. 2016;12(2):633–40.

Lim CC, Yoon J, Gerald LB, Ault AP, Heo S, Bell ML. Harmful algal bloom aerosols and human health. EBioMedicine. 2023;93:104604.

MacKeigan PW, Zastepa A, Taranu ZE, Westrick JA, Laing A, Pick FR, Beisner BE, Gregory-Eaves I. Microcystin concentrations and congener composition in relation to environmental variables across 440 north-temperate and Boreal lakes. Sci Total Environ. 2023;884:163811.

Madigan MT, Bender KS, Buckley DH, Sattley WM, Stahl DA. Ecological diversity in bacteria. In: Brock biology of microorganisms. 16th ed. Harlow: Pearson Education; 2022. p. 517–21.

Mahmood NA, Carmichael WW. The pharmacology of anatoxin-a(s), a neurotoxin produced by the freshwater cyanobacterium *Anabaena flos-aquae* NRC 525-17. Toxicon. 1986;24(5):425–34.

Massey IY, Yang F. A mini review on microcystins and bacterial degradation. Toxins (Basel). 2020;12(4):268.

Melaram R, Newton AR, Chaffin J. Microcystin contamination and toxicity: implications for agriculture and public health. Toxins. 2022;14(5):350.

Nienaber MA, Steinitz-Kannan M. A guide to Cyanobacteria: identification and impact. Lexington, KY: University Press of Kentucky; 2018. p. 27–37.

Nugumanova G, Ponomarev ED, Askarova S, Fasler-Kan E, Barteneva NS. Freshwater cyanotoxins, cyanopeptide and neurodegenerative diseases. Toxins (Basel). 2023;15(3):233.

Preece EP, Hardy FJ, Moore BC, Bryan M. A review of microcystin detections in estuarine and marine waters: environmental implications and human health risks. Harmful Algae. 2017 Jan;61:31–45.

Rastogi RP, Madamwar D, Incharoensakdi A. Bloom dynamics of Cyanobacteria and their toxins: environmental health Impcats and mitigation strategies. Front Microbiol. 2015;6:1254.

Roy-Lachapelle A, Solliec M, Bouchard ME, Sauve S. Detection of cyanotoxins in algae dietary supplements. Toxins (Basel). 2017;9(3):76.

Stewart I, Schluter PJ, Shaw GR. Cyanobacterial lipopolysaccharides and human health—a review. Environ Health. 2006;5:7. PMID: 16563160.

Stewart I, Carmichael WW, Sadler R, McGregor GB, Reardon K, Eaglesham GK, Wickramasinghe WA, Seawright AA, Shaw GR. Occupational and environmental Hazard assessments for the isolation, purification and toxicity testing of cyanobacterial toxins. Environ Health. 2009;8:52.

Su RC, Lad A, Breiddenbach JD, Kleinhenz AL, Modyanov N, Malhotra D, Haller ST, Kennedy DJ. Assessment of diagnostic biomarkers of liver injury in the setting of microcystin-LR (MC-LR) hepatotoxicity. Chemosphere. 2020;257:127111.

Testai E. Saxitoxins or paralytic shellfish poisons. In: Chorus I, Welker M, editors. Toxic cyanobacteria in water. Abington: CRC Press; 2021. p. 94–108.

Testai E, Scardala S, Vuchi S, Buratti FM, Funari E. Risk to human health associated with the environmental occurrence of cyanobacterial neurotoxic alkaloids Anatoxins and Saxitoxins. Crit Rev Toxicol. 2016;46(5):385–419.

United States Environmental Protection Agency (EPA). Drinking Water Health Advisory for the cyanobacterial toxin Cylindrospermopsin; 2015a. https://www.epa.gov/sites/default/files/2017-06/documents/cylindrospermopsin-report-2015.pdf. Accessed 9 Aug 2023.

United States Environmental Protection Agency (EPA). Drinking Water Health Advisory for the cyanobacterial microcystins toxins; 2015b. https://www.epa.gov/sites/default/files/2017-06/documents/microcystins-report-2015.pdf. Accessed 9 Aug 2023.

United States Environmental Protection Agency (EPA). Health effects support document for the cyanobacterial toxin Anatoxin-A; 2015c. https://www.epa.gov/sites/default/files/2017-06/documents/anatoxin-a-report-2015.pdf. Accessed 9 Aug 2023.

United States Environmental Protection Agency (EPA). Health effects support document for the cyanobacterial toxin microcystins; 2015d. https://www.epa.gov/sites/default/files/2017-06/documents/microcystins-support-report-2015.pdf. Accessed 9 Aug 2023.

United States Environmental Protection Agency (EPA). Cyanotoxins: drinking water advisories; 2016a. https://www.epa.gov/sites/default/files/2016-11/documents/cyanotoxins_-_drinking_water_advisories.pdf. Accessed 9 Aug 2023.

United States Environmental Protection Agency (EPA). Method 546: determination of total microcystins and nodularins in drinking water and ambient water by Adda enzyme-linked immunosorbant assay; 2016b. https://www.epa.gov/sites/default/files/2016-09/documents/method-546-determination-total-microcystins-nodularins-drinking-water-ambient-water-adda-enzyme-linked-immunosorbent-assay.pdf. Accessed 28 Nov 2023.

United States Environmental Protection Agency (EPA). Recommended human recreational ambient water quality criteria or swimming advisories for microcystins and cylindrospermopsin; 2019. https://www.epa.gov/sites/default/files/2019-05/documents/hh-rec-criteria-habs-document-2019.pdf. Accessed 9 Aug 2023.

Welker M. Cyanobacterial lipopolysaccharides (LPS). In: Chorus I, Welker M, editors. Toxic cyanobacteria in water. Abington: CRC Press; 2021. p. 137–48.

World Health Organization (WHO). Guidelines for drinking-water quality, fourth edition, incorporating the first addendum; 2017. https://cdn.who.int/media/docs/default-source/wash-documents/water-safety-and-quality/dwq-guidelines-4/gdwq4-with-add1-title.pdf?sfvrsn=97cdca01_3. Accessed 13 Nov 2023.

World Health Organization (WHO). Cyanobacterial toxins: cylindrospermopsin; 2020. https://iris.who.int/bitstream/handle/10665/338063/WHO-HEP-ECH-WSH-2020.4-eng.pdf?sequence=1&isAllowed=y. Accessed 13 Nov 2023.

Yunes JS. Cyanobacterial toxins. In: Mishra AK, Tiwari DN, Rai AN, editors. Cyanobacteria: from basic science to applications. London: Academic Press; 2019. p. 449–53.

Zhang S, Liu H, Du X, Chen X, Petlulu P, Tian Z, Shi L, Zhang B, Yuan S, Guo X, Wang Y, Guo H, Zhang H. A new Idenity of microcystins: environmental endocrine disruptors? An evidence-based review. Sci Total Environ. 2022;851(Pt 2):158262.

Zurawell RW. Toxic cyanobacteria. In: Bartram J, editor. Routledge handbook of water and health. Abingdon: Routeledge; 2017. p. 98–9.

17 Mycotoxins, Endotoxins, and Agricultural Respiratory Disorders

Jason Dietz

Mycotoxins

Background

For all of the research dedicated to viruses and bacteria and their role in human health, a comparatively trivial amount of time has been dedicated to an entire kingdom of life forms: fungi. Fungi go by many scientific and colloquial names including mushrooms, molds, mildew, and yeast, and they are ubiquitous in the environment. Physicians and other healthcare practitioners are familiar with infectious *mycoses*—histoplasmosis, coccidioidomycosis, and others—that threaten the human host through active replication. Willingly or unwittingly, humans can be afflicted by *mycetismi* (mushroom poisonings) when they consume mushrooms, the fruiting bodies of fungi that make their appearance on hiking trails and dinner plates. Finally, as the focus of this chapter, there are the *mycotoxicoses*. These are constellations of signs and symptoms that arise in humans and animals exposed to secondary metabolites of fungi (Smith and Moss 1985; Pitt 2000). These metabolites are low-molecular-weight compounds that are not necessary for the fungus to live but serve a secondary purpose in inhibiting growth from other organisms, sometimes inadvertently affecting humans and livestock. It is only in the past few decades that a deeper understanding of these compounds has taken shape, with dramatic implications for public health around the world.

Lacking in chlorophyll, fungi are classified as either saprophytes or parasites, deriving their nutrients by feeding on the organisms around them. Although fungi can grow on almost any substrate, the species and mycotoxins of interest here are primarily pathogens of plants, gaining access to the human host through inadvertent consumption (Austwick 1975). But the relationship is not always detrimental. Penicillin, discovered in black mold in 1928, as well as statins, cyclosporin, and ergot alkaloids all have utility as human pharmaceuticals.

Mycotoxins are very stable compounds and they are, by any practical constraint, impossible to remove once they have contaminated a food (Lee and Ryu 2017). Good agricultural practices are the primary defense (Murphy et al. 2006). Fungicidal compounds are not effective, acknowledging that the toxin can persist in the absence of living fungal colonies. There is nothing that protects products labeled as "organic" from being equally affected. Changes in weather patterns, particularly the degree of rainfall and humidity, can affect fungal growth. To this end, modern seed hybrids that mature earlier and permit multiple crops serve to reduce the accumulation of some mycotoxins (Pitt and Miller 2017).

J. Dietz (✉)
Division of Medical Toxicology, Ronald O. Perelman Department of Emergency Medicine, NYU Grossman School of Medicine, New York, NY, USA

W. J. Meggs, R. L. Langley (eds.), *Farm Toxicology*, https://doi.org/10.1007/978-3-031-80441-0_17

While it is comparatively easy to assess the nutritional value of food, the concept of "safety" is far more open-ended, and the testing needed is far more complex. The hesitancy of many national and international organizations to offer harmonized concentration limits and guidelines illustrates how difficult it can be to link an exposure to the human health effects. Although in vitro and in vivo research can demonstrate mutagenic and carcinogenic potential, every population around the world is exposed to these ubiquitous toxins at some level. There is insufficient data about the effects of chronic, low-level exposure, just as there is a paucity of data about the additive or sometimes antagonistic effects of different mycotoxins contaminating the same food supply.

Toxicity

With hundreds of mycotoxins identified and countless new compounds remaining to be elucidated, it is neither feasible nor clinically relevant to provide an exhaustive list. Total estimates of the number of compounds vary widely because so much remains to be studied, driven forward in spurts in response to disease outbreaks (Cimbalo et al. 2020). The main mycotoxins of interest come from strains of three specific fungal genera: *Penicillium*, *Aspergillus*, and *Fusarium* (Pandey et al. 2023). Unfortunately, the specific mycotoxin cannot always be identified just by knowing the genus and species of the fungus. Many different species of fungi are capable of producing an identical mycotoxin, and a single species can produce more than one mycotoxin.

Despite the "toxin" in the name, not all mycotoxins have proven adverse effects on humans or agricultural animals (Gruber-Dorninger et al. 2017). The World Health Organization (WHO), the Food and Agricultural Organization (FAO), and the International Agency for Research on Cancer (IARC) have attempted to maintain surveys of available data, but monographs and publications are often many years out of date. Unlike other compounds leading to human diseases, much of the data about mycotoxins are dispersed in chemical and biochemical journals or agricultural publications. Country-specific agricultural organizations impose guidelines or regulations that establish maximum concentrations in the food supply, but this is based more on perceived risks in nonrepresentative animal models rather than human disease outcomes. In the United States, given that the major intersection with human disease comes from the consumption of contaminated food, regulation falls primarily within the scope of the Food and Drug Administration (FDA). The U.S. Department of Agriculture (USDA) also has programs to monitor for aflatoxins in various legumes and grains and an official understanding with the FDA that it will report to them the samples that exceed established action levels (Dohlman 2003).

Aflatoxins are probably the best-known and most carefully researched of all the mycotoxins. There were reports of human cancer linked to contaminated peanuts nearly 100 years ago in Africa and adverse effects on human health for centuries prior to that, but the discovery of aflatoxins occurred in more recent times. As with many of the mycotoxins, it was driven by an outbreak. Nearly 100,000 turkeys became ill and died in 1959 and, despite a thorough investigation of known infectious etiologies, a cause could not be found. Ultimately, it was peanut meal contaminated with *Aspergillus* that had caused the disease in the turkey poults (Bennett and Klich 2003). This set in motion an entirely new era of research.

Aflatoxins are actually a family of compounds, the first four—B_1, B_2, G_1, and G_2—were named for their florescent blue and green color on thin-layer chromatography (Murphy et al. 2006). The mycotoxin-producing fungus can grow on many different products including groundnuts, corn, wheat, and coffee. Other aflatoxin compounds, such as M_1, were named for their presence in milk, which hints at the implications for public health. AFB_1 is regarded as the most toxic and, unfortunately, is also the compound present in the highest concentrations in contaminated foodstuffs (Lee and Ryu 2017).

Aflatoxin is a potent carcinogen and a major risk factor for the development of primary hepatocellular carcinoma. In the international setting, comorbid hepatitis B, HIV, and malnutrition augment the underlying risk. The IARC has published multiple monographs on this toxin, and it has been identified as a class 1 carcinogen since 1987 (IARC 2012).

Ochratoxin A, derived from species of *Aspergillus* and *Penicillium*, remains a compound of interest to regulatory agencies even though its linkage to a peculiar human disease has since been disproven. Balkan endemic nephropathy is a tubulointerstitial kidney disease that was once prevalent in rural areas of Bulgaria, Romania, and (former) Yugoslavia (Pitt and Miller 2017). Families and even whole towns were afflicted by chronic renal failure, sometimes in association with atypical presentations of transitional cell carcinoma. The disease led to a great deal of fear because it afflicted very specific regions, and a single causative agent could not be found. Ochratoxin A was thought to be the missing link, led by considerable circumstantial evidence and plausible biochemical effects. It is only in the past 20 years that aristolochic acid from plants (and sometimes found as a contaminant in Chinese herbal medicines) was found to be the more probable etiology (Bui-Klimke and Wu 2014). Nonetheless, ochratoxin A can contaminate an incredible diversity of agricultural products including cereal grains, cocoa, coffee beans, nuts, and fruits (Lee and Ryu 2017). With confirmed teratogenic, neurotoxic, and immunosuppressive effects in animal models, it remains a mycotoxin of significant interest. It is only categorized as a "possible" human carcinogen by the IARC. There are no FDA action levels or guidance for food contamination in the United States.

Zearalenone is included in lists of mycotoxins, but it is an outlier; its structure and activity are that of a nonsteroidal estrogen. It affects a variety of livestock, most notably prepubertal swine. The physiological changes seen in pigs include vulval and breast enlargement, infertility, small litter sizes, and low birth weights. Given its role as an endocrine disrupter, it is not surprising that there are similar concerns with regard to human health. Many small-scale studies and historical reviews have tried to demonstrate a causal relationship to precocious puberty in young girls (Massart and Saggese 2010), but these studies have neither the sample size nor the epidemiological rigor to provide definitive answers. To date, there have been no reports of acute poisoning in humans and no studies of human carcinogenicity (IARC 2012). Although at one time a major contaminant of the corn supply in North America, it is hypothesized that the use of hybrid corn varietals with shorter maturation periods has served to inhibit the *Fusarium* fungal growth (Pitt and Miller 2017).

Patulin is a contaminant in a wide variety of foodstuffs, most often recognized as blue mold. Following the discovery of penicillin, there was a robust investigation into other fungal metabolites and a search for the next antibiotic. Labs around the world pursued the goal, and their parallel and disjointed efforts led to a confusing proliferation of names for this chemical including penicidin, claviformin, clavacin, mycoin c, and expansin (Singh 2012). Although the chemical possesses growth-suppressing activity against a variety of bacteria, viruses, and protozoa, it was considered too toxic to use in animals and, in the 1960's, was reclassified as a mycotoxin. The focus of most investigations has centered on fruits, particularly apple juice and unfermented apple cider (Zhong et al. 2018). The IARC, in a monograph dating back to 1986, found inadequate evidence to make a formal evaluation on the carcinogenicity of patulin in humans. Nonetheless, the frequency of this contaminant in apple products, particularly those consumed by infants and young children, has led many countries to impose regulations or guidelines that limit the total concentration.

Treatment

The primary care provider benefits from an awareness of these toxins, but it is often difficult to make the diagnosis of a mycotoxin-associated disease. Consultation with an occupational/environmental physician or medical toxicologist is recommended. Outbreaks related to affected crops require the coordination of public health and agricultural agencies who already work to provide surveillance of many of the grains that are imported into the United States.

Respiratory Conditions

The agricultural workplace is filled with inhalation hazards (Donham and Thelin 2016). While the focus to this point has been on fungi and their mycotoxins, they are far from being the only trigger for respiratory inflammation. Employees come to the worksite with predisposing conditions such as asthma, obesity, or a history of smoking. Once on the job, they are exposed to a variety of organic materials, which include endotoxin (lipopolysaccharides found in gram-negative bacteria), wood dust, and animal hair and excrement, as well as pesticides, machinery exhaust, nitrogen oxides, and countless other inorganic dusts and fumes.

It can be challenging for the rural healthcare practitioner, in a single visit or with a single test, to distinguish an acute, self-limited case from one that might portend a worse long-term prognosis. All of these diagnoses are defined by a careful occupational history, often with the aid of imaging studies and pulmonary function tests. The benefit of repeat assessment over time should not be underestimated.

Work-Related Asthma

Introduction

The terminology can be confusing because work-related asthma can encompass patients with de novo asthma attributable to the workplace (occupational asthma) as well as those with preexisting reactive airway disease who experience worsening of their symptoms due to workplace triggers (work-aggravated asthma) (Tarlo et al. 2008). The core definition of asthma remains the same as it would in any other context, but occupational asthma is attributable to a specific occupational environment and not to stimuli encountered outside of the workplace. Although it can be difficult to disentangle work-related asthma from the much larger baseline prevalence of reactive airway disease in a population, this condition still ranks as one of the most common chronic occupational lung diseases.

Adult-onset asthma should always include a detailed occupational history, and the practitioner needs to have some familiarity with common sensitizers and triggers (Tarlo et al. 2009). If multiple patients are simultaneously presenting with new, acute symptoms and there is concern for a chemical irritant, regional poison control centers (national number: 1-800-222-1222) can offer targeted guidance.

Toxicity

The list of possible irritants extends into the hundreds of different chemicals and proteins. One often cited occupational respiratory syndrome is byssinosis, or cotton worker's lung. Textile workers can be at varying degrees of risk depending on their role in the cleaning and carding of cotton, as can workers exposed to flax or hemp dust. Cotton dust, specifically the endotoxin component of the bacteria associated with cotton dust, is able to trigger airway inflammation and an obstructive pattern on spirometry (Rylander et al. 1989). Affected individuals present with cough, chest tightness, and wheezing, often within a few hours of each repeated exposure. While this disease is of diminished importance in the developed world, in the setting of both increased awareness and increased mechanization of the cotton industry, that might be changing. Although hemp production is limited, commercial cultivation of the same cannabis plant continues to accelerate across the United States under conflicting state guidance. In the absence of unifying federal regulations, this occupational exposure might not receive the research, awareness, and workplace protections that it otherwise deserves (Couch et al. 2019; Sack et al. 2023).

Diagnosis

The initial workup is consistent with any new diagnosis of asthma but requires the healthcare provider to consider a causative occupational exposure. Pulmonary function tests are performed, ideally at the end of the workweek (Tarlo et al. 2009). Classic occupational symptoms often improve over the weekend or during holidays and other prolonged absences from the worksite. The National Institute for Occupational Safety and Health (NIOSH) has an online decision tree to aid in the diagnosis of work-related asthma (NIOSH 2023). This is a broad term that requires: (1) a healthcare professional's diagnosis of asthma and (2) an association between the symptoms of asthma and the work. The correct diagnosis can have ramifications on a worker's compensation claim and, therefore, confirmatory testing can extend beyond the purview of the primary care provider.

Treatment

A diagnosis of occupational asthma does not necessitate a change in occupation, particularly if the symptoms can be well-controlled with medication. Ideally, the patient should have their specific tasks and exposures modified at the worksite, but this can be challenging depending on the size of the employer, particularly while the diagnostic workup is ongoing.

Organic Dust Toxic Syndrome (ODTS)

Introduction

Organic dust toxic syndrome (also referred to as silo unloader's syndrome, atypical farmer's lung, precipitin-negative farmer's lung, pulmonary mycotoxicosis, grain fever, mill fever, humidifier fever, or toxic pneumonitis) is a common, noninfectious, self-limited, inhalational syndrome. The presentation is described as "flu-like" and prominently features fever, chills, malaise, and myalgias, in addition to other symptoms such as dry cough, dyspnea, chest tightness, headache, and nausea (Seifert et al. 2003). Symptom-onset follows exposure to high concentrations of organic dust. Farmers often report that they are completing an unusual work task, such as unloading a silo or disposing of moldy hay, that leads to uncommonly high dust exposure. Signs and symptoms begin within a few hours of the exposure and often come to a resolution in less than 48 h although the syndrome can persist for up to a week (Von Essen et al. 1990). Individuals can have more than one attack of ODTS, but these episodes can be years apart (Rask-Andersen 1989).

Toxicity

There are many theories regarding the etiology of the syndrome, and a single causative agent has not been found in all circumstances. The multitude of overlapping names hints at some of the proposed theories and the connection to different occupations. Organic dusts implicated in the syndrome often derive from animal feeds spoiled by molds, as well as hay and corn silage, wood-chip shaving, and mulch.

Modernization of farm practices, guided by economies of scale, has led to the formation of concentrated animal feed operations (CAFOs) that aggregate expanding populations of livestock onto increasingly small footprints of land. While confined spaces augment business efficiencies, they also expose workers to increasing concentrations of stored animal feed and animal waste. There appears to be a dose–response relationship in ODTS. Higher concentrations of particulate organic matter, for a more sustained duration, increase the likelihood of developing the syndrome. Clusters of cases can present on the same day from the same work site. This is distinct from the pulmonary hypersensitivities that require individual predisposition paired with a prolonged sensitization. Patients who develop ODTS generally do not have underlying atopy.

Diagnosis

Clinical and occupational history are the primary guides for the diagnosis as there are no confirmatory investigations. Given the short duration of the illness and the nonspecific symptoms, many patients never seek physician input or might conflate the presentation with a viral malady. Practitioners who work in rural areas might place this diagnosis higher on the differential, but it remains a diagnosis of exclusion. The chest X-ray is classically reported as normal although mild interstitial infiltrates can be seen.

Treatment

In the vast majority of cases, symptoms will be mild to moderate, and treatment focuses on supportive care. For the small subset of patients that present with significant respiratory symptoms, hospitalization can be required to address hypoxia and respiratory distress.

Hypersensitivity Pneumonitis (Farmer's Lung)

Introduction

Hypersensitivity pneumonitis (also referred to as extrinsic allergic alveolitis) is an inflammatory and sometimes fibrotic lung disease that occurs when the immune system, particularly the T-cell-mediated component, has an aberrant response to an environmental antigen.

The many colloquial names that have been bestowed on this condition allude to some of the respective triggers. Farmer's lung, mushroom worker's lung, compost lung, potato riddler's lung, and riding school lung give some color to the disease. However, as varied as they sound, they are not diagnostic of a single fungal or animal-protein antigen exposure, and they often share overlapping risk factors. In rural areas, a diagnosis of hypersensitivity pneumonitis might reflexively be labeled as "farmer's lung" because of the broad familiarity with the term, but a more detailed search for the causative trigger should be sought.

Toxicity

Fungal spores can contain allergens, which are different from mycotoxins. The spores sensitize the immune system (an indirect injury) rather than serving as the direct compound or metabolite capable of inducing the damage. For farmer's lung in particular, both *Aspergillus* spp. and thermophilic actinomycetes have been implicated. Many individuals are exposed to the same antigens, but only a small subset will develop the illness, and an even smaller subset will progress to the advanced stages of fibrosis.

Diagnosis

There is not a gold-standard diagnostic test for hypersensitivity pneumonitis. A definitive diagnosis, even among pulmonologists, can be challenging. Only in recent years have two major pulmonary organizations released guidelines with more rigorous diagnostic criteria, in the hope of both aiding future research and improving clinical prognostication (Raghu et al. 2020; Fernández Pérez et al. 2021).

Acute hypersensitivity pneumonitis, much like the preceding pathologies, can present with an acute, flu-like illness. Repeated exposure can then lead to a more chronic disease, with associated hypoxemia, restrictive patterns on pulmonary function testing, and often radiographic evidence of interstitial changes.

Apart from the history and physical exam, a plain chest radiograph is often the first test used in the evaluation of symptomatic patients. It can be obtained rapidly, which is of value when the pulmonary findings might otherwise improve or resolve on the order of days to weeks. The presence of fibrosis portends a worse prognosis, independent of specific etiology.

Nonspecific markers of inflammation remain equally nonspecific in this setting although erythrocyte sedimentation rate and C-reactive protein can be elevated, particularly during the acute presentation of an illness. A peripheral blood count can show leukocytosis, driven by an elevated neutrophil count without eosinophilia.

Serum antibodies are of variable utility, and a negative result can rarely be used to rule out a given etiology. Equally problematic, similar levels of serum antibodies have been found in individuals with similar exposures but who do not progress to any apparent illness.

Treatment

Glucocorticoids are a commonly offered therapy, particularly in the acute setting, but the evidence is more equivocal about whether their continued utilization helps resolve radiographic findings or reverse existing changes in pulmonary function testing (Mönkäre and Haahtela 1987). In farmer's lung, specifically, there can be a more rapid initial resolution of radiographic findings, but one study found no clinical differences between the treated and untreated groups at 6 months of follow-up (Kokkarinen et al. 1992).

More advanced workups can be delegated to specialty consults who can consider bronchioalveolar lavage, tissue biopsy, or other invasive testing in situations where diagnostic certainty can have significant implications for prognosis. Delayed presentations or those following a chronic time course can be difficult to distinguish from idiopathic pulmonary fibrosis or sarcoidosis.

References

Austwick PKC. Mycotoxins. Br Med Bull. 1975;31:222.

Bennett JW, Klich M. Mycotoxins. Clin Microbiol Rev. 2003;16(3):497–516.

Bui-Klimke T, Wu F. Evaluating weight of evidence in the mystery of Balkan endemic nephropathy. Risk Anal. 2014;34(9):1688–705.

Cimbalo A, Alonso-Garrido M, Font G, Manyes L. Toxicity of mycotoxins in vivo on vertebrate organisms: a review. Food Chem Toxicol. 2020;137:111161.

Couch JR, Grimes GR, Wiegand DM, Green BJ, Glassford EK, Zwack LM, et al. Potential occupational and respiratory hazards in a Minnesota cannabis cultivation and processing facility. Am J Ind Med. 2019;62(10):874–82.

Dohlman E. Mycotoxin hazards and regulations impacts on food and animal feed crop trade. In: International trade and food safety: economic theory and case studies. Economic Research Service/USDA. International Trade and Food Safety/AER-828; 2003. p. 97–108.

Donham K, Thelin A. Agricultural respiratory diseases. In: Agricultural medicine rural occupational and environmental health, safety, and prevention. 2nd ed. Wiley Blackwell; 2016. p. 95–154.

Fernández Pérez ER, Travis WD, Lynch DA, Brown KK, Johannson KA, Selman M, et al. Diagnosis and evaluation of hypersensitivity pneumonitis. Chest. 2021;160(2):e97–156.

Gruber-Dorninger C, Novak B, Nagl V, Berthiller F. Emerging mycotoxins: beyond traditionally determined food contaminants. J Agric Food Chem. 2017;65(33):7052–70.

International Agency for Research on Cancer (IARC). In: Pitt JI, Wild CP, Baan RA, Gelderblom WCA, Miller JD, Riley RT, Wu F, editors. Improving public health through mycotoxin control, vol. 158. Lyon: IARC Scientific Publication; 2012.

Kokkarinen JI, Tukiainen HO, Terho EO. Effect of corticosteroid treatment on the recovery of pulmonary function in farmer's lung. Am Rev Respir Dis. 1992;145(1):3–5.

Lee HJ, Ryu D. Worldwide occurrence of mycotoxins in cereals and cereal-derived food products: public health perspectives of their co-occurrence. J Agric Food Chem. 2017;65(33):7034–51.

Massart F, Saggese G. Oestrogenic mycotoxin exposures and precocious pubertal development. Int J Androl. 2010;33(2):369–76.

Mönkäre S, Haahtela T. Farmer's lung—a 5-year follow-up of eighty-six patients. Clin Exp Allergy. 1987;17(2):143–51.

Murphy PA, Hendrich S, Landgren C, Bryant CM. Food mycotoxins: an update. J Food Sci. 2006;71(5):51. https://doi.org/10.1111/j.1750-3841.2006.00052.x.

NIOSH (National Institute for Occupational Safety and Health). WRA State Reporting Guidelines [Internet]. 2023. https://www.cdc.gov/niosh/topics/surveillance/ords/statesurveillance/reportingguidelines-wra.html.

Pandey AK, Samota MK, Kumar A, Silva AS, Dubey NK. Fungal mycotoxins in food commodities: present status and future concerns. Front Sustain Food Syst. 2023;7:1162595.

Pitt JI. Toxigenic fungi and mycotoxins. Br Med Bull. 2000;1:184.

Pitt JI, Miller JD. A concise history of mycotoxin research. J Agric Food Chem. 2017;65(33):7021–33.

Raghu G, Remy-Jardin M, Ryerson CJ, Myers JL, Kreuter M, Vasakova M, et al. Diagnosis of hypersensitivity pneumonitis in adults: an official ATS/JRS/ALAT clinical practice guideline. Am J Respir Crit Care Med. 2020;202(3):e36–69.

Rask-Andersen A. Organic dust toxic syndrome among farmers. Occup Environ Med. 1989;46(4):233–8.

Rylander R, Bake B, Fischer JJ, Helander IM. Pulmonary function and symptoms after inhalation of endotoxin. Am Rev Respir Dis. 1989;140(4):981–6.

Sack C, Simpson C, Pacheco K. The emerging spectrum of respiratory diseases in the U.S. cannabis industry. Semin Respir Crit Care Med. 2023;44(03):405–14.

Seifert SA, Essen SV, Jacobitz K, Crouch R, Lintner CP. Organic dust toxic syndrome: a review. J Toxicol Clin Toxicol. 2003;41(2):185–93.

Singh J. Mechanism of antifungal action of Patulin. Champaign, IL: University of Illinois Urbana-Champaign; 2012.

Smith JE, Moss MO. Mycotoxins: formation, analysis, and significance. Chichester; New York: Wiley; 1985. p. 148.

Tarlo SM, Balmes J, Balkissoon R, Beach J, Beckett W, Bernstein D, et al. Diagnosis and management of work-related asthma. Chest. 2008;134(3):1S–41S.

Tarlo SM, Cartier A, Lemière C. On behalf of the Canadian thoracic society asthma committee. Work-related asthma: a case-based guide. Can Respir J. 2009;16(6):e57–61.

Von Essen S, Robbins RA, Thompson AB, Rennard SI. Organic dust toxic syndrome: an acute febrile reaction to organic dust exposure distinct from hypersensitivity pneumonitis. J Toxicol Clin Toxicol. 1990;28(4):389–420.

Zhong L, Carere J, Lu Z, Lu F, Zhou T. Patulin in apples and apple-based food products: the burdens and the mitigation strategies. Toxins. 2018;10:475.

Venomous Animals

18

Benjamin German

Introduction

Envenomation, also called envenoming, by snakes and other animals is a common problem in agricultural settings. Envenomation occurs when an organism delivers venom, a toxic biologic substance, to another organism. Venom can be used for predation by incapacitating prey and can also aid in digestion. Venom can also serve a defensive purpose by causing harm to predators or other threats. Some animals, like honeybees, only use venom for defense.

Most venoms are mixtures of enzymes and other proteins that work in synergy to cause damage to the target organism Laustsen 2016). Some venoms also contain smaller bioactive molecules like histamine and serotonin (Habermann 1972). A given venom has typically evolved over time to specifically target the biology of prey items and/or threats (Ward-Smith et al. 2020; Holding et al. 2016).

In contrast to other poisons, venom requires a delivery mechanism to be transferred to the victim. Examples of venom delivery systems include snake or arthropod fangs, scorpion or wasp stingers, and venomous projections from the bodies of caterpillars. Venomous animals are found nearly worldwide in various forms with increasing diversity in tropical areas.

B. German (✉)
Emergency Medicine, WakeMed Health and Hospitals, Raleigh, NC, USA

Farmers are disproportionately burdened by envenomation, particularly in the developing world. Venomous animals often inhabit agricultural settings where conflict with humans can occur. Agricultural activities also tend to occur in remote areas and prolonged transport to medical care can be an issue. Furthermore, hospitals or clinics in the developing world often lack supplies and appropriately trained personnel, leading to inconsistent envenomation care (Chippaux 2017).

An additional barrier in some areas is a mistrust of western medicine and a pattern of first seeking care from a traditional or faith healer (Schioldann et al. 2018). Traditional healers are often more affordable and more readily available than hospital care. Traditional medicine techniques, however, are often ineffective in helping serious envenomations and can cause additional harm (Fig. 18.4b, c). This leads to delays in victims receiving definitive care and can worsen outcomes (Schioldann et al. 2018; Steinhorst et al. 2021). Additionally, for minor envenomations, traditional medicine seems to work because the victim survives and recovers, as they would without treatment. This reinforces the practice of first seeking care from a traditional healer (Steinhorst et al. 2021).

The total global burden of envenomations can only be roughly estimated. Some regions, like North America, Europe, Australia, and parts of Asia have systems in place for collecting data on

W. J. Meggs, R. L. Langley (eds.), *Farm Toxicology*, https://doi.org/10.1007/978-3-031-80441-0_18

envenomations. Many parts of the world, however, do not have the means to track envenomations and significant data gaps exist (Farooq et al. 2022; World Health Organization 2019; Warrell and Williams 2023). The best data available is for snakebites. The World Health Organization (WHO), which has designated snakebite envenomation (SBE) a neglected tropical disease, estimates that 1.8–2.7 million people are envenomated by snakes, and 81,000 to 138,000 die from snakebite every year (World Health Organization 2019).

Types of Venomous Animals

Vertebrates

Snakes

There are nearly 4000 species of snakes in the world, with about 600 venomous species (Warrell and Williams 2023). Snakes have adapted to utilize many different habitats, including forests, deserts, grasslands, wetlands, and even the open ocean. Snakes are found in nearly every part of the world except for very cold areas and certain islands. Snakes are ectothermic animals and increase in number and species diversity in warmer regions (Gutiérrez et al. 2017).

Of the medically important venomous snakes, most deliver venom through modified hollow front teeth called fangs. The venom is produced in glands in the head and channeled through ducts to the fangs. When these snakes bite, muscles compress the glands and venom is expelled into the wounds through the fangs. Important families of front-fanged snakes include Viperidae (vipers, Fig. 18.1), Elapidae (cobras, kraits, mambas, coral snakes, Australian snakes, sea snakes, Fig. 18.2), and Atractaspididae (stiletto snakes). A few members of the family Colubridae are also capable of delivering dangerous venom through grooved upper teeth in the rear of the mouth, such as the boomslang (*Dispholidus typus*) (Weinstein et al. 2022).

Snakes often thrive in agricultural areas, where they feed upon prey such as rodents, which are attracted to crops and human habitation. In many parts of the developing world, farming is hands-on and labor-intensive, which increases the potential for human-snake conflict (Fig. 18.3a). Impoverished populations are heavily impacted by snakebite in these regions, due to their subsistence occupations, often porous housing structures, and lack of access to healthcare (White 2018). High-risk agricultural activities include tea cultivation, latex rubber collection, and sugar cane cultivation (Gutiérrez et al. 2017). Farmers in any region with venomous snakes, however, are at risk for snakebite envenomation.

Prevention Most snakebites occur to the upper and lower extremities and involve a person placing their hands or feet near an unseen snake. Awareness and vigilance in areas with snakes is essential as many snakes have excellent camouflage (Fig. 18.3b). Protective footwear, like boots, can prevent some lower extremity envenomations. Many snakes are nocturnal and handheld lighting is important when walking at night. Since the bulk of the global burden of snakebite occurs in developing regions, however, sturdy footwear, flashlights, or batteries are often unavailable to those with the greatest need. Many tropical areas also experience a rainy season when farming and snakes are most active (Akani et al. 2013). Subsistence farmers frequently wear sandals, or go barefooted, to avoid soaked footwear and this provides no protection against snakebite.

Pathophysiology of Snake Envenomation

Snake venoms are complex mixtures of bioactive substances, and an individual venom contains numerous proteins, including enzymes and inhibitors. Snake venom typically consists of 90–95% protein by dry weight (Oliveira et al. 2022). Major classes of snake venom enzymes include metalloproteinases, other proteinases, phospholipases, hyaluronidases, and acetylcholinesterases (Oliveira et al. 2022; Mackessy 2021). Major classes of nonenzymatic snake venom proteins include alpha neurotoxins, cardiotoxins, and myotoxins (Oliveira et al. 2022; Mackessy 2021). Numerous unique snake venom toxins have been identified, with new toxins often being isolated

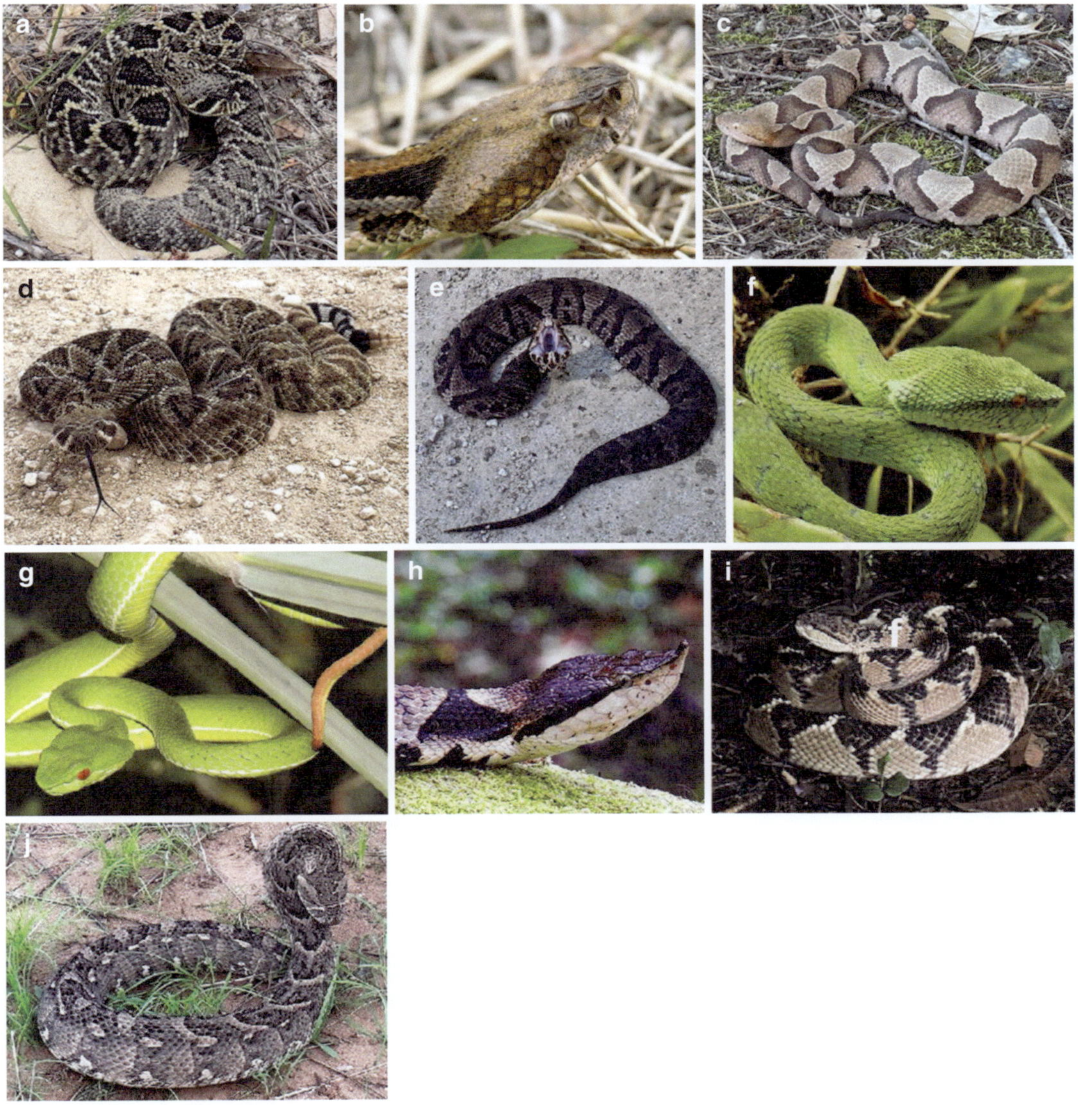

Fig. 18.1 Viperid snakes. Selected viperid snakes from different regions. *Crotalus adamanteus* (eastern diamondback rattlesnake, Florida, US; part **a**), *Crotalus horridus* (timber rattlesnake, North Carolina, US; part **b**), *Agkistrodon contortrix* (eastern copperhead, North Carolina, US; part **c**), *Crotalus atrox* (western diamondback rattlesnake, Texas, US; part **d**), *Agkistrodon piscivorous* (eastern cottonmouth, Florida, US; part **e**), *Tropidolaemus subannulatus* (Bornean keeled pit viper, Borneo, Malaysia; part **f**), *Deinagkistrodon acutus* (Chinese moccasin, Taiwan; part **g**), *Trimeresurus stejnegeri* (bamboo viper, Taiwan; part **h**), *Lachesis muta* (South American bushmaster, Peru; part **i**), *Bitis arietans* (puff adder, Guinea, Africa; part **j**). (Images **a**–**g**, **j** courtesy of B.T.G, images **h**, **i** courtesy of B.N.)

and characterized (Oliveira et al. 2022). Grouping toxins by clinical effects is helpful when discussing the diagnosis and management of snake envenomations. Most snake venom toxins can be classified as having neurotoxic, hemotoxic, or cytotoxic effects (Oliveira et al. 2022).

Neurotoxins

Neurotoxic venom proteins interfere with nervous system function. The family Elapidae contains the most significantly neurotoxic species. Some snakes from other families, such as certain rattlesnakes in the family Viperidae, can produce

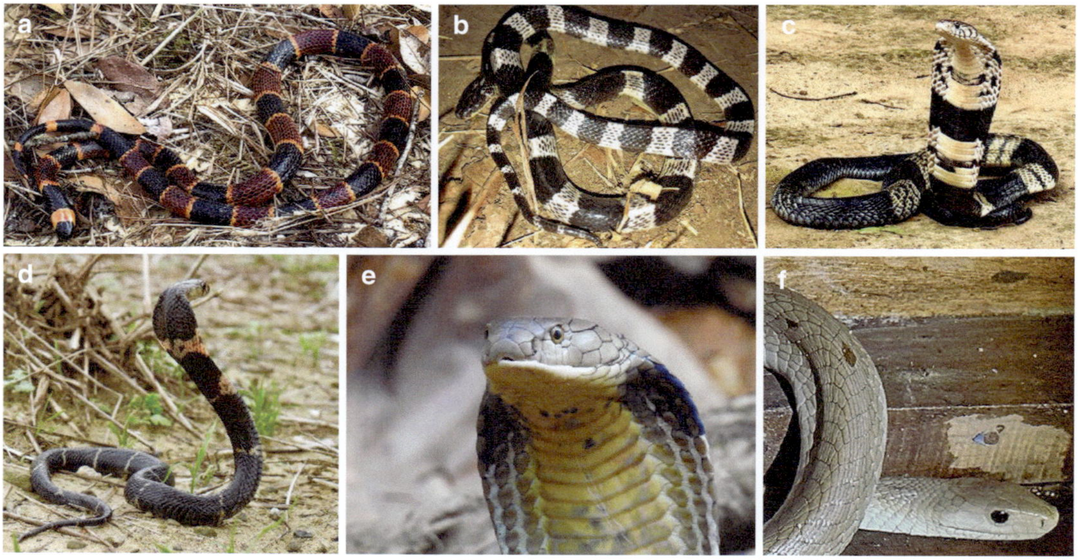

Fig. 18.2 Elapid snakes. Selected elapid snakes from different regions. *Micrurus fulvius* (eastern coral snake, Florida, US; part **a**), *Bungarus candidus* (Malayan krait, Bali, Indonesia; part **b**), *Naja savannula* (West African banded cobra, Guinea, Africa; part **c**), *Naja atra* (Chinese cobra, Taiwan; part **d**), *Ophiophagus hannah* (king cobra, Bali, Indonesia; part **e**), *Dendroaspis polylepis* (black mamba, Guinea, Africa; part **f**). (Images **a**, **c**–**f** courtesy of B.G, image **b** courtesy of B.N.)

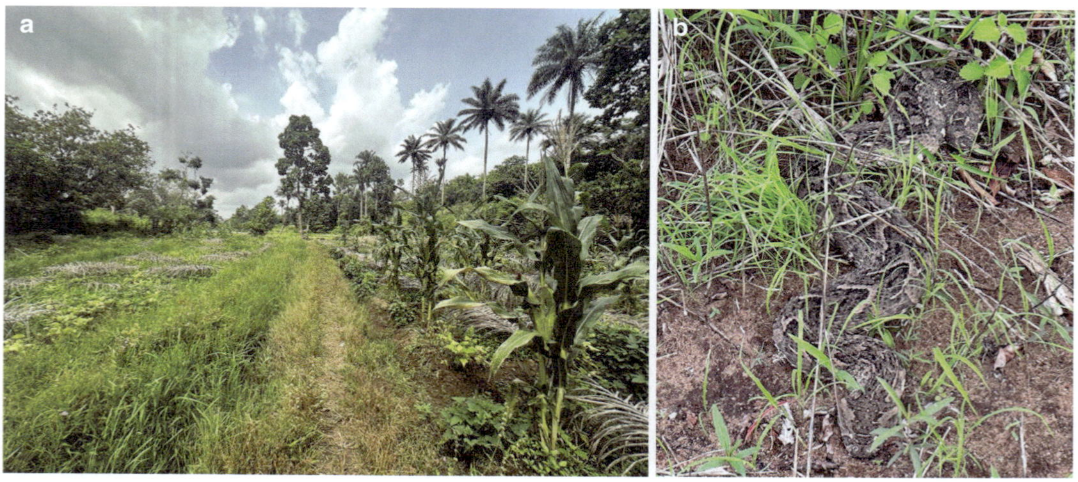

Fig. 18.3 Rural mixed agricultural area in Guinea, Africa. Several venomous snake species inhabit this area, including mambas, cobras, vipers, and stiletto snakes. Many snake envenomations occur in similar situations throughout the world (part **a**). *Bitis arietans* (puff adder) in ambush position awaiting prey in Guinea, Africa (part **b**). Many venomous snakes, particularly vipers, are cryptic and easy to overlook, which leads to accidental snakebite. (Images **a**, **b** courtesy of B.G.)

neurotoxic effects as well (Levine et al. 2023; Silva et al. 2016).

Snake neurotoxins can cause inhibition or excitation at the neuromuscular junction, in addition to other neurotoxic effects (Oliveira et al. 2022; Mackessy 2021). Most inhibitory proteins work by antagonizing the effects of acetylcholine and are designed to paralyze prey thereby aiding in capture and ingestion. Common inhibitory toxins include alpha neurotoxins, which act at the postsynaptic membrane, and beta neurotoxins, which act at the presynaptic membranes (Mackessy 2021). American coral snakes (genus *Micrurus*) and Asian kraits (genus Bungarus) are examples of neurotoxic snakes whose venom produces inhibitory effects. In human victims, these venoms cause muscular weakness. When the weakness affects the respiratory musculature, death from asphyxiation can occur.

Other snakes, such as the African mambas (genus *Dendroaspis*), can produce mixed excitatory and inhibitory effects. Mambas produce low molecular weight excitatory proteins called dendrotoxins, which bind voltage-gated potassium channels in neurons (Quarch et al. 2017). The effect is a release of acetylcholine into the neuromuscular junction, which causes excitatory symptoms like muscle fasciculations (Quarch et al. 2017). Mamba venom also has proteins that agonize muscarinic acetylcholine receptors and can cause SLUDGE (Salivation, Lacrimation, Urination, Defecation, Gastrointestinal upset, Emesis) symptoms (Jolkkonen et al. 1995; Greene et al. 2023). These snakes also possess potent postsynaptic nicotinic acetylcholine receptor antagonists which cause muscle weakness (Jolkkonen et al. 1995; Greene et al. 2023). The combined effect of mamba venom is a severe envenomation picture characterized by excitatory and muscarinic SLUDGE symptoms followed by descending paralysis. These bites are often fatal if not aggressively treated (Erulu 2018).

Hemotoxins

Hemotoxic venom proteins target components of the circulatory system, including blood cells, blood vessels, platelets, and coagulation factors. The effect of these toxins is a disruption of hemostasis, which manifests clinically as bleeding problems, swelling, and the sequelae of intravascular fluid loss (Gutiérrez et al. 2017). Examples of snake hemotoxins include metalloproteinases, other proteinases, and phospholipases (Oliveira et al. 2022; Mackessy 2021). Some of these proteins activate coagulation while others inhibit coagulation. When the coagulation cascade is inappropriately activated, microthrombi generation can cause factor consumption and eventual depletion (Berling and Isbister 2015). Severe and life-threatening bleeding can result. Thrombotic complications can also occur, and ischemic strokes, pulmonary emboli, and myocardial infarction have been reported acutely with hemotoxic envenomations (Paul et al. 2014; Bart et al. 2016; Rathnayaka et al. 2022).

Hemotoxins can also directly attack blood vessels, which causes fluid extravasation, local tissue injury, hypovolemia, hypotension, and shock in severe cases (Gutiérrez et al. 2017; Baldo et al. 2010). Some venom components can also directly lower blood pressure (Gutiérrez et al. 2017). Most viperid snakes, such as rattlesnakes and other vipers, produce venoms containing hemotoxins (Bart et al. 2016). Certain Australian elapids also produce hemotoxic venom proteins and severe bleeding can occur in bites from these snakes (Berling et al. 2015).

Cytotoxins

Cytotoxic proteins cause direct damage to cells and tissue. Tissue necrosis and permanent limb dysfunction or limb loss can result, and this is a major cause of long-term morbidity in snakebites (Gutiérrez et al. 2017; Oliveira et al. 2022; World Health Organization 2010a). Cytotoxic proteins can also directly affect cardiac tissue, renal tissue, and other organ systems (Gutiérrez et al. 2017; Oliveira et al. 2022; World Health Organization 2010a). Many viperid snakes can produce cytotoxic effects as can several elapid species, such as spitting cobras (genus *Naja*) and certain Australian elapids (World Health Organization 2010a). Phospholipases, through their effects on cell membranes, are an important cause of cytotoxicity (Hiu and Yap 2020). Hyaluronidases and other enzymatic toxins attack the extracellular matrix, which promotes venom spread and further potentiates tissue injury (Girish et al. 2002).

Factors Affecting Envenomation Severity

The clinical effects of snake envenomation are determined by several factors, including the composition of the venom, the amount of venom injected, the size and other characteristics of the victim, the anatomic site of injection, and the depth of venom injection.

Venom composition is most affected by the species of snake. Expected effects from a North American rattlesnake bite include local tissue injury, coagulopathy, and in severe cases, hemodynamic compromise. In contrast, a North American coral snake envenomation may produce few local or hematologic changes, but descending paralysis progressing to respiratory failure may result. These snakes produce different toxins with different actions. Intraspecific venom variation also occurs, however, and venom composition can differ significantly even between members of the same species (Smith and Mackessy 2016). An example is the Mojave rattlesnake, *Crotalus scutulatus*, which is native to the southwestern United States and northern Mexico. Certain populations of this snake produce a neurotoxin, called Mojave Toxin, which inhibits acetylcholine release from the presynaptic membrane (Ludolph 2023). Other populations of these snakes do not produce neurotoxic effects.

The amount of venom injected is generally impossible to determine in the clinical setting, but a greater amount of venom generally produces a more severe envenomation (Hayes et al. 2002; Hayes 2005; Corbit and Hayes 2016; Janes et al. 2010). A common myth is that juvenile snakes are more dangerous than adults. While small snakes can still produce severe envenomations, a larger snake typically yields more venom, has longer fangs, and a more powerful bite; the likely result is a more severe envenomation (Hayes et al. 2002; Hayes 2005; Corbit and Hayes 2016; Janes et al. 2010). Sometimes victims receive more than one bite, which will also increase the amount of venom injected. Venomous snakes can deliver venom in each of multiple bites (Hayes et al. 2002).

The depth of venom injection and the anatomic site of injection also affects envenomation severity (Gutiérrez et al. 2017). Venom injected into muscle tissue may increase the risk of compartment syndrome, which while rare in snakebite, can cause severe morbidity including permanent limb dysfunction and loss (Warrell and Williams 2023; Gutiérrez et al. 2017; World Health Organization 2010a; Toschlog et al. 2013). Intravascular envenomation is rare but can produce rapid and devastating systemic envenomation (Naik 2023).

The anatomic site of venom injection also influences the clinical severity. Most snakebites occur on the extremities, particularly the hands and feet, but bites to the head, neck, and trunk also occur. Head and neck bites are particularly dangerous as they can cause swelling which compromises the airway. Envenomation directly into a digit can cause severe local tissue damage, permanent dysfunction, and can result in loss of the digit (Toschlog et al. 2013).

Victim characteristics are also important. Due to their smaller mass, pediatric patients are at greater risk of complications from snake envenomation (Le Geyt et al. 2021). Older patients with significant comorbidities are also at higher risk (Feitosa et al. 2015). For example, patients with underlying heart, lung, kidney, liver, or other organ system dysfunction may be more susceptible to the toxic venom effects. Pharmaceuticals taken by the victim, such as anticoagulants, antihypertensives, and other medications can also potentially worsen an envenomation.

Clinical Management of Snake Envenomation

Antidotes

Antivenom Since a given snake venom contains hundreds of individual proteins, neutralizing toxic venom effects involves inhibiting the action of as many of the toxic proteins as possible. Antivenoms have long been the definitive treatment for snake envenomation (Warrell and Williams 2023; Gutiérrez et al. 2017). This section discusses snake antivenoms, but the principles apply to all antivenoms.

Antivenoms were first developed in the late 1800s and came into wider use in the 1950s (Pucca et al. 2019). Antivenoms are traditionally made by immunizing host animals, such as horses or sheep, with whole venom from a relevant snake or group of selected snakes (Gutiérrez et al. 2017; Pucca et al. 2019). The host animal generates antibodies against the venom proteins. Host animal serum is then collected and the venom-specific antibodies in the serum constitute the antivenom. The antibodies combat venom toxicity by binding and inactivating venom proteins.

Early antivenoms consisted of whole animal serum containing the venom-specific antibodies as well as many other nonessential proteins. Given the broad range of foreign proteins found in whole serum, allergic reactions were common with early antivenoms and were a significant risk of antivenom administration (Pucca et al. 2019). In the later twentieth century, evolving molecular techniques led to purer antivenom products. A notable development was the enzyme digestion of antibodies to separate the F(ab′) or F(ab′)2 fragments from the Fc fragment (Pucca et al. 2019). After digestion, the Fc fragment is discarded leaving only the antigen-binding antibody fragments in the product. Affinity purification of the venom-binding fragments was another significant development (Russell et al. 1985). This technique allows non-venom-binding antibodies to be discarded. This process yields an antivenom product that contains essential venom-binding antibodies, reduces the nonessential protein content, and decreases the risk of hypersensitivity reactions (Pucca et al. 2019).

Antivenoms can be monovalent (effective against venom from one species of snake), or polyvalent (effective against the venoms of multiple snakes). Monovalent antivenoms have been used to treat envenomations from species whose bites are relatively rare but serious enough to warrant treatment. Examples of monovalent antivenoms include African boomslang (*D. typus*) antivenom, Thai king cobra (*Ophiophagus hannah*) antivenom, and North American coral snake (*Micrurus fulvius*) antivenom.

A polyvalent antivenom neutralizes venom from several different snake species. These antivenoms are made to cover specific geographic areas that are inhabited by multiple venomous species. In areas with multiple venomous species, a polyvalent antivenom simplifies envenomation treatment by negating the need to know the identity of the biting snake (Ratanabanangkoon 2023). Examples of polyvalent snake antivenoms include Crotalidae Polyvalent Immune F(ab′), used for North American pit viper envenomations, and Inoserp PAN-AFRICA antivenom, used for multiple sub-Saharan African snake species.

Given the global diversity of snake venoms and the unique protein structures of the venom components, it is currently impractical to create a single antivenom that would protect against all the medically significant venomous snakes in the world. Regional approaches are still used.

Multiple different antivenoms are currently used globally. The choice of antivenoms depends on the geographic region and which products are available (Warrell and Williams 2023; Gutiérrez et al. 2017). In developing regions, antivenom may not be readily available. Most modern antivenoms are F(ab′)2 products (Gutiérrez et al. 2017). Some are F(ab′), such as Crotalidae Polyvalent Immune F(ab′), which is used for North American pit viper envenomation. Other antivenoms are whole IgG products (World Health Organization 2010b). Each antivenom has its own efficacy and side effect profile. Purified F(ab′) or F(ab′)2 products generally carry a lower risk of adverse reaction, but immediate and delayed hypersensitivity reactions are a risk with any antivenom due to the presence of foreign proteins (Asita de Silva et al. 2016).

Clinicians should become familiar with the available antivenom products in their region, their indications, dosage, administration protocol, and side effect profile. If antivenom is not available, the clinician should work with their hospital and public health authorities, or nongovernmental organizations to procure appropriate products which cover the dangerous species native to their area.

Monoclonal Antibodies Monoclonal antibodies generated against individual snake venom toxins have proven effective in treating venom toxicity in animal models but are not currently being used to treat human envenomations at scale (Ledsgaard et al. 2023; Laustsen et al. 2017). In the future, it may be possible to create antivenoms that consist of mixtures of monoclonal antibodies directed against multiple toxins (Laustsen et al. 2017).

Small Molecules Recently, investigators have been evaluating small molecule compounds as venom enzyme inhibitors. Some of these compounds have shown promise in protecting against the toxic effects of certain venom components in animal studies. Varespladib, a phospholipase A2 inhibitor has shown effectiveness against certain snake venoms in animal studies and is currently undergoing human trials (Lewin et al. 2016). Another study evaluated the combination of marimastat, a metalloproteinase inhibitor, and varespladib in mice injected with venom from three medically significant viper species from different continents. The combination of drugs was shown to prevent lethality in the animal model (Albulescu et al. 2020).

Acetylcholinesterases Neostigmine has been used to reverse the effects of certain neurotoxic snake envenomations (Gutiérrez et al. 2017; World Health Organization 2010b, 2016; Vital Brazil and Vieira 1996). By inhibiting the action of acetylcholinesterase, neostigmine increases the availability of acetylcholine in the neuromuscular junction and can reverse muscular weakness (Dawson 2003). It is important to note that this is usually a temporary effect and, while it may improve or delay weakness in some patients, Neostigmine does not replace antivenom (Warrell and Williams 2023; Gutiérrez et al. 2017; Ralph et al. 2022). Neostigmine is thought to work better when used in envenomations from snakes with postsynaptic toxins (Gutiérrez et al. 2017). If neostigmine is used, atropine should be concurrently administered to protect against muscarinic overstimulation from excess acetylcholine (Warrell and Williams 2023; Gutiérrez et al. 2017; Ralph et al. 2022). Atropine is also used to counteract the direct muscarinic effects of certain snakes, like African mambas (genus *Dendroaspis*) (Greene et al. 2023).

Clinical Management of Snakebite

First Aid for Snakebite

Over time, various methods have been tried to treat snakebite in the field. Incising the bite site, suction, tourniquets or other constriction bands, topical and oral herbal preparations, electric shock, and other treatments have been used. Many of these measures have not shown efficacy and can be harmful (Parker-Cote and Meggs 2018).

In case of a snake envenomation, help should be summoned as quickly as possible with the goal of rapidly transporting the victim to the closest medical facility. Ideally, the facility will have antivenom capability. In the United States and some other regions, antivenom is readily available, but this is not the case in many developing parts of the world (Chippaux 2017; World Health Organization 2019). Prolonged transport to medical care is a common problem in many of these areas. All potential snake envenomations should receive a medical evaluation as soon as possible. Some snakebites may initially produce minimal symptoms only to worsen hours later.

The victim should be reassured and kept calm. The bitten area and the patient should be kept as immobile as possible. Bitten limbs should be kept at or below the level of the heart in the field (Gold et al. 2004). Exertion should be minimized, unless active travel is necessary. Reducing limb movement may help slow venom spread (World Health Organization 2010a). Significant elevation in the field could increase the rate of venom spread while a dependent limb could increase tissue damage.

The wound may be washed with soap and water to remove residual venom from the skin. The time of the bite should be marked on the skin at the bite site. Constrictive clothing, watches, jewelry, or other items should be removed from the bitten area (World Health Organization 2010a). Other more aggressive interventions to the bitten area should be avoided. Incision, suction, arterial tourniquets, ice, heat, electric shock, chemical agents, and other similar local measures should not be used due to ineffectiveness and the potential to cause harm (Parker-Cote and Meggs 2018). If a constriction band has already been applied, leave it in place unless it is noted that arterial flow to the extremity is compromised (Watt et al. 1988). If a hospital is very close, an arterial tourniquet can be left in place for a short period of time, but it should otherwise be loosened to permit arterial flow (Fig. 18.4a). Abrupt removal of a constriction device can cause rapid worsening of an envenomation with possible life-threatening effects (Watt et al. 1988).

An exception for serious neurotoxic snakebites is the pressure immobilization bandage (PIB) technique. This technique was first developed in Australia, home to many neurotoxic elapid snakes. The technique involves wrapping a bitten extremity with a bandage and then immobilizing the extremity with a splint (Sutherland et al. 1979). The goal is to compress the lymphatic vessels and minimize muscular contraction in the extremity to delay venom egress to the central circulation (Parker-Cote and Meggs 2018). The bandage is applied tightly enough to compress the lymphatics, but not so tight as to affect venous or arterial blood flow (Sutherland et al. 1979; German et al. 2005).

To apply a PIB, an elastic bandage is started at the bite site and then wrapped circumferentially all the way to the proximal extent of the extremity. Splinting material is then applied over the bandage to limit movement (Parker-Cote and Meggs 2018). The bandage is kept in place until the victim reaches definitive medical care with antivenom capability. Once applied, a PIB should not be removed until definitive care is available.

The PIB technique should only be considered for snakebites from dangerously neurotoxic species, such as mambas, kraits, certain cobras, Australian elapids, and coral snakes (World Health Organization 2010b; Parker-Cote and Meggs 2018; German et al. 2005). The technique may worsen local tissue damage if utilized for bites from species with hemotoxic or cytotoxic venom, which includes most vipers, spitting cobras, and stiletto snakes (World Health Organization 2010b; Parker-Cote and Meggs 2018).

Food or drink should not be given by mouth to a snakebite victim in the field. Neurotoxic envenomations can cause descending paralysis affecting the muscles of airway maintenance, swallowing, and respiration. Nausea and vomiting are also common with serious snake envenomations (Gutiérrez et al. 2017; World Health Organization 2010a).

EMS, if available, should obtain IV access and carefully monitor airway, breathing, and circulatory function (Benjamin et al. 2020). Cardiac and pulse oximetry monitoring should be performed, if available. IV fluid can be helpful for volume expansion and may support hemodynamics while also serving to dilute venom components in the circulation. Antivenom is not typically administered in the field except in very rare circumstances and the focus should be on getting the patient to a higher level of medical care as rapidly as possible.

Hospital Evaluation and Management of Snakebite

Initial Evaluation and Stabilization

When a snakebite patient arrives at a medical facility, the clinician should rapidly assess airway, breathing, and circulation (ABC) and immediately address life threats. Intravenous (IV) or intraosseus (IO) access should be obtained, and crystalloid fluid should be started with the goal of euvolemia and normotension (Benjamin et al. 2020). Cardiac monitoring, pulse oximetry, blood pressure monitoring, and respiratory rate/effort monitoring should be performed (Fig. 18.4a, d). End-tidal carbon dioxide monitoring (ETCO2) can be useful to monitor for hypercapnia from compromised respiration (Tednes and Slesinger 2023). Signs of airway compromise from neurotoxicity or angioedema should be identified and treated aggressively. Supplemental oxygen should be given for airway concerns or hypoxia. Body and head positioning along with oral suction can help temporize a patient's airway prior to antivenom and further airway management. For airway compromise or respiratory distress, early placement of an endotracheal or supraglottic tube and mechanical ventilation should be performed, if possible. In austere settings, bag valve mask respiration may be the only option (World Health Organization 2010a). Single breath count (SBC) testing is an easy way to evaluate respiratory function. The test involves asking the patient to take a deep breath and then count out loud from one to the highest number they can reach. A normal SBC is near 50. SBC less than 20 is indicative of significant respiratory compromise and the need for artificial ventilation (Benjamin et al. 2020; Rega et al. 2010).

Anaphylactic or anaphylactoid reactions do occasionally occur from snake venom itself and these reactions should be treated like other severe allergic reactions with IM epinephrine (Benjamin et al. 2020; Hogan and Dire 1990). Any snakebite patient who presents with sudden cardiovascular collapse, severe angioedema, or other signs of severe allergy should be given epinephrine in addition to antivenom (Benjamin et al. 2020). It is important to note any signs of neurotoxicity, hemorrhage, respiratory compromise, cardiac issues, or other signs of severe or systemic envenomation.

Hemotoxic/cytotoxic bites are very painful, and analgesia should be provided early with acetaminophen, opioids, or ketamine (Warrell and Williams 2023; Gutiérrez et al. 2017; Brandehoff et al. 2020). Aspirin and NSAIDs should be avoided due to potential worsening of coagulopathy (World Health Organization 2010a). If tourniquets, constriction bands, a PIB, or other similar compressive items are present they should be left in place until IV or IO access has been obtained, critical care equipment is at the bedside, and antivenom is available (World Health Organization 2010a). Abruptly removing a constricting device can cause rapid clinical worsening due to the release of sequestered venom (Watt et al. 1988). If signs of envenomation are present, consider beginning antivenom administration before loosening or removing a constriction device (Fig. 18.4a).

Prophylactic antibiotics are not typically needed for snakebites unless the bite site has been incised and/or contaminated with foreign material that increases the risk of infection (World Health Organization 2010b, 2016). Tetanus vaccination should be updated, if indicated.

History

A history should be conducted to ascertain the circumstances of the snakebite. The time the bite occurred, bite location, number of bites, baseline health of the victim, comorbidities, medications, allergies, and tetanus vaccination status should be documented. The identification of culprit snake species may be helpful but is not essential. In many cases the species is unknown, and the clinical envenomation syndrome will determine treatment. Patients and families should be discouraged from capturing snakes or bringing

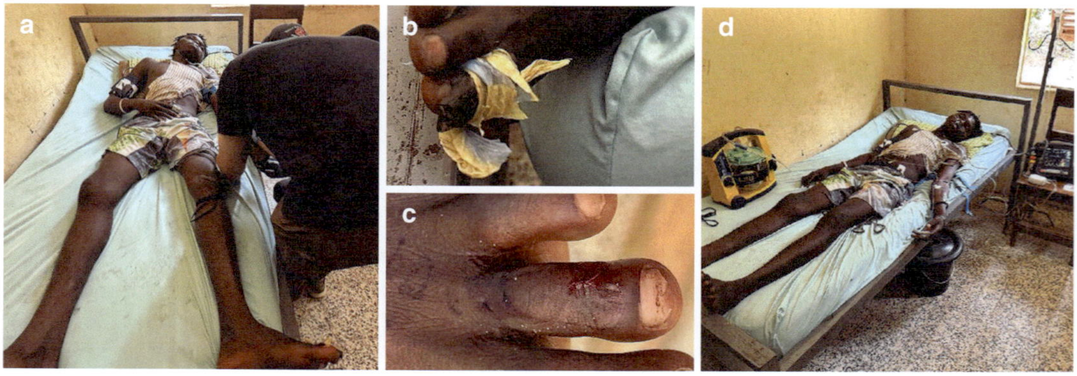

Fig. 18.4 A patient bitten by a neurotoxic cobra (*Naja savannula*) undergoing initial stabilization in a snakebite clinic operated by the Asclepius Snakebite Foundation in Guinea, Africa (part **a**). Note the constriction bands on the right leg, which were left in place while IV access was obtained. The bands were gradually loosened and removed after antivenom was administered. The patient initially visited a traditional healer who made an incision over the bite and tied a "black stone" or piece of charred cow bone to the wound (part **b**). After the black stone was removed, the incision was visible (part **c**). The patient's weakness was closely monitored while awaiting response to antivenom (part **d**). The patient began to regain strength about 45 min after antivenom was infused and artificial ventilation was avoided. He continued to improve over the next 24 h and was discharged with his family after 36 h. (Images **a**–**d** courtesy of B.G.)

snakes to the hospital as this can lead to secondary bites. Even decapitated snake heads or "dead" snakes can bite and cause severe envenomation (Willhite et al. 2018).

Physical Examination

After initial evaluation, stabilization, and history, a thorough physical examination should be performed from head to toe. The clinician should note evidence of neurotoxicity, including cranial nerve impairment, speech or swallowing problems, respiratory weakness, muscle fasciculations, muscarinic SLUDGE signs, and mental status changes such as somnolence or agitation. Cardiopulmonary examination should focus on heart rate and rhythm, signs of hypoperfusion, and assessing for wheezing, pulmonary edema, or other respiratory issues. Signs of coagulopathy or clinical bleeding should be noted. Check for petechiae, hemorrhagic bullae, gingival bleeding, GI bleeding, hematuria, or other bleeding. Abdominal tenderness or distention can indicate intraperitoneal bleeding (World Health Organization 2010a, 2016; Kassegne et al. 2020).

The bitten area should be examined, and the number of punctures noted. It is important to note, however, that envenomation can occur without visible wounds (Norris and Dart 1989). Retained fangs or teeth are occasionally noted in the wound and these should be removed with forceps. If not done in the field, the bite site should be marked with a pen and the most proximal extent of local findings (tenderness, redness, swelling, ecchymosis) should be marked with the time on the skin. The area should be examined initially every 15–30 min and re-marked if progression of local signs is occurring (Benjamin et al. 2020).

Laboratory Studies

If laboratory capability exists then the following tests should be sent: complete blood count (CBC), hemoglobin level if CBC is not available, comprehensive metabolic panel (CMP), prothrombin time (PT), international normalized ratio (INR), partial thromboplastin time (PTT), fibrinogen, creatine kinase (CK), and urinalysis (UA) (Warrell and Williams 2023; Gutiérrez et al. 2017; World Health Organization 2010b, 2016; Benjamin et al. 2020). In the absence of a laboratory, the 20-min whole blood clotting test (20MWBCT) can be performed to assess for coagulopathy (Warrell and Williams 2023; Gutiérrez et al. 2017; World Health Organization 2010b, 2016; Benjamin et al. 2020).

The 20MWBCT is performed by drawing a few mL of blood and placing it in a clean, dry glass tube or other small glass container. The blood is then left for 20 min undisturbed after which time, the container is rotated on its side to check for clotting (Fig. 18.5). Unclotted blood indicates coagulopathy (Warrell and Williams 2023; Gutiérrez et al. 2017; World Health Organization 2010b, 2016; Benjamin et al. 2018, 2020). Urine can also be grossly inspected for abnormally dark coloration, which can indicate myoglobinuria or hemolysis (World Health Organization 2010b).

Arterial or venous blood gas studies can be helpful in evaluating acid-base balance and hypercarbia from respiratory compromise. Lactic acid levels, if available, can be used to assess tissue perfusion and effectiveness of resuscitation in critical envenomations.

The goals of the initial evaluation are to address immediate life threats, begin monitoring, obtain IV access, obtain a relevant history, and perform a physical examination. This will achieve initial stabilization and provide the information to determine the clinical envenomation syndrome that is occurring and assess the need for antivenom and other therapies.

Clinical Envenomation Syndromes and Treatment

Clinical Envenomation Syndromes

The clinical envenomation syndrome produced by a venomous snakebite is determined primarily by the composition of the venom. Due to the diversity of toxins found in snake venoms, mixed syndromes can also. For example, bites from the coastal taipan (*Oxyuranus scutellatus*) from Australia and New Guinea can produce both life-threatening neurotoxic and hemotoxic effects (White 2003). Most snake envenomations, however, will produce one of the following syndromes.

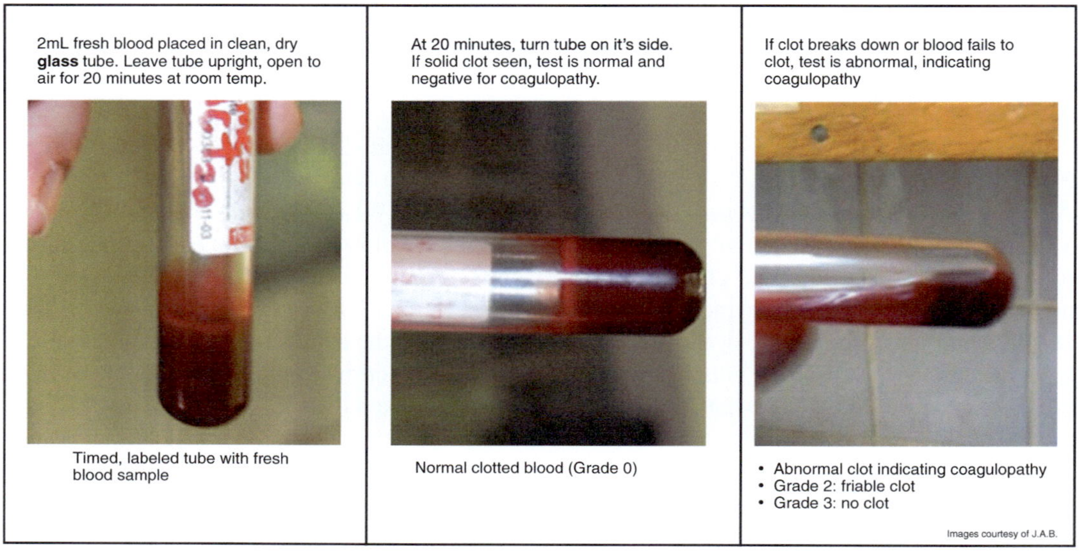

Fig. 18.5 20 Minute whole blood clotting test (20WBCT). (Images courtesy of J.A.B.)

Neurotoxic Envenomations

Envenomations from neurotoxic snakes may have minimal local findings. There may not be significant swelling, redness, ecchymosis, tenderness, or other local findings (Norris and Dart 1989; White 2003). This is particularly true with snakes such as mambas, certain neurotoxic cobras, kraits, and coral snakes (Norris and Dart 1989; White 2003). Some other snakes, such as certain vipers, and some Australian elapids, produce mixed syndromes that can present with signs of local tissue damage and coagulopathy along with neurotoxicity (Levine et al. 2023; Silva et al. 2016; White 2003). Any bite from a potentially neurotoxic snake must be monitored closely with frequent reassessments. Depending on the species and other factors, the neurotoxicity may not become evident for many hours after the bite (Corbett and Clark 2017).

Signs of a neurotoxic envenomation syndrome include bilateral ptosis, disconjugate gaze, nystagmus, facial weakness, speech abnormalities, dysphagia, drooling, tachypnea or bradypnea, accessory respiratory muscle use, mental status changes, skeletal muscle weakness, muscle fasciculations or myokymia, ataxia, and muscarinic SLUDGE symptoms (Warrell and Williams 2023; Gutiérrez et al. 2017; Jolkkonen et al. 1995; Greene et al. 2023; World Health Organization 2010b, 2016; Benjamin et al. 2020). Any signs of neurotoxicity warrant aggressive airway and respiratory support and the administration of antivenom (Warrell and Williams 2023; Gutiérrez et al. 2017; World Health Organization 2010b; Benjamin et al. 2020). For envenomations producing muscarinic signs, consider dosing with atropine 0.5 mg IV/IO (Benjamin et al. 2020). Atropine can be re-dosed every 5 min, as needed, to the resolution of wheezing, rales, and oral hypersecretion (Benjamin et al. 2020). Pediatric patients can receive 0.01–0.02 mg/kg atropine to a maximum dose of 0.5 mg (Benjamin et al. 2020).

The administration of an anticholinesterase, such as neostigmine, may help transiently reverse muscle weakness by increasing the available acetylcholine in the synapse. Neostigmine may be more effective in reversing the effects of alpha neurotoxins than beta neurotoxins (Warrell and Williams 2023; Gutiérrez et al. 2017; World Health Organization 2016; Ralph et al. 2022). Atropine is typically administered just before neostigmine to counteract muscarinic cholinergic effects (Greene et al. 2023; Benjamin et al. 2020). Neostigmine is dosed with 1 mg IV/IO with 0.5 mg atropine in adults. Neostigmine is dosed 0.025–0.04 mg/kg in pediatric patients to a maximum dose of 0.5 mg with atropine 0.01–0.02 mg/kg to a maximum dose of 0.5 mg (Benjamin et al. 2020). Patients with a positive response to neostigmine may need to be re-dosed every 1–4 h for refractory symptoms, unless intubation and ventilation are performed, or antivenom is clearly reversing neurotoxicity (Benjamin et al. 2020). Maximum doses of neostigmine in 24 h are 10 mg for adults and 5 mg for pediatric patients (Benjamin et al. 2020). Redosing with atropine may also be required if cholinergic symptoms develop. Patients with no initial improvement with neostigmine should not receive additional doses (Benjamin et al. 2020). While neostigmine can be a useful adjunct for neurotoxic weakness, antivenom remains the definitive treatment for all serious snake envenomations (Warrell and Williams 2023; Gutiérrez et al. 2017).

Some patients with neurotoxic envenomations, particularly from snakes with postsynaptic toxins, may exhibit weakness that is not easily reversed by antivenom or neostigmine (Warrell and Williams 2023). This likely occurs from destruction of presynaptic terminals by beta neurotoxins (Warrell and Williams 2023). Antivenom administration is still important to bind free toxins, but these patients may still require intubation and artificial ventilation, sometimes for prolonged periods (Warrell and Williams 2023; World Health Organization 2010b, 2016).

Hemotoxic/Cytotoxic Envenomation

Hemotoxic and cytotoxic envenomations often have similar initial clinical presentations. Envenomations from hemotoxic/cytotoxic snakes will typically have local pain and tenderness that may initially seem out of proportion to the appearance of the bite. These venoms cause severe pain when attacking tissue (World Health Organization 2010b). Worsening pain is suggestive of a progressing envenomation and often precedes other signs. Other signs of hemotoxic/cytotoxic envenomation include tenderness, erythema, swelling, oozing of fluid or blood from punctures, gingival bleeding, ecchymosis, bullae, lymphangitis, and regional lymphadenopathy (Warrell and Williams 2023; Gutiérrez et al. 2017; World Health Organization 2010b, 2016).

The primary differentiator between hemotoxic and cytotoxic envenomation is the presence of coagulopathy and/or significant bleeding, which occur in hemotoxic envenomations, but are not typically seen with primarily cytotoxic snakes (World Health Organization 2010b). Figures 18.6 and 18.7 illustrate local signs of tissue damage from hemotoxic/cytotoxic envenomation.

Envenomations from many viper species, some Australian elapids, and a few rear-fanged snakes can cause severe coagulopathy which leads to clinically significant bleeding (Warrell and Williams 2023; Gutiérrez et al. 2017; World Health Organization 2010a, 2016).

Bleeding can manifest in various ways, including hematemesis, hemoptysis, hematochezia, intraperitoneal bleeding, hematuria, and intracranial bleeding (Warrell and Williams 2023; Gutiérrez et al. 2017; World Health Organization 2010a, 2016).

Bleeding can result from either direct or consumptive coagulopathy. Thrombosis can also occur, and rare cases of ischemic stroke, pulmonary emboli, and myocardial infarction have occurred in hemotoxic snake envenomations (Paul et al. 2014; Bart et al. 2016; Rathnayaka et al. 2022).

Antivenom is the first-line treatment for coagulopathy and bleeding (Warrell and Williams 2023; Gutiérrez et al. 2017; World Health Organization 2010b, 2016; Ralph et al. 2022). Adequate antivenom treatment for coagulopathy can be assessed by trending platelets, coagulation studies, and/or the 20WBCT, which should be improving (World Health Organization 2010b, 2016; Ralph et al. 2022). In some cases, transfusion of blood, platelets, and clotting factors is performed for uncontrolled life-threatening bleeding that is refractory to antivenom (World Health Organization 2010b, 2016). However, caution should be exercised with giving blood products prior to adequate antivenom administration, as unbound venom components will degrade

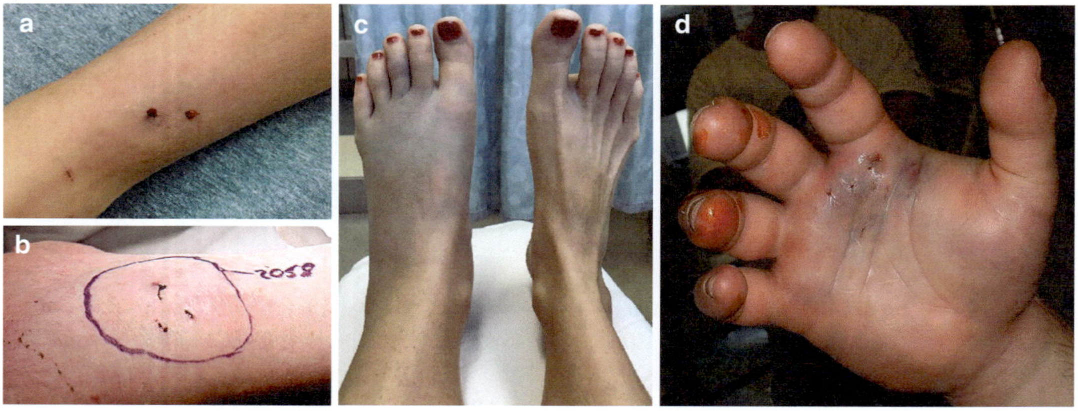

Fig. 18.6 Tissue injury from hemotoxic/cytotoxic envenomation. Examples of local tissue injury from hemotoxic/cytotoxic snake envenomations. Puncture marks with bloody oozing soon after a bite from *Agkistrodon contortrix* (eastern copperhead) (part **a**). *Agkistrodon contortrix* (eastern copperhead) bite to ankle region with three punctures; area of swelling and tenderness is marked with the time (part **b**). *Agkistrodon contortrix* bite to left lower extremity with bruising and swelling progressing up the leg (part **c**). *Agkistrodon piscivorous* (eastern cottonmouth) envenomation in patient who sustained three bites to the palm (part **d**). (Images courtesy of B.G.)

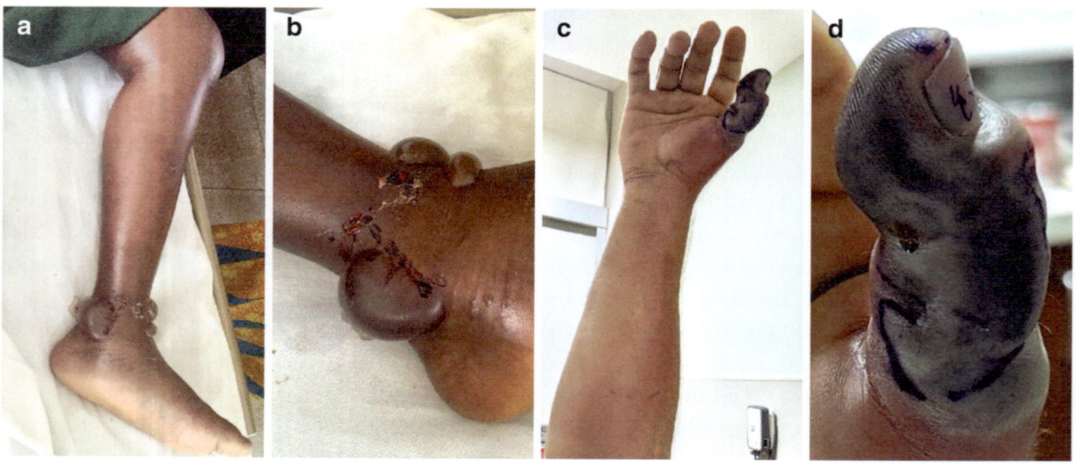

Fig. 18.7 Tissue injury from hemotoxic/cytotoxic envenomation. *Bitis arietans* (puff adder) envenomation in a child from Africa showing bleb formation soon after the bite (parts **a**, **b**). *Agkistrodon contortrix* (eastern copperhead) bite to the thumb showing local hemorrhage and cytotoxic effects with swelling extending to the arm (parts **c**, **d**). Tissue damage is best mediated through early antivenom administration, elevation of the injured area, and wound care. Effects such as these may still result in necrosis requiring surgical debridement and further care. (Images courtesy of B.G.)

new blood products (Warrell and Williams 2023). Blood products carry their own risks, including allergic reactions, infectious agents (particularly in the developing world), and other transfusion-associated problems (Warrell and Williams 2023; Zeng et al. 2022).

Swelling is usually extra compartmental and true compartment syndrome is rare in snake envenomation (World Health Organization 2010a; Toschlog et al. 2013; Hsu et al. 2015). It does occur, however, and the clinician should be familiar with diagnosing this condition. Once the victim is in the hospital and IV access is obtained, it is advised to elevate the extremity above the level of the heart as strictly as possible to help reduce tissue pressure. Elevation and adequate antivenom administration are first-line therapies for limb swelling and usually obviate the need for acute surgical management (Toschlog et al. 2013). Fasciotomy is rarely necessary for snake envenomation. In cases where clinical concern for compartment syndrome remains after elevation and antivenom administration, a surgeon should be consulted, and compartment pressures should be measured to assess the need for fasciotomy (World Health Organization 2010b, 2016; Toschlog et al. 2013). Antivenom and elevation should be continued while awaiting surgical consultation.

Bites directly into a digit are at risk for severe localized tissue damage and can lead to digit loss. Again, antivenom and elevation are first-line treatment, and surgical care is rarely needed. Compartment pressures are not measured directly in a digit and alternate methods must be used to assess perfusion. Doppler demonstration of pulseless in an envenomed digit warrants surgical consultation (Toschlog et al. 2013). Decompression of an envenomated digit by digital dermotomy can reduce pressure in the digit and potentially prevent ischemic damage (Toschlog et al. 2013; Watt 1985).

Venom Ophthalmia

Spitting cobras (genus *Naja*), and Rhinkals snakes (genus *Hemachatus*) are capable of accurately spraying cytotoxic venom directly into the eyes of potential threats. The venom is destructive to ocular tissues and causes immediate burning pain, redness, lacrimation, and photophobia (World Health Organization 2010a; Benjamin et al. 2020; Chang et al. 2020; Hansen et al. 1994; Chu et al. 2010). The treatment is prompt and aggressive eye irrigation with water, milk, or other available nontoxic aqueous solution (World Health Organization 2010b; Benjamin et al. 2020; Chang et al. 2020; Hansen et al. 1994; Chu et al. 2010). Topical ophthalmic anesthetic drops and vasoconstrictors are helpful with this process (World Health Organization 2010b; Benjamin et al. 2020; Chang et al. 2020). If the venom is not removed, corneal erosion and ulceration can occur leading to scarring and blindness (World Health Organization 2010b; Chang et al. 2020). Antivenom is not indicated for ocular venom exposure unless the victim has received a bite from the snake as well (World Health Organization 2010b; Benjamin et al. 2020). After thorough eye irrigation has been completed, the eyes should be examined with fluorescein using a slit lamp to detect corneal injury. Antibiotic eye drops or ointment are indicated until symptoms resolve (World Health Organization 2010b; Benjamin et al. 2020). Patients with evidence of corneal injury require daily rechecks for resolution (World Health Organization 2010b; Benjamin et al. 2020).

Dry Bites

On occasion, a venomous snake will bite, but no venom will be injected. These bites are frequently called "dry bites." A true dry bite should only be suspected if no signs or symptoms of envenomation are noted after an extended period of observation with frequent reassessments (Gutiérrez et al. 2017; World Health Organization 2010b; Pucca et al. 2020). Asymptomatic snakebites should be observed in a medical setting until the clinician is confident that no envenomation has occurred. In developed regions with lab testing capabilities, reliable transportation to the hospital, and a responsible patient who will return for signs of worsening, an observation period of 8–12 h is sufficient for bites from hemotoxic/cytotoxic snakes (Lavonas et al. 2011). If no signs or symptoms occur within the period, the patient may be discharged with education and instructions to return to the hospital for any signs of worsening. In developing regions or austere environments, or when a bite from a neurotoxic snake is possible, the observation period should be 24 h with monitoring and frequent reassessments (Warrell and Williams 2023; Gutiérrez et al. 2017; World Health Organization 2010a; Benjamin et al. 2020).

Indications for Antivenom

Any snake envenomation producing life-threatening signs, significant organ dysfunction, coagulopathy, threat to limb integrity, or evidence of progressive tissue damage, should be treated with antivenom (Warrell and Williams 2023;

Gutiérrez et al. 2017; World Health Organization 2010b, 2016; Ralph et al. 2022; Lavonas et al. 2011). Severity grading systems have been used for various groups of snakes in different regions, but come with limitations given the dynamic and progressive nature of snake envenomation. It is strongly advised that any clinician who may be in the position to treat snake envenomation become familiar with the antivenom products in their area. The preparation, dosing, administration, and side effect profiles of the antivenoms should be reviewed.

Antivenom Administration

Antivenoms are typically packaged in vials or ampoules in powder or liquid formulations. Lyophilized powder formulations are more stable than liquid products but must be resuspended in sterile saline or sterile water prior to administration (World Health Organization 2010a, b, 2016). Antivenoms are only administered by intravenous (IV) or intraosseus (IO) route and not by intramuscular (IM) injection or other routes (Warrell and Williams 2023; Gutiérrez et al. 2017; Benjamin et al. 2020). After resuspension, antivenom is typically diluted in a bag of sterile saline for infusion (World Health Organization 2010b; Benjamin et al. 2020). Antivenom is usually started as a bolus dose given over 30–60 min (World Health Organization 2010b). The number of vials administered in the initial dose depends on the clinical envenomation syndrome and the antivenom being used. Envenomations that present with severe effects may need a higher initial bolus dose (Lavonas et al. 2011; "CroFab" package insert 2023).

The infusion is typically started slowly over 10–15 min while closely monitoring for early hypersensitivity reaction (World Health Organization 2010b, 2016). If no signs of adverse reaction are noted, then the infusion rate can be increased to complete the dose. For severe life-threatening envenomations, the resuspended antivenom can be drawn into a syringe from the vials and given by slow IV push while monitoring for adverse reactions (World Health Organization 2010b; Benjamin et al. 2020). Antivenom dosing is the same in pediatric and adult patients (World Health Organization 2010b, 2016; Le Geyt et al. 2021). In pediatric patients receiving large amounts of antivenom, fluid volume can be a problem and the antivenom may need to be concentrated in a smaller volume (Le Geyt et al. 2021).

The goal is to achieve "control" of the envenomation syndrome (Benjamin et al. 2020; Dart et al. 2001). Control, broadly defined, is the halting or reversal of venom effects (Seifert et al. 2022; Dart et al. 2001). Control in a hemotoxic/cytotoxic envenomation means that signs of ongoing tissue damage are halted, clinical bleeding is halted, and coagulation studies and other labs are clearly improving toward normal (Benjamin et al. 2020; Lavonas et al. 2011; Seifert et al. 2022). Labs or 20WBCT should be repeated every 2 h until significant improvement is noted (Benjamin et al. 2020). Tissue damage that has already occurred is unlikely to be reversed by antivenom (Ho et al. 2021). The goal is to prevent additional damage.

For a neurotoxic envenomation, control means that neurotoxic signs are clearly improving or normalizing. Some neurotoxic effects, however, can be difficult to completely reverse with antivenom (Warrell and Williams 2023; Gutiérrez et al. 2017; Silva et al. 2017). Presynaptic toxic effects may be resistant to antivenom due to the irreversible damage done to presynaptic membranes (Warrell and Williams 2023; Gutiérrez et al. 2017; Silva et al. 2017). Severely neurotoxic patients may require intubation and artificial ventilation in conjunction with antivenom (Warrell and Williams 2023; Gutiérrez et al. 2017; Benjamin et al. 2020; Silva et al. 2017).

After the initial bolus dose of antivenom, the patient should be examined carefully and repeat lab studies checked to assess for control. If signs of envenomation progression persist, the antivenom is re-dosed until control is achieved (World Health Organization 2010b, 2016; Benjamin et al. 2020; Lavonas et al. 2011). Snake envenomations are dynamic and frequent clinical and lab reassessments are necessary until control has been achieved and maintained. The natural course of envenomation is to worsen over time until the toxic proteins are neutralized.

Early Antivenom Reactions

Signs of early reactions include coughing, throat clearing, wheezing, angioedema, generalized erythema, urticaria, tachycardia, fever, and hypotension (Warrell and Williams 2023; Gutiérrez et al. 2017; World Health Organization 2010b, 2016; Benjamin et al. 2020). Early reactions usually occur in the first hour of antivenom administration. If signs of allergic reaction are noted, the infusion should be immediately stopped. The patient should be treated with IM epinephrine and IV or IM antihistamines (Warrell and Williams 2023; Gutiérrez et al. 2017; World Health Organization 2010b, 2016; Benjamin et al. 2020; Clark et al. 2002). Epinephrine doses should be repeated, as needed, until the reaction subsides. Once the allergic reaction resolves, the antivenom infusion can be resumed. For severe allergic reactions, or persistent allergic symptoms, an epinephrine infusion can be concurrently administered with antivenom if the envenomation syndrome itself is life-threatening (Benjamin et al. 2020; Clark et al. 2002).

The only effective pretreatment to prophylaxis against early antivenom reactions is epinephrine, which may be administered by subcutaneous (SC) or IM route prior to starting the antivenom infusion (Premawardhena et al. 1999; de Silva et al. 2011). Epinephrine pretreatment may be considered for patients with significant prior allergic history, who have had a prior reaction to antivenom, or for antivenom products with higher risks of hypersensitivity reaction. These conditions are not absolute contraindications to antivenom administration; however, fear of a reaction should not prevent an envenomated patient from being treated (Benjamin et al. 2020). Pretreatment with antihistamines and corticosteroids have not shown efficacy in preventing early reactions but are often used as adjuncts (de Silva et al. 2011).

Serum Sickness

Serum sickness is a delayed hypersensitivity reaction that occurs due to the formation of immune complexes in the body after antivenom administration (Warrell and Williams 2023; Gutiérrez et al. 2017; World Health Organization 2010b, 2016). The antivenom and venom proteins are foreign to the body and can elicit a delayed immune response. Serum sickness typically occurs many days or even weeks after treatment with antivenom. Serum sickness symptoms include fever, malaise, myalgia, arthralgia, rash, and lymphadenopathy (Warrell and Williams 2023; Gutiérrez et al. 2017; World Health Organization 2010b, 2016). Mild cases of serum sickness can be treated supportively with antihistamines and NSAIDs. Severe cases with high fever, renal involvement (elevated creatinine or proteinuria), or severe pain, can be treated with oral corticosteroids, NSAIDs, and antihistamines (Warrell and Williams 2023; Gutiérrez et al. 2017; World Health Organization 2010b, 2016). Avoid NSAIDs in patients with renal impairment or who have evidence of recurrent coagulopathy following snake envenomation (World Health Organization 2010b, 2016).

Post-Emergency Care

Once the initial treating clinician is confident that control of the envenomation syndrome has been achieved and any adverse effects have also been resolved, the patient should be kept in the emergency department for observation or admitted to the hospital. Serial reexaminations should be performed to assess for recurrent venom effects and additional antivenom given as needed. For patients with significant laboratory abnormalities or coagulopathy, labs or 20WBCT should be rechecked at hours 2, 4, 6, 12, and 24 (Benjamin et al. 2020). Delayed coagulopathy can occur after antivenom treatment and patients with evidence of coagulopathy while in the hospital should be discharged with bleeding precautions and asked to return on days 2–3 and 5–7 for lab rechecks (Lavonas et al. 2011). If recurrent coagulopathy is identified, then additional antivenom is indicated (Lavonas et al. 2011). Patients with neurotoxic envenomations should be monitored in the hospital until all significant neurotoxic effects have resolved.

Hospital Discharge Criteria

After control of an envenomation syndrome has been maintained for 24 h and the patient is clearly improving, certain criteria should be met before discharge. All life-threatening venom effects should be resolved, including active bleeding, clinically significant lab abnormalities, and neurotoxicity that affects respiration and mobility. Hemotoxic/cytotoxic envenomations with significant swelling that impacts mobility may require assistance in the form of crutches or other mobility aids. Continued elevation of an affected extremity at home should be emphasized. Compression wraps or stockings for edema may be considered in the post-acute setting but should not be used until the clinician is confident acute venom effects are resolved. Fully treated envenomations with evidence of necrosis may require surgical debridement in the hospital and/or later at wound check visits. Extensive necrosis can necessitate the amputation of digits or limbs leading to permanent disability (Warrell and Williams 2023; Gutiérrez et al. 2017; World Health Organization 2010b, 2016). While not indicated on a routine basis early in snakebite, broad-spectrum antibiotics should be given if necrosis or any signs of infection develop (Warrell and Williams 2023; Gutiérrez et al. 2017; World Health Organization 2010b, 2016; Wagener et al. 2017).

Snakebite Treatment Pathways

A single global treatment algorithm that includes all available antivenom products does not exist, but there are several useful regional protocols. The clinician should refer to their institutional or regional protocol, if one exists, for information on antivenom dosing and administration. Regional poison centers should also be consulted, if available.

The United States military published a Joint Trauma Systems clinical practice guideline entitled "Global Snake Envenomation Management," which covers all regions of the world where snakebite is a problem (Benjamin et al. 2020). This excellent guideline covers the major envenomation syndromes, with multiple treatment algorithms, and recommended antivenoms for different regions. The "Unified Treatment Algorithm for Crotaline Snakebites in the United States" covers native US pit vipers, which cause the majority of snake envenomations in the country (Lavonas et al. 2011).

Global Pathway

A global pathway for the hospital management of snakebites is included here and summarizes the clinical information presented in the text (Fig. 18.8). This pathway starts with the initial assessment and stabilization and lists initial critical actions. An observation pathway for possible dry bites is included. For bites with signs of envenomation, the pathway diverges based on the clinical syndrome. The left branch covers neurotoxic envenomations, and the right branch covers hemotoxic/cytotoxic envenomations. While some hemotoxic/cytotoxic envenomations can produce neurotoxicity and vice versa, most snake envenomations will be predominated by one syndrome. Given that neurotoxic effects can compromise respiration, airway management is emphasized in the neurotoxic pathway. Hemotoxic/cytotoxic envenomations can threaten life or limb by coagulopathy, bleeding, shock, and tissue damage. Accordingly, these issues are emphasized in the hemotoxic/cytotoxic pathway. Envenomations are dynamic conditions and due to the unique combination of factors present in an individual case, frequent reassessment is required and changes in the patient's condition warrant reconsideration of the treatment plan. This pathway does not replace the advice of a local snakebite expert or local protocols and is meant to serve as a guideline.

Other Terrestrial Vertebrates

Lizards

There are two medically significant venomous lizards in the world, the Gila monster *Heloderma suspectum* (Fig. 18.9) and the Mexican beaded lizard *Heloderma horridum*. These closely related lizards live in the southwestern United States and along the west coast of Mexico to northern Guatemala. Helodermid lizards are large with powerful jaws, a strong bite, and venom glands located in the lower jaw. Bites from these lizards are rare and usually occur when a person is handling or disturbing the animals. The venom causes severe pain, which can last hours to days. There are reports of more serious effects, such as airway edema, cardiovascular

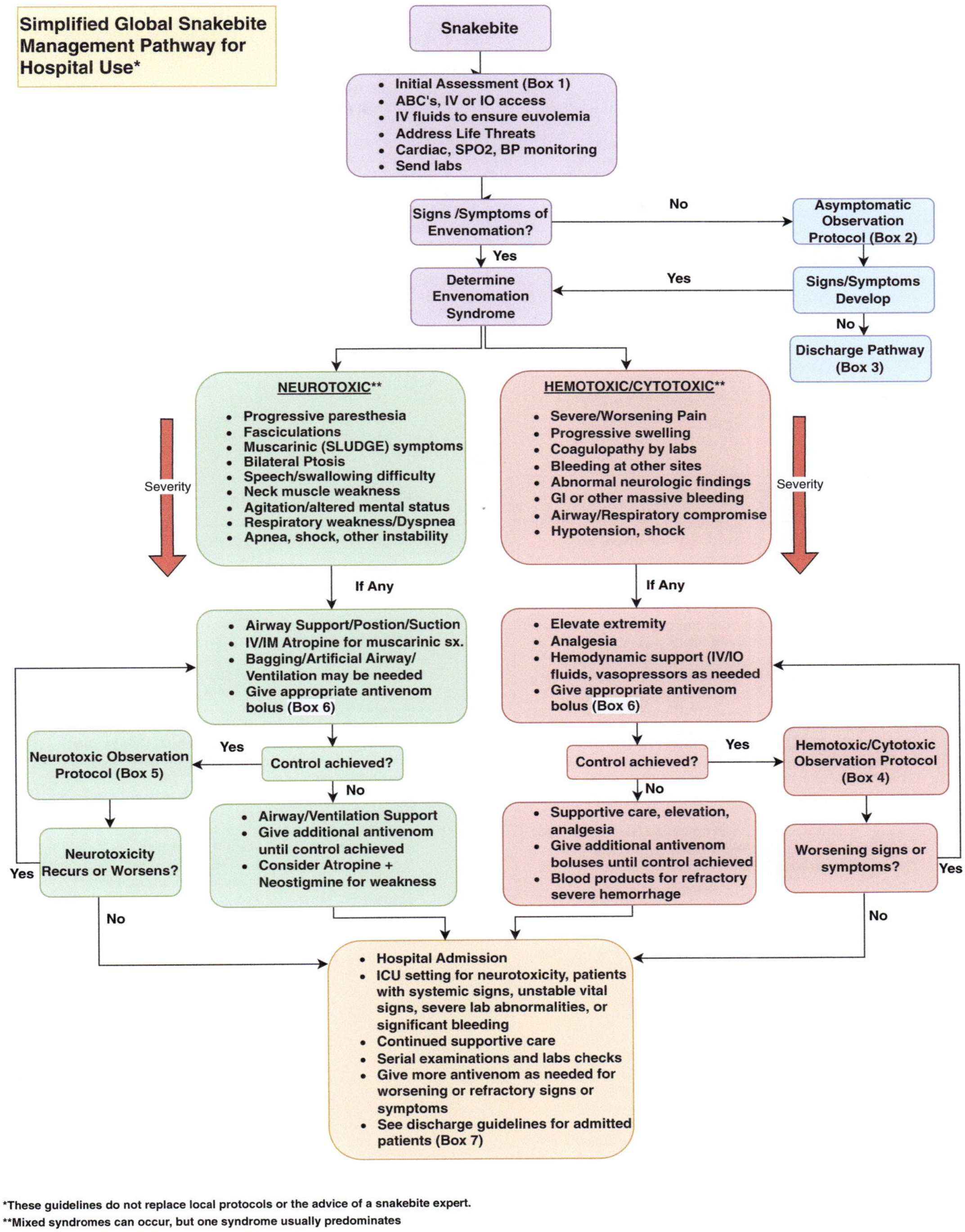

Fig. 18.8 Simplified global snakebite management pathway for hospital use

Box 1. Initial Hospital Snakebite Evaluation

1. ABC/IV. Rapidly assess Airway, Breathing, and Circulation. Obtain IV or IO access.
2. Airway compromise/respiratory distress: supplemental O2, position patient to optimize airway, suction, and prepare for intubation.
3. Treat hypotension with IV crystalloid boluses.
4. Anaphylactoid reactions from venom (rare): IM epinephrine, IV or IM antihistamines, and IV or IM corticosteroids.
5. Tourniquet in place: do not remove abruptly. Wait until IV access, and critical care equipment and antivenom are available. Then gradually loosen incrementally while watching for venom effects.
6. Perform history and physical examination.
7. Mark and time the bite site. Check every 15-30 minutes to assess for developing local signs of envenomation (tenderness, swelling, redness, bruising, etc..) and re-mark/time if worsening noted.

Box 2. Asymptomatic Observation Protocol

1. Mark/time the bite site. Check every 15-30 minutes to assess for developing local signs of envenomation (tenderness, swelling, redness, bruising, blisters) and re-mark/time as needed.
2. Monitor for neurotoxic symptoms.
3. Trend vital signs.
4. Patients with known or potential bites from neurotoxic snakes should be observed for 24 hours.
5. Most hemotoxic/cytotoxic snakebites will declare themselves over several hours. Patients with asymptomatic bites from these snakes can be discharged after 8-12 hours if NO signs of envenomation are noted, they receive education and return precautions, AND they are able to return easily to the hospital. ALL other patients should be observed for 24 hours.
6. Check lab studies to assess for coagulopathy (PT, INR, PTT, CBC) or perform 20MWBCT* at hrs.
7. If ANY progressive signs of envenomation develop or evidence of coagulopathy is seen during the observation period, then return to the envenomation pathway.

*20 Minute whole blood clotting test

Box 3. Discharge Criteria for Asymptomatic Patients

1. Patients who have no signs of envenomation during their observation period may be discharged.
2. Known or suspected bites from neurotoxic snakes require 24 hours of observation.
3. Other snakebites can be discharged after 8-12 hours if completely asymptomatic, lab studies are normal, they have been educated and given return precautions, and they can return easily for worsening. If no to any, then observe 24 hours or return to envenomation pathway.
4. If any evidence of worsening signs or symptoms, patient should not be discharged.
5. Tetanus vaccination should be updated before discharge.
6. Prophylactic antibiotics are not indicated.

Box 4. Hemotoxic/Cytotoxic Observation Protocol

1. Patient has received antivenom and control has been achieved. Pain, swelling, and other local signs should not be worsening. Perform full reassessments at hours 2, 4, 6, 12, and 24
2. Maintain strict elevation of the bitten limb.
3. Administer analgesics (opioids, acetaminophen, ketamine) as needed. Pain is often severe.
4. For limb swelling, continue strict elevation. If there is concern for compartment syndrome (rare), measure compartment pressures and/or consult a surgeon. Antivenom and elevation remain first-line treatment, but surgery is sometimes needed.
5. Abnormal vital signs should be improving with antivenom and supportive care. Continue IV fluids to maintain euvolemia.
6. Recheck labs or 20MWBCT at hours after antivenom administered. Laboratory abnormalities should be improving. Coagulation studies or 20MWBCT should trend toward normal.
7. If control is maintained, patient should be admitted to the hospital for monitoring, pain control, elevation, and wound care.
8. In case of worsening local signs, severe refractory pain, any systemic signs, worsening vital signs, worsening lab studies, or clinical bleeding, return to the envenomation pathway.

*20 Minute whole blood clotting test

Box 5. Neurotoxic Observation Protocol

1. The patient has received antivenom and control has been achieved. Neurotoxic symptoms should have abated, or are clearly improving.
2. Maintain vigilant airway and ventilatory support. Watch carefully for airway, swallowing, or breathing compromise.
3. Continue IV fluids to maintain euvolemia.
4. Elevate the bitten area if there are concurrent local signs of envenomation.
5. Pain is often not as severe as with hemotoxic/cytotoxic envenomations. Use caution with opioids or other medications that may cause respiratory depression.
6. Delayed worsening of the neurotoxic syndrome can occur despite initial control. All patients with neurotoxic envenomations should be observed a minimum of 24 hours in an ICU setting.
7. If any worsening clinical trends are noted, return to the envenomation pathway and give additional antivenom. Neostigmine with atropine may also be considered for refractory weakness.

Fig. 18.8 (continued)

Box 6. Antivenom Administration

1. Use the proper antivenom for the geographic region where the bite occurred. If no antivenom is available, contact your Poison Center or Public Health Agency.
2. Test doses of serum or antivenom are not needed.
3. Resuspend, dilute, and administer the antivenom as directed by the package insert. Start the infusion slowly over 15 minutes. If tolerated, increase infusion rate to complete infusion in 1 hour.
4. If allergy to antivenom occurs, stop the infusion, treat with IM epinephrine, IV/IM antihistamines, and IV/IM corticosteroids.
5. Infusion may be restarted after allergic reaction resolves if benefits outweigh risks. Epinephrine infusion concurrent with antivenom can be used.
6. For severe envenomations presenting with shock, severe neurotoxicity, or other severe life-threats, antivenom bolus may be slow-pushed via syringe over several minutes.
7. Antivenom redosing is frequently needed, so monitor the patient closely for signs of worsening or refractory envenomation.
8. Serum sickness may occur days to weeks after antivenom administration. Care is supportive.

Box 7. Discharge Criteria for Admitted Patients

1. For patients who have been admitted to the hospital after receiving antivenom
2. Patients should have clearly improving trajectory
3. Vital signs normal
4. Neurotoxicity resolved
5. Coagulopathy corrected and labs near normal
6. No evidence of bleeding
7. Pain controlled
8. Mobility issues addressed
9. Wound care performed with plan going forward for continued care
10. Patient education performed. Return precautions given.
11. Follow up plan in place for continued outpatient care
12. Patients treated for coagulopathy should return in 5-7 days for recheck of labs (CBC, PT, INR, fibrinogen), if possible.
13. Bleeding precautions (no contact sports, elective surgery, etc..) for 2 weeks after discharge in patients treated for coagulopathy

Fig. 18.8 (continued)

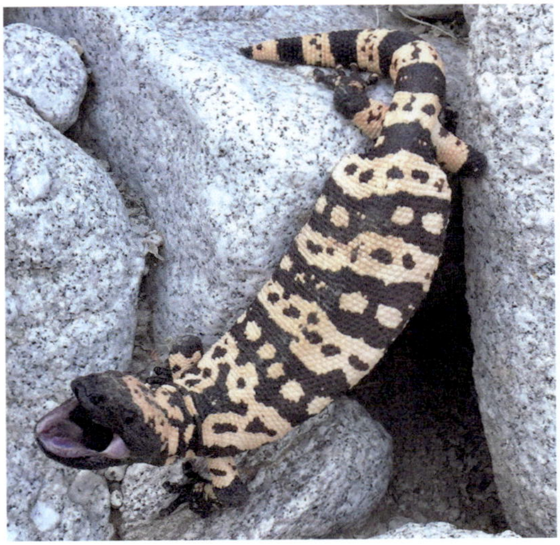

Fig. 18.9 *Heloderma suspectum* (Gila monster) from Arizona, US. These lizards have powerful bites and their long sharp teeth introduce venomous oral secretions into the wound. Bites to humans are rare and usually occur during handling of the animals. No commercial antivenom exists and treatment is supportive. (Image courtesy of B.G.)

effects, and neurotoxicity, but death is extremely rare (Chippaux and Amri 2021; French et al. 2015) There was a death reported in Colorado, USA in 2024 from a pet Gila monster bite (AP News 2024). Treatment consists of dislodging the lizard as quickly as possible to prevent additional venom absorption, wound cleansing, analgesia, and supportive care. Airway management, fluid resuscitation, and cardiovascular support may be required in rare severe cases (Chippaux and Amri 2021; French et al. 2015). No commercial antivenom exists for lizard envenomations.

Invertebrates

Arthropods

The phylum Arthropoda is an ancient and massive taxon. Most arthropods are harmless to humans, but there are several groups capable of causing human envenomation. Important groups of venomous arthropods include arachnids (spiders, scorpions, ticks, mites), centipedes, and insects (bees, wasps, ants, caterpillars, and others). Arthropods primarily deliver venom by biting or stinging.

Biting arthropods include spiders and centipedes. These animals have modified mouthparts or *chelicerae* connected to venom glands, which function as fangs. Spiders and centipedes primarily use their venom to immobilize, kill, and digest prey. Their bite and venom serve a secondary defensive purpose against threats.

Stinging arthropods include scorpions, bees, wasps, ants, and caterpillars. Scorpions have a stinger connected to venom glands at the tip of the tail. Like spiders and centipedes, the venom is used primarily to capture and kill prey but serves a defensive purpose as well.

Bees, wasps, and ants are insects in the order Hymenoptera and have stingers, consisting of a modified ovipositor, or egg-laying appendage. Only female members of Hymenoptera can deliver a sting.

Caterpillars are the larval form of butterflies and moths and are classified in the order Lepidoptera. Certain caterpillar species can cause envenomation through *setae* or spines that are connected to venom glands. Caterpillars sting for defensive purposes.

Spiders

There are 50,000 known species of spider in the world and nearly all have venom. Very few spiders, however, are medically significant (Isbister and Fan 2011). There are two genera that cause the bulk clinically significant spider envenomations worldwide, *Latrodectus* (widow spiders), which cause neurotoxic effects, and *Loxosceles* (brown spiders), which can cause dermonecrotic lesions, and rarely hemolysis and coagulopathy. Other spiders can cause significant clinical effects, such as *Atrax robustus* (Sydney funnel-web spider) from Australia, and *Phoneutria* species (wandering spiders) from South America.

Latrodectus. Widow spiders, of which there are several different species, are common throughout North America but are also found on every other continent, excluding Antarctica (Graudins 2003). These spiders are typically shiny black with red markings, but some color variation occurs globally, depending on the species (Fig. 18.10a). They tend to be secretive, often building small, tangled webs under or near their hiding places. Wood piles, rock piles, crawlspaces, crop fields, barns, garages, and similar situations are common places to find these spiders. They are most active at night. Bites to humans usually occur when a spider is accidentally disturbed in its web, or when a spider hides in footwear or other clothing that is subsequently donned. *Latrodectus* venom contains neurotoxic proteins, including alpha-latrotoxin, and the envenomation syndrome, called Latrodectism, is characterized by the effects of excessive acetylcholine release from presynaptic neuron terminals (Graudins 2003; Caruso et al. 2021; Maretić 1983). The result is pain, muscle spasm, and autonomic symptoms like hypertension, tachycardia, and diaphoresis (Graudins 2003; Caruso et al. 2021; Maretić 1983).

Clinical Presentation

A patient may see the spider or bring it with them when they present for treatment, in which case efforts should be made to identify the spider. In other cases, the patient may not realize they were bitten, and the clinician must recognize the envenomation syndrome. A *Latrodectus* spider bite may initially cause little to no pain and many bites may not be immediately recognized. When symptoms worsen, sometimes hours later, the syndrome may not be recognized as Latrodectism (Graudins 2003; Caruso et al. 2021; Maretić 1983). However, many patients do initially feel a biting or stinging sensation, leading to the discovery of the spider (Graudins 2003). Many *Latrodectus* bites do not ultimately cause significant envenomation symptoms (Graudins 2003; Caruso et al. 2021; Maretić 1983; Monte et al. 2011). Envenomation typically manifests within an hour of the bite with local erythema, pain, diaphoresis, and piloerection (Graudins 2003; Caruso et al. 2021; Maretić 1983). Swelling or other signs of tissue injury are usually absent. Envenomation symptoms tend to spread from the bitten area and steadily worsen over hours.

Systemic symptoms include hypertension, tachycardia, generalized diaphoresis, diffuse muscle spasms, vomiting, and fever (Graudins 2003; Caruso et al. 2021; Maretić 1983). Severe facial muscle spasms may occur along with hypersalivation and lacrimation from acetylcholine overstimulation (Maretić 1983). In some cases, abdominal muscle spasms and rigidity can mimic an acute abdomen (Graudins 2003; Caruso et al. 2021; Maretić 1983; Monte et al. 2011). The pain, diaphoresis, and hypertension that occur can mimic cardiac presentations, but can also rarely cause serious cardiac problems. Takotsubo cardiomyopathy and other myocardial dysfunction have occurred in *Latrodectus*

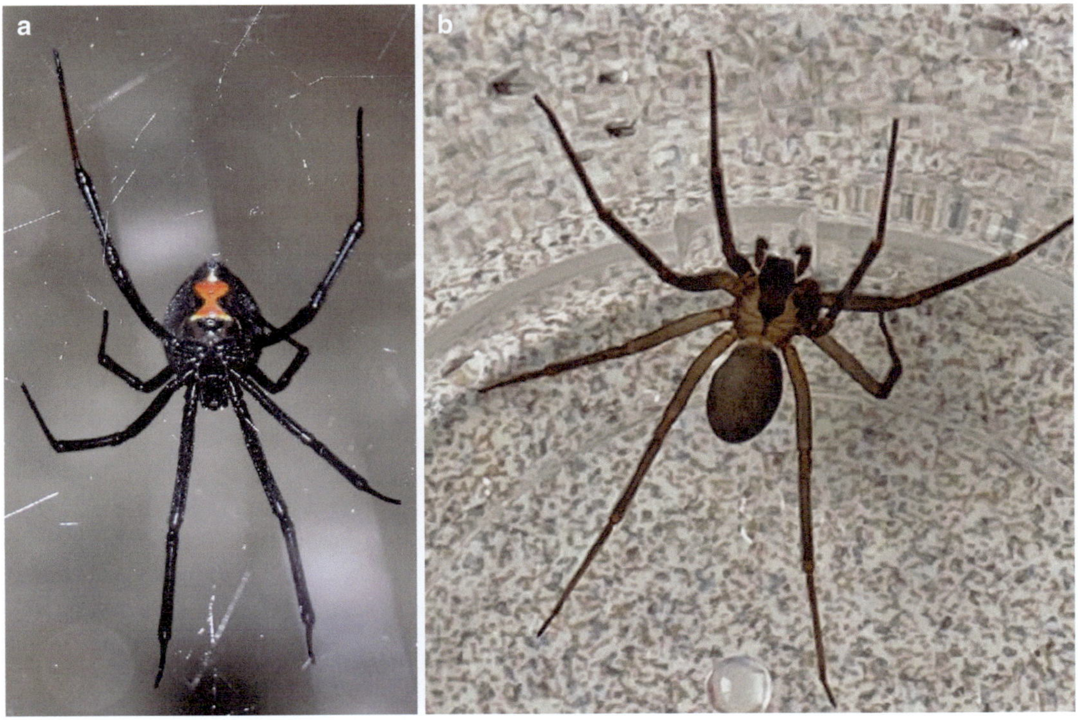

Fig. 18.10 *Latrodectus hesperus* (western black widow), California, US, with characteristic reddish ventral markings (part **a**). Markings on other widow spiders vary, but the body morphology remains similar. *Loxosceles reclusa* (brown recluse spider), Kentucky, US. Note the violin-shaped marking on the thorax (part **b**). (Images **a**, **b** courtesy of B.G)

envenomations (Fusto et al. 2020; Pereañez et al. 2022; Dendane et al. 2012). Muscular overstimulation can lead to rhabdomyolysis (Graudins 2003; Caruso et al. 2021; Maretić 1983). Priapism has also been described as a complication (Caruso et al. 2021; Hoover and Fortenberry 2004; Quan and Ruha 2009). Latrodectism in pregnant patients can cause uterine cramping, mimic preeclampsia, and can even pose a risk to the pregnancy (Sherman et al. 2000). The syndrome tends to peak at 24 h and can last for days, causing great discomfort to the patient (Graudins 2003). Death is extremely rare in Latrodectism but has occurred (Caruso et al. 2021).

Diagnosis hinges upon a history of known or possible *Latrodectus* bite coupled with the clinical features of Latrodectism. A history of moving wood, harvesting crops, reaching into dark places, or putting on footwear or other clothing prior to the onset of symptoms should raise clinical suspicion. Localized pain, muscle spasm, and diaphoresis that progress to involve other body regions in a hypertensive, tachycardic patient should place Latrodectism among the differential diagnoses. Most laboratory studies will be unrevealing, but CK level, metabolic panel, and urinalysis should be checked in cases where rhabdomyolysis is a concern.

Latrodectism Treatment

Initial care for a known or suspected *Latrodectus* bite involves assessing the ABCs and stabilizing life threats. Tetanus vaccination should be updated. Antibiotics are not indicated. Asymptomatic patients may be observed for 4–6 h and discharged if symptoms remain absent or mild. IV access should be obtained in patients with worsening or severe pain, unstable vital signs, or other severe symptoms. IV fluids, pain medication, and antiemetics should be used initially for symptom relief.

Many therapies have been tried for Latrodectism over time, but few have proved universally effective (Graudins 2003; Caruso et al. 2021; Monte et al. 2011; Ryan et al. 2017; Clark et al. 1992). Intravenous calcium gluconate, opioids, benzodiazepines, muscle relaxers, and anti-inflammatory drugs have all been used widely with variable results (Isbister and Fan 2011; Graudins 2003; Caruso et al. 2021; Maretić 1983; Monte et al. 2011; Ryan et al. 2017). Calcium gluconate has not proved to be efficacious in improving symptoms or shortening duration (Caruso et al. 2021; Monte et al. 2011; Clark et al. 1992). Opioids are frequently used for severe pain and benzodiazepines are used for muscle spasm and the combination has shown improved symptom relief (Clark et al. 1992). Caution should be exercised when co-administering these agents due to the potential for respiratory depression and patients should not be discharged with prescriptions for both.

Several antivenoms exist for Latrodectism, including products made for use in the US, Australia, Mexico, South America, and Africa. Antivenom is the only treatment that neutralizes the venom toxins and provides rapid, lasting relief (Graudins 2003; Monte et al. 2011; Ryan et al. 2017; Clark et al. 1992). The available antivenom products are either whole IgG or F(ab)2 equine products. Antivenom is typically administered IV by slow infusion while monitoring for early hypersensitivity reaction (Graudins 2003). The usual starting dose is one vial with redosing, as needed, for refractory symptoms (Graudins 2003; Clark et al. 1992; Heard et al. 1999). Antivenom rapidly relieves pain and the other symptoms of Latrodectism, often within an hour (Graudins 2003; Caruso et al. 2021; Clark et al. 1992). Antivenom can limit the need for additional medications and help some patients avoid hospitalization (Monte et al. 2011; Clark et al. 1992). Antivenom administration should be considered for patients with severe or refractory pain, significant systemic signs of envenomation, evidence of cardiopulmonary instability, complications such as priapism, and in pregnant patients with significant abdominal pain or symptoms mimicking preeclampsia (Graudins 2003; Caruso et al. 2021; Monte et al. 2011; Hoover and Fortenberry 2004; Ryan et al. 2017; Clark et al. 1992).

Many clinicians are hesitant to use *Latrodectus* antivenom due to the fear of hypersensitivity reaction (Graudins 2003; Caruso et al. 2021; Monte et al. 2011; Murphy et al. 2011). A 2011 review of the National Poison Data System in the US by Monte et al. revealed that between 2000 and 2008, antivenom was used in 3.78% of 9872 cases of *Latrodectus* envenomation, but use increased to 20% in severe cases (Monte et al. 2011). In the same study, 3.5% of patients receiving antivenom had an adverse reaction; there were no deaths (Monte et al. 2011). As with any antivenom product, hypersensitivity reactions do occur. There have been two fatalities documented from *Latrodectus* antivenom administration (Caruso et al. 2021; Clark et al. 1992; Murphy et al. 2011). Both fatal cases involved asthmatic patients (Caruso et al. 2021; Clark et al. 1992; Murphy et al. 2011). Caution should be exercised when considering antivenom for patients with asthma or a significant allergic history. Pretreatment with epinephrine has been shown to significantly reduce the rate of immediate hypersensitivity reaction with certain snake antivenoms and may be considered prior to *Latrodectus* antivenom administration in higher-risk patients (Premawardhena et al. 1999; de Silva et al. 2011). If a hypersensitivity reaction occurs during antivenom infusion, the infusion should be stopped immediately and the patient treated with IM or SC epinephrine, IV or IM antihistamines, and IV or IM corticosteroids.

Patients may be discharged when their symptoms are well-controlled, including after they have received antivenom (Clark et al. 1992). Patients with persistent severe symptoms, uncontrolled pain, hypersensitivity reactions, or other complications require extended observation or admission. Consider consulting a medical toxicologist, or other envenomation specialist, if available, to assist with treatment decisions.

Other Neurotoxic Spiders

Other medically important neurotoxic spiders include the Australian funnel-web spiders (*Atrax* species) and the wandering or banana spiders of Central and South America (*Phoneutria* species). These spiders can produce severe neurotoxic symptoms and have been known to cause death. Like the Latrodectus spider, these other spiders produce venom containing small molecular weight toxins that affect ion channels and neurotransmitter release. Regional antivenoms exist for these spiders and may be considered along with aggressive supportive care.

Loxosceles. *Loxosceles* spp. spiders are the most well-known and problematic necrotizing spiders and can be naturally found in the temperate and tropical regions of the Americas, Africa, and Europe, but these spiders have also been introduced to many other regions of the world (Gomez and Wasserman 2003; Nentwig et al. 2017). They are small, brown spiders and many have a characteristic violin-shaped mark on the thorax (Fig. 18.10b). *Loxosceles* are active hunters for insect prey and can achieve high population densities in certain situations, such as barns, woodpiles, and other undisturbed areas but they also enter human habitation, which is how many bites occur, especially in the developing world.

Loxosceles venom has cytotoxic and hemotoxic properties and contains various proteins, including the enzyme sphingomyelinase D, which causes the characteristic dermonecrotic lesions (Gomez and Wasserman 2003; Chaves-Moreira et al. 2017; Futrell 1992). The local effects of *Loxosceles* venom are tissue damage, thrombosis, ischemia, and neutrophil aggregation and degranulation (Gomez and Wasserman 2003; Chaves-Moreira et al. 2017; Futrell 1992). The combination of these processes leads to tissue necrosis (Gomez and Wasserman 2003; Chaves-Moreira et al. 2017; Futrell 1992). The venom can also produce a systemic syndrome that is marked by hemolysis and coagulopathy and can lead to severe anemia, renal failure, and other life-threatening problems (Gomez and Wasserman 2003; Chaves-Moreira et al. 2017; Futrell 1992; da Silva et al. 2004; Algren et al. 2011; Rogers et al. 2011).

Most *Loxosceles* bites produce mild localized effects and many probably go unrecognized (Futrell 1992; da Silva et al. 2004). Many patients may not feel the initial bite, but some may feel a sharp sensation. If envenomation occurs, local erythema, irritation, itching, central blanching, and mild swelling may be noted within a few hours of the bite (Gomez and Wasserman 2003; Futrell 1992; Hogan et al. 2004; Algren et al. 2011; Rogers et al. 2011; Stoecker et al. 2017). Most bites do not progress to necrosis and even fewer cases of systemic Loxoscelism develop (Gomez and Wasserman 2003; Futrell 1992; Hogan et al. 2004). If the syndrome does progress, local pain, tenderness, and mild swelling develop over 1–3 days. Early bulla formation, ecchymosis, and gravity-dependent spread of the lesion are classic early findings (Algren et al. 2011). The lesion then typically ulcerates and transitions to an eschar that may take weeks or months to heal and can leave significant scarring.

The diagnosis of *Loxosceles* envenomations can be difficult and they are thought to be overdiagnosed by patients and clinicians. Many different processes can produce ulcerative skin lesions that can be misdiagnosed as a "spider bite." Cutaneous infections, inflammatory processes, autoimmune conditions, and other etiologies that produce ulcerative skin lesions can mimic a dermonecrotic spider bite. Caution should be exercised when making the diagnosis of *Loxosceles* spider bite when a spider is not visualized, or other history is not strongly suggestive of spider exposure. Stoecker et al. developed a mnemonic device to assist in the diagnosis of *Loxosceles* bites in the United States, called NOT RECLUSE, which is summarized below (Stoecker et al. 2017).

- **N** (numerous)—Usually only one lesion is present.
- **O** (occurrence)—Bites usually occur when the spider is disturbed.
- **T** (timing)—Most bites happen between April and October.
- **R** (red center)—Recluse bites typically have a pale center.
- **E** (elevated)—Recluse bites are usually flat. Elevation >1 cm suggests against *Loxosceles* bite.
- **C** (chronic)—*Loxosceles* bites nearly always heal within 3 months.
- **L** (large)—Bites are rarely >10 cm in size.
- **U** (ulcerates too early)—Bites typically do not ulcerate before 7 days.
- **S** (swollen)—There is usually not significant swelling unless the bite is on the feet or face.
- **E** (exudative)—*Loxosceles* bites are not exudative.

The treatment of the dermonecrotic lesions of *Loxosceles* envenomation is largely supportive. Various therapies have been tried including corticosteroids, dapsone, antibiotics, antihistamines, vasodilators, hyperbaric oxygen, and surgical debridement problems (Gomez and Wasserman 2003; Chaves-Moreira et al. 2017; Futrell 1992; da Silva et al. 2004; Algren et al. 2011). None of these measures has shown efficacy in altering the course of *Loxosceles* dermonecrotic lesions. (Gomez and Wasserman 2003; Chaves-Moreira et al. 2017; Futrell 1992; da Silva et al. 2004; Algren et al. 2011).

Systemic manifestations of *Loxosceles* envenomation are rare, but potentially life-threatening, particularly in pediatric patients (Rosen et al. 2012; McDade et al. 2010). Hemolysis, coagulopathy, renal failure, and shock can occur (de Souza et al. 2008). Corticosteroids have been shown to decrease the hemolytic process and help prevent progression to renal failure (Gomez and Wasserman 2003; Chaves-Moreira et al. 2017; Futrell 1992; da Silva et al. 2004; Algren et al. 2011). In cases of severe hemolysis, transfusion of packed red cells and other blood products may be necessary problems (Gomez and Wasserman 2003; Chaves-Moreira et al. 2017; Futrell 1992; da Silva et al. 2004; Algren et al. 2011; Rogers et al. 2011).

Antivenoms for *Loxosceles* spiders have been produced in countries like Brazil and Mexico and have shown some efficacy in reducing the likelihood of necrosis when given early (Malaque et al. 2022). Antivenom may also improve the course of systemic Loxoscelism and the coagulopathic/hemolytic effects if given early. Early diagnosis of the syndrome and availability of antivenom are challenges.

Scorpions

Scorpions are ancient arthropods that can be found on every continent except Antarctica. There are over 2200 scorpion species in the world, but only around 100 species are considered medically significant (Ward et al. 2018). Scorpions have pincers on the anterior body for grasping prey and a stinger at the end of the tail. The stinger is connected to a venom sac in the last segment of the tail. Scorpions primarily use their venom for killing and digesting prey, but the stinging apparatus is also well-equipped to deliver defensive stings.

Scorpions can be found in diverse habitats including desert, grassland, forest, islands, urban, and agricultural areas. They are generally secretive and nocturnal. Most scorpion stings occur when the animal is disturbed and typical scenarios include stepping on them with bare feet, picking up objects sheltering scorpions, or donning clothing that conceals a scorpion.

Most scorpion stings produce immediate burning pain. Mild localized redness and swelling can occur but are usually not dramatic. Pain and other local symptoms can last from minutes to hours, and sometimes longer. Scorpions of the genus Hemiscorpius, in the Middle East, possess cytotoxic venom that causes a syndrome similar to Loxoscelism characterized by local tissue necrosis, hemolysis, coagulopathy, and renal failure (Mostafazadeh et al. 2017). Several scorpion species possess potent neurotoxins that can cause severe envenomation in humans that occasionally results in death. Most neurotoxic scorpions are found in the family Buthidae, which includes the Arizona bark scorpion (*Centruroides sculpturatus*) of the southwestern US and the deathstalker scorpions (*Leiurus* species) of the Middle East.

The dangerous neurotoxic scorpions, like neurotoxic spiders, produce low molecular weight protein toxins that affect ion movement across cell membranes. Sodium, potassium, and calcium channels are most affected (Isbister and Bawaskar 2014; Rowe et al. 2011; Boyer-Hassen 2003; Quintero-Hernández et al. 2013). Some toxins produce the effect of keeping sodium channels open thereby prolonging action potentials leading to nerve and muscle overstimulation (Boyer-Hassen 2003; Quintero-Hernández et al. 2013). Other toxins block potassium cellular reentry in a synergistic manner (Quintero-Hernández et al. 2013). This mechanism potentiates pain, which can be prolonged in neurotoxic scorpion stings, and is thought to cause the more severe effects of scorpion envenomation, including acetylcholine overstimulation, catecholamine release, cardiotoxicity, and neurologic dysfunction (Isbister and Bawaskar 2014; Boyer-Hassen 2003; Rowe et al. 2011)).

Diagnosis of a scorpion sting relies on a history suggestive of scorpion exposure or a witnessed sting that is followed by characteristic symptoms. Since most scorpions are not dangerously venomous, most stings will produce mild symptoms such as local pain and mild local inflammation. A puncture wound may not be seen. Many other biting and stinging arthropods produce similar symptoms and if a scorpion is not seen, it may be impossible to determine the culprit. In most cases, tetanus vaccination, local wound care, and analgesia are the only measures needed. In areas inhabited by more dangerous scorpions, patients should be observed to ensure that more severe symptoms do not develop.

Neurotoxic scorpion venom effects include local and regional pain/paresthesia, vital sign abnormalities, systemic neurologic abnormalities, muscular overstimulation leading to rhabdomyolysis, autonomic dysfunction, pancreatitis, cardiopulmonary compromise, and death in some cases (Isbister and Bawaskar 2014; Boyer-Hassen 2003; Dehghani et al. 2023; Sofer et al. 1991). The most common effects are local and regional pain and paresthesia which can last for hours to days. In more severe cases, patients exhibit systemic signs such as tachycardia, hypertension, hyperthermia, muscle hyperactivity/spasm, cranial nerve abnormalities such as disconjugate eye movements or hypersecretion, diaphoresis, agitation, vomiting, wheezing, pulmonary edema, and respiratory failure (Isbister and Bawaskar 2014; Boyer-Hassen 2003). Children are much more vulnerable to the effects of neurotoxic scorpions and have the highest risk of severe envenomation (Boyer-Hassen 2003). The elderly and those with preexisting cardiopulmonary disease are also at greater risk.

Laboratory studies are not needed for mild envenomations with only local symptoms. For more severe envenomations, obtain complete blood count, comprehensive metabolic panel, creatine kinase, and urinalysis. Lipase level should be considered if significant abdominal pain is present. If vital signs are abnormal, obtain an electrocardiogram, chest X-ray, and start cardiac monitoring and continuous pulse oximetry.

Treatment of scorpion envenomation begins with addressing life threats and providing supportive care. As with any envenomation, immediate hypersensitivity reaction to scorpion venom can occur and should be treated with standard measures, including epinephrine, antihistamines, and corticosteroids. Analgesia and anxiolysis are important considerations. Use caution when administering sedating medications if airway or respiratory concerns are present. Topical lidocaine has shown efficacy in reducing the pain associated with scorpion stings (Aksel et al. 2015). Local wound care consists of cleansing with soap and water. Antibiotics are not indicated in the acute setting. Several regional antivenoms are available for scorpion envenomation. Antivenom is not indicated for stings with only local symptoms. For patients with more severe systemic symptoms, antivenom should be considered along with aggressive supportive care. A local or regional expert should be consulted early in cases of systemic toxicity. In cases with severe neurotoxicity or cardiopulmonary compromise, airway protection and mechanical ventilation may be needed.

In the rare case of a cytotoxic scorpion envenomation, which would likely only occur naturally in the Middle East, antivenom should be considered early. Close monitoring of blood counts and coagulation parameters should be done, particularly in children. Plasmapheresis has been shown to improve the course of severe cytotoxic scorpion stings in Iran (Mostafazadeh et al. 2017).

Centipedes

Centipedes are venomous arthropods found in many regions of the world. Centipedes can cause envenomation by biting with modified chelicerae that function as fangs. Typical effects of centipede envenomation include pain, redness, and local swelling. Immediate and delayed hypersensitivity reactions can occur and should be treated with standard measures (Fung et al. 2011). Severe or life-threatening envenomation is very rare and usually, supportive care and analgesia are the only measures needed. There is no commercial antivenom for centipedes.

Insects

Hymenoptera

The order Hymenoptera contains bees, wasps, and ants. Many species can deliver venomous stings. Hymenoptera are found nearly worldwide and are a common cause of human envenomation. Many of these insects are social and live in nests or hives. Multiple stings can occur when members of a colony feel threatened. These insects thrive in agricultural settings and some, such are bees, are essential pollinators for agricultural crops and agricultural workers are particularly at risk of envenomation.

Like other venoms, Hymenoptera venoms are mixtures of various toxic substances. Low molecular weight toxins, such as histamine, serotonin, and other biologic amines are common (Habermann 1972). These agents cause pain, inflammation, and vasodilation. Toxic alkaloids are present in certain venoms and can cause tissue damage and other effects. Various enzymes and other proteins are also found in the venom. Many venom components are antigenic and can cause hypersensitivity reactions, which are the major cause of mortality from insect stings.

Most insect stings cause local pain, itching, swelling, and redness. Pain can be severe. Immediate hypersensitivity reactions can cause life-threatening anaphylaxis and death can occur from a single sting. Delayed hypersensitivity reactions can also occur. These are characterized by progressive redness, swelling, induration, itching, and pain that progress from the sting site to a larger area (Severino et al. 2009). These reactions are called large local reactions. These reactions can closely mimic cellulitis. Certain insects, such as fire ants, contain toxic alkaloids which produce localized tissue damage and necrosis. Stings initially develop a pustular appearance and then progress to necrotic lesions over several days before healing.

Massive envenomation can occur when a victim is stung repeatedly by large numbers of insects. Massive envenomation with systemic toxicity generally occurs when stings number more than 50 (Vetter et al. 1999; Chen et al. 2020). Higher numbers of stings generally produce more severe effects. Massive Hymenoptera envenomation tends to occur with victims who are unable to rapidly escape the reach of the insects. Very young or elderly patients, intoxicated patients, or immobilized persons are at increased risk of massive envenomation. In massive envenomation, the vasoactive substances in the venom can cause hypotension and shock. Rhabdomyolysis, acute kidney injury, respiratory failure, cardiac dysfunction, seizures, coagulopathy, and death can result (Vetter et al. 1999; Chen et al. 2020).

Field treatment for Hymenoptera stings starts with evacuating the area and avoiding additional stings. Some insects, like honeybees, leave the stinger in the victim's skin. The stinger is still connected to the venom sac, which can introduce additional venom. Stingers should be removed as quickly as possible by scraping or pulling. If symptoms remain limited to local pain and other signs of inflammation, immediate hospital care is not needed. Patients with a history of hypersensitivity reactions to insect stings should receive a medical evaluation. Ideally, people with a history of hypersensitivity reaction to stings should carry antihistamines and an epinephrine auto-injector with them.

Patients with signs or symptoms of anaphylaxis, other systemic symptoms (confusion, dyspnea, vomiting, syncope), massive envenomation, or a history of severe reactions to stings should seek medical attention as quickly as possible. In the hospital setting, IV access and cardiac/respiratory monitoring performed. Life threats should be addressed with a focus on airway management and the rapid administration of epinephrine for anaphylactic symptoms or cardiopulmonary instability. Repeated doses of epinephrine and epinephrine infusion may be needed in severe cases. Antihistamines and corticosteroids should be administered. IV crystalloid fluid should be administered to optimize euvolemia and as needed for hypotension. Patients with severe reactions or massive envenomation should receive laboratory studies including complete blood count, basic metabolic panel, liver panel, and urinalysis. Prothrombin time, international normalized ratio, fibrinogen, and creatine kinase should be considered for massive envenomations. Significant laboratory abnormalities should be followed up with repeat labs to determine the trajectory.

Patients with successfully treated anaphylaxis should be monitored for 4–6 h after resolution of all signs and symptoms before discharge is considered. All patients with anaphylaxis should be prescribed epinephrine for out-of-hospital use. Patients with complicated or refractory anaphylaxis, continued systemic symptoms, significant laboratory abnormalities, and patients with massive envenomation should be admitted to the hospital for continued monitoring and treatment.

Patients with severe anaphylaxis, shock, or organ dysfunction may require intubation and mechanical ventilation along with aggressive IV fluids and vasopressor agents. Patients with severe kidney injury require the involvement of a nephrologist.

Large local reactions can be treated with topical or oral corticosteroids, antihistamines, and nonsteroidal anti-inflammatory drugs. If infection is suspected, antibiotics should be given. Tetanus vaccination should be updated for all patients.

Serum sickness can occur after Hymenoptera stings due to the antigenic effects of the foreign proteins in the venom. Treatment is the same for other causes of serum sickness and focuses on the alleviation of symptoms by treating with corticosteroids, antihistamines, and anti-inflammatory drugs.

Patients with a severe reaction to an insect sting should be referred to an allergist to consider venom immunotherapy.

Caterpillars

Most caterpillar envenomations produce local symptoms including pain, irritation, erythema, and minor tissue damage consisting of blisters, ulcers, or other wounds. Treatment for minor caterpillar envenomations consists of removing the spines, cleansing the area, providing analgesia, and performing basic wound care. Sticky tape or forceps can be used to remove spines.

Certain caterpillar species can produce more severe and even life-threatening envenomations. Caterpillars in the genus *Lonomia*, which are primarily found in South America, can produce systemic venom effects including, coagulopathy, hemorrhage, acute kidney injury, shock, and death. There is an antivenom for Lonomia envenomations produced by Instituto Butantan in Brazil. This is the only caterpillar antivenom in existence.

Severe caterpillar envenomations are only described from Latin America and typically involve stings by multiple caterpillars. Treatment is supportive with fluid resuscitation, management of coagulopathy, and the administration of antivenom.

References

Akani GC, Ebere N, Franco D, et al. Correlation between annual activity patterns of venomous snakes and rural people in The Niger Delta, southern Nigeria. J Venom Anim Toxins Incl Trop Dis. 2013;19:2. https://doi.org/10.1186/1678-9199-19-2.

Aksel G, Güler S, Doğan NÖ, Çorbacioğlu ŞK. A randomized trial comparing intravenous paracetamol, topical lidocaine, and ice application for treatment of pain associated with scorpion stings. Hum Exp Toxicol. 2015;34(6):662–7. Epub 2014 Oct 10. https://doi.org/10.1177/0960327114551394.

Albulescu LO, Xie C, Ainsworth S, et al. A therapeutic combination of two small molecule toxin inhibitors provides broad preclinical efficacy against viper snakebite. Nat Commun. 2020;11:6094. https://doi.org/10.1038/s41467-020-19981-6.

Algren DA, et al. Pearls about loxoscelism. Ann Emerg Med. 2011;57(4):419–20; author reply 420-1. https://doi.org/10.1016/j.annemergmed.2010.10.020.

AP News. Colorado man died from pet Gila monster's venomous bite, autopsy shows. New York, NY: Associated Press; 2024.

Asita de Silva H, et al. Adverse reactions to snake antivenom, and their prevention and treatment. Br J Clin Pharmacol. 2016;81(3):446–52. https://doi.org/10.1111/bcp.12739.

Baldo C, et al. Mechanisms of vascular damage by hemorrhagic snake venom metalloproteinases: tissue distribution and in situ hydrolysis. PLoS Negl Trop Dis. 2010;4:e727. https://doi.org/10.1371/journal.pntd.0000727.

Bart G, et al. Bilateral pulmonary embolism following a viper envenomation in France: a case report and review. Medicine. 2016;95(19):e2798. https://doi.org/10.1097/MD.0000000000002798.

Benjamin JM, et al. Delayed double reading of whole blood clotting test (WBCT) results at 20 and 30 minutes enhances diagnosis and treatment of viper envenomation. J Venom Anim Toxins Incl Trop Dis. 2018;24:14. https://doi.org/10.1186/s40409-018-0151-1.

Benjamin JM, Brandehoff N, Wilson B, et al. Global snake envenomation management (CPG ID: 81). In: Joint Trauma System Clinical Practice Guidelines (CPGs); 2020. p. 1–89.

Berling I, Isbister GK. Hematologic effects and complications of snake envenoming. Transfus Med Rev. 2015;29(2):82–9. https://doi.org/10.1016/j.tmrv.2014.09.005.

Berling I, et al. Intracranial haemorrhages associated with venom induced consumption coagulopathy in Australian snakebites (ASP-21). Toxicon. 2015;102:8–13. https://doi.org/10.1016/j.toxicon.2015.05.012.

Boyer-Hassen L. Scorpion envenomation. In: Dart RC, editor. Medical toxicology. 3rd ed. Philadelphia, PA: Lippincott Williams & Wilkins; 2003. p. 1603–5.

Brandehoff N, et al. Ketamine for pain control of snake envenomation in Guinea: a case series. Toxicon. 2020;187:82–5. https://doi.org/10.1016/j.toxicon.2020.08.020.

Caruso MB, Lauria PSS, de Souza CMV, Casais-E-Silva LL, Zingali RB. Widow spiders in the new world: a review on *Latrodectus* Walckenaer, 1805 (Theridiidae) and latrodectism in the Americas. J Venom Anim Toxins Incl Trop Dis. 2021;27:e20210011. PMID: 34745240; PMCID: PMC8553018. https://doi.org/10.1590/1678-9199-JVATITD-2021-0011.

Chang K-C, et al. Venom Ophthalmia and ocular complications caused by snake venom. Toxins. 2020;12(9):576. https://doi.org/10.3390/toxins12090576.

Chaves-Moreira D, et al. Highlights in the knowledge of brown spider toxins. J Venom Anim Toxin Includ Trop Dis. 2017;23(6):8. https://doi.org/10.1186/s40409-017-0097-8.

Chen TH, Liao WT, Chen CS, Lin PC, Wu MY. An envenoming syndrome from massive *Vespa* stings induces multiple organ failure. Insects. 2020;11(4):219. PMID: 32252275; PMCID: PMC7240471. https://doi.org/10.3390/insects11040219.

Chippaux JP. Snakebite envenomation turns again into a neglected tropical disease! J Venom Anim Toxins Incl Trop Dis. 2017;23:38. https://doi.org/10.1186/s40409-017-0127-6.

Chippaux J-P, Amri K. Severe *Heloderma* spp. envenomation: a review of the literature. Clin Toxicol. 2021;59(3):179–84. https://doi.org/10.1080/15563650.2020.1853145.

Chu ER, Weinstein SA, White J, Warrell DA. Venom ophthalmia caused by venoms of spitting elapid and other snakes: report of ten cases with review of epidemiology, clinical features, pathophysiology and management. Toxicon. 2010;56(3):259–72. https://doi.org/10.1016/j.toxicon.2010.02.023.

Clark RF, Wethern-Kestner S, Vance MV, Gerkin R. Clinical presentation and treatment of black widow spider envenomation: a review of 163 cases. Ann Emerg Med. 1992;21(7):782–7. https://doi.org/10.1016/s0196-0644(05)81021-2.

Clark RF, et al. Immediate and delayed allergic reactions to Crotalidae polyvalent immune fab (ovine) antivenom. Ann Emerg Med. 2002;39(6):671–6. https://doi.org/10.1067/mem.2002.123134.

Corbett B, Clark RF. North American Snake envenomation. Emerg Med Clin North Am. 2017;35(2):339–54. https://doi.org/10.1016/j.emc.2016.12.003.

Corbit AG, Hayes WK. Factors that influence the clinical severity of venomous snakebites in southern California. Toxicon. 2016;117:106.

CroFab. CroFab [Package Insert]. West Conshohocken, PA: BTG International; 2023.

da Silva PH, et al. Brown spiders and loxoscelism. Toxicon. 2004;44(7):693–709. https://doi.org/10.1016/j.toxicon.2004.07.012.

Dart RC, et al. A randomized multicenter trial of crotalinae polyvalent immune fab (ovine) antivenom for the treatment for crotaline snakebite in the United States. Arch Intern Med. 2001;161(16):2030–6. https://doi.org/10.1001/archinte.161.16.2030.

Dawson AH. Cholinergic drugs. In: Dart RC, editor. Medical toxicology. 3rd ed. Philadelphia, PA: Lippincott Williams & Wilkins; 2003. p. 567–71.

de Silva HA, et al. Low-dose adrenaline, promethazine, and hydrocortisone in the prevention of acute adverse reactions to antivenom following snakebite: a randomised, double-blind, placebo-controlled trial. PLoS Med. 2011;8(5):e1000435. https://doi.org/10.1371/journal.pmed.1000435.

de Souza AL, Malaque CM, Sztajnbok J, Romano CC, Duarte AJ, Seguro AC. Loxosceles venom-induced cytokine activation, hemolysis, and acute kidney injury. Toxicon. 2008;51:151–6.

Dehghani R, Ghorbani A, Varzandeh M, Karami-Robati F. Toxicity mechanism of dangerous scorpion stings in Iran. J Arthropod Borne Dis. 2023;17(2):105–19. PMID: 37822761; PMCID: PMC10562200. https://doi.org/10.18502/jad.v17i2.13616.

Dendane T, Abidi K, Madani N, Benthami A, Gueddari FZ, Abouqal R, Zeggwagh AA. Reversible myocarditis after black widow spider envenomation. Case Rep Med. 2012;2012:794540. Epub 2012 Jan 26. PMID: 22319538; PMCID: PMC3272799. https://doi.org/10.1155/2012/794540.

Erulu VE, et al. Revered but poorly understood: a case report of *Dendroaspis polylepis* (black mamba) envenomation in Watamu, Malindi Kenya, and a review of the literature. Trop Med Infect Dis. 2018;3(3):104. PMID: 30274500; PMCID: PMC6161185. https://doi.org/10.3390/tropicalmed3030104.

Farooq H, et al. Snakebite incidence in rural sub-Saharan Africa might be severely underestimated. Toxicon. 2022;219:106932. https://doi.org/10.1016/j.toxicon.2022.106932.

Feitosa EL, et al. Older age and time to medical assistance are associated with severity and mortality of snakebites in the Brazilian Amazon: a case-control study. PLoS One. 2015;10(7):e0132237. https://doi.org/10.1371/journal.pone.0132237.

French R, et al. Gila monster (Heloderma suspectum) envenomation: descriptive analysis of calls to United States poison centers with focus on Arizona cases. Clin Toxicol. 2015;53(1):60–70. https://doi.org/10.3109/15563650.2014.988791.

Fung HT, Lam SK, Wong OF. Centipede bite victims: a review of patients presenting to two emergency departments in Hong Kong. Hong Kong Med J. 2011;17(5):381–5.

Fusto G, Bennardo L, Duca ED, et al. Spider bites of medical significance in the Mediterranean area: misdiagnosis, clinical features and management. J Venom Anim Toxin Includ Trop Dis. 2020;26:e20190100. PMID: 33061945; PMCID: PMC7534902. https://doi.org/10.1590/1678-9199-jvatitd-2019-0100.

Futrell JM. Loxoscelism. Am J Med Sci. 1992;304:261–7.

German BT, Hack JB, Brewer KL, Meggs WJ. Pressure-immobilization bandages delay toxicity in a porcine model of eastern coral snake (*Micrurus fulvius fulvius*) envenomation. Ann Emerg Med. 2005;45:603–8. https://doi.org/10.1016/j.annemergmed.2004.11.025.

Girish KS, Jagadeesha DK, Rajeev KB, Kemparaju K. Snake venom hyaluronidase: an evidence for isoforms and extracellular matrix degradation. Mol Cell Biochem. 2002;240(1–2):105–10. https://doi.org/10.1023/a:1020651607164.

Gold BS, Barish RA, Dart RC. North American snake envenomation: diagnosis, treatment, and management. Emerg Med Clin N Am. 2004;22:423–43. https://doi.org/10.1016/j.emc.2004.01.007.

Gomez HF, Wasserman GS. Recluse spider and other necrotizing arachnids. In: Dart RC, editor. Medical toxicology. 3rd ed. Philadelphia, PA: Lippincott Williams & Wilkins; 2003. p. 1596–602.

Graudins A. Widow spider envenomation: latrodectism. In: Dart RC, editor. Medical toxicology. 3rd ed. Philadelphia, PA: Lippincott Williams & Wilkins; 2003. p. 1592–5.

Greene SC, et al. Captive black mamba (Dendroaspis Polylepis) bite leading to respiratory failure. J Emerg Med. 2023;64(3):311–4. https://doi.org/10.1016/j.jemermed.2023.01.011.

Gutiérrez J, Calvete J, Habib A, et al. Snakebite envenoming. Nat Rev Dis Primers. 2017;3:17063. https://doi.org/10.1038/nrdp.2017.63.

Habermann E. Bee and wasp venoms. Science. 1972;177(4046):314–22. http://www.jstor.org/stable/1734340.

Hansen EA, Stein EA, Mader TH, Mazzoli RA. Spitting cobra ophthalmia in United Nations forces in Somalia. Am J Ophthalmol. 1994;117(5):671. https://doi.org/10.1016/s0002-9394(14)70078-9.

Hayes WK, et al. Defensive bites by rattle snakes (genus *Crotalus*): venom expenditure, envenomation severity, and the importance of snake size. In: Program and abstracts of the biology of the rattlesnakes symposium, vol. 2. Loma Linda, CA: Loma Linda University; 2005. p. 31.

Hayes WK, et al. Factors that influence venom expenditure in viperids and other snake species during predatory and defensive contexts. In: Biology of the Vipers. Eagle Mountain, UT: Eagle Mountain Publishing; 2002. p. 207–33.

Heard K, O'Malley GF, Dart RC. Antivenom therapy in the Americas. Drugs. 1999;58(1):5–15. https://doi.org/10.2165/00003495-199958010-00002.

Hiu JJ, Yap MKK. Cytotoxicity of snake venom enzymatic toxins: phospholipase A2 and l-amino acid oxidase. Biochem Soc Trans. 2020;48(2):719–31. https://doi.org/10.1042/BST20200110.

Ho C-H, et al. Analysis of the necrosis-inducing components of the venom of *Naja atra* and assessment of the neutralization ability of freeze-dried antivenom. Toxins. 2021;13(9):619. https://doi.org/10.3390/toxins13090619.

Hogan DE, Dire DJ. Anaphylactic shock secondary to rattlesnake bite. Ann Emerg Med. 1990;19(7):814–6. https://doi.org/10.1016/s0196-0644(05)81710-x.

Hogan CJ, et al. Loxoscelism: old obstacles, new directions. Ann Emerg Med. 2004;44(6):608–24. https://doi.org/10.1016/j.annemergmed.2004.08.028.

Holding ML, Biardi JE, Gibbs HL. Coevolution of venom function and venom resistance in a rattlesnake predator and its squirrel prey. Proc Biol Sci. 2016;283(1829):20152841. PMID: 27122552; PMCID: PMC4855376. https://doi.org/10.1098/rspb.2015.2841.

Hoover NG, Fortenberry JD. Use of antivenin to treat priapism after a black widow spider bite. Pediatrics. 2004;114(1):e128–9. https://doi.org/10.1542/peds.114.1.e128.

Hsu C-P, et al. Predictors of the development of post-snakebite compartment syndrome. Scand J Trauma Resusc Emerg Med. 2015;23(97):11. https://doi.org/10.1186/s13049-015-0179-y.

Isbister GK, Bawaskar HS. Scorpion envenomation. N Engl J Med. 2014;371(5):457–63. https://doi.org/10.1056/NEJMra1401108.

Isbister GK, Fan HW. Spider bite. Lancet. 2011;378(9808):2039–47. https://doi.org/10.1016/S0140-6736(10)62230-1.

Janes DN, Bush SP, Kolluru GR. Large snake size suggests increased snakebite severity in patients bitten by rattlesnakes in southern California. Wilderness Environ Med. 2010;21:120–6.

Jolkkonen M, et al. Muscarinic toxins from the black mamba Dendroaspis polylepis. Eur J Biochem. 1995;234(2):579–85. https://doi.org/10.1111/j.1432-1033.1995.579_b.x.

Kassegne I, et al. Severe snakebite envenomation revealed by an acute abdomen. J Surg Case Rep. 2020;2020(6):rjaa148. https://doi.org/10.1093/jscr/rjaa148.

Laustsen AH. Toxin synergism in snake venoms. Toxin Rev. 2016;35:165–70. https://doi.org/10.1080/15569543.2016.1220397.

Laustsen AH, Johansen KH, Engmark M, Andersen MR. Recombinant snakebite antivenoms: a cost-competitive solution to a neglected tropical disease? PLoS Negl Trop Dis. 2017;11:e0005361.

Lavonas EJ, et al. Unified treatment algorithm for the management of crotaline snakebite in the United States: results of an evidence-informed consensus workshop. BMC Emerg Med. 2011;11(2):3. https://doi.org/10.1186/1471-227X-11-2.

Le Geyt J, Pach S, Gutiérrez JM, et al. Paediatric snakebite envenoming: recognition and management of cases. Arch Dis Child. 2021;106:14–9.

Ledsgaard L, Wade J, Jenkins TP, et al. Discovery and optimization of a broadly-neutralizing human monoclonal antibody against long-chain α-neurotoxins from snakes. Nat Commun. 2023;14:682. https://doi.org/10.1038/s41467-023-36393-4.

Levine M, et al. Neurotoxicity associated with the southern Pacific rattlesnake (*Crotalus helleri*). Ann Emerg Med. 2023;81(3):318–22. https://doi.org/10.1016/j.annemergmed.2022.08.020.

Lewin M, et al. Varespladib (LY315920) appears to be a potent, broad-Spectrum, inhibitor of Snake venom phospholipase A2 and a possible pre-referral treatment for envenomation. Toxins. 2016;8(9):248. https://doi.org/10.3390/toxins8090248.

Ludolph AC. Mojave toxin. In: Spencer PS, Schaumburg HH, Ludolph AC, editors. Experimental and clinical neurotoxicology. 2nd ed. New York, NY: Oxford Academic; 2023. Accessed 19 Dec 2023. p. 31. https://doi.org/10.1093/oso/9780195084771.003.0306.

Mackessy SP, editor. Handbook of venoms and toxins of reptiles. 2nd ed. Boca Raton, FL: CRC; 2021. https://doi.org/10.1201/9780429054204.

Malaque CMS, et al. Impact of antivenom administration on the evolution of cutaneous lesions in loxoscelism: a prospective observational study. PLoS Negl Trop Dis. 2022;16(10):e0010842. https://doi.org/10.1371/journal.pntd.0010842.

Maretić Z. Latrodectism: variations in clinical manifestations provoked by Latrodectus species of spiders. Toxicon. 1983;21(4):457–66. https://doi.org/10.1016/0041-0101(83)90123-x.

McDade J, et al. Brown recluse spider (Loxosceles reclusa) envenomation leading to acute hemolytic anemia in six adolescents. J Pediatr. 2010;156(1):155–7. https://doi.org/10.1016/j.jpeds.2009.07.021.

Monte AA, Bucher-Bartelson B, Heard KJ. A US perspective of symptomatic Latrodectus spp. envenomation and treatment: a National Poison Data System review. Ann Pharmacother. 2011;45(12):1491–8. Epub 2011 Nov 24. https://doi.org/10.1345/aph.1Q424.

Mostafazadeh B, Gorbani A, Mogaddaspour M, Khoddami Vishteh HR. The effect of plasmapheresis on treating disseminated intravascular coagulation (DIC) caused by a Hemiscorpius lepturus (Gadim) sting. Clin Toxicol (Phila). 2017;55(8):902–7. Epub 2017 May 11. https://doi.org/10.1080/15563650.2017.1324164.

Murphy CM, Hong JJ, Beuhler MC. Anaphylaxis with Latrodectus antivenin resulting in cardiac arrest. J Med Toxicol. 2011;7(4):317–21. https://doi.org/10.1007/s13181-011-0183-1.

Naik SB. Intravenous snake bite: a catastrophic snake envenomation. Ann Afr Med. 2023;22(3):239–45. https://doi.org/10.4103/aam.aam_9_23.

Nentwig W, et al. Distribution and medical aspects of Loxosceles rufescens, one of the most invasive spiders of the world (Araneae: Sicariidae). Toxicon. 2017;132:19–28. https://doi.org/10.1016/j.toxicon.2017.04.007.

Norris RL, Dart RC. Apparent coral snake envenomation in a patient without visible fang marks. Am J Emerg Med. 1989;7(4):402–5. https://doi.org/10.1016/0735-6757(89)90047-8.

Oliveira AL, et al. The chemistry of snake venom and its medicinal potential. Nat Rev Chem. 2022;6(7):451–69. https://doi.org/10.1038/s41570-022-00393-7.

Parker-Cote J, Meggs WJ. First aid and pre-hospital management of venomous snakebites. Trop Med Infect Dis. 2018;3(2):45. https://doi.org/10.3390/tropicalmed3020045.

Paul G, Paul BS, Puri S. Snake bite and stroke: our experience of two cases. Indian J Crit Care Med. 2014;18(4):257–8. https://doi.org/10.4103/0972-5229.130585.

Pereañez JA, et al. Tako-tsubo cardiomyopathy in clinical toxinology: a systematic review. Toxicon. 2022;219:106929. https://doi.org/10.1016/j.toxicon.2022.09.015.

Premawardhena AP, et al. Low dose subcutaneous adrenaline to prevent acute adverse reactions to antivenom serum in people bitten by snakes: randomised, placebo-controlled trial. BMJ. 1999;318(7190):1041–3.

Pucca MB, et al. History of envenoming therapy and current perspectives. Front Immunol. 2019;10(1598):10. https://doi.org/10.3389/fimmu.2019.01598.

Pucca MB, et al. Current knowledge on Snake dry bites. Toxins. 2020;12(11):668. https://doi.org/10.3390/toxins12110668.

Quan D, Ruha AM. Priapism associated with Latrodectus mactans envenomation. Am J Emerg Med. 2009;27(6):759.e1–2. https://doi.org/10.1016/j.ajem.2008.10.033.

Quarch V, Brander L, Cioccari L. An Unexpected Case of Black Mamba (*Dendroaspis polylepis*) Bite in Switzerland. Case Rep Crit Care. 2017;2017:5021924. Epub 2017 Jul 31. PMID: 28831315; PMCID: PMC5555024. https://doi.org/10.1155/2017/5021924.

Quintero-Hernández V, Jiménez-Vargas JM, Gurrola GB, Valdivia HH, Possani LD. Scorpion venom components that affect ion-channels function. Toxicon. 2013;76:328–42. Epub 2013 Jul 26. PMID: 23891887; PMCID: PMC4089097. https://doi.org/10.1016/j.toxicon.2013.07.012.

Ralph R, Faiz MA, Sharma SK, Ribeiro I, Chappuis F. Managing snakebite. BMJ. 2022;376:e057926. https://doi.org/10.1136/bmj-2020-057926.

Ratanabanangkoon K. Polyvalent snake antivenoms: production strategy and their therapeutic benefits. Toxins. 2023;15(9):517. https://doi.org/10.3390/toxins15090517.

Rathnayaka RMMKN, Ranathunga PEAN, Kularatne SAM. Acute myocardial infarction after Russell's viper (*Daboia russelii*) bite. Am J Cardiol. 2022;175:175–8. https://doi.org/10.1016/j.amjcard.2022.04.013.

Rega PP, Bork CE, Burkholder-Allen K, Bisesi MS, Gold JP. Single-breath-count test: an important adjunct in the triaging of patients in a mass-casualty incident due to botulism. Prehosp Disaster Med. 2010;25(3):219–22. https://doi.org/10.1017/S1049023X00008062.

Rogers KM, et al. Systemic loxoscelism in the age of community-acquired methicillin-resistant Staphylococcus aureus. Ann Emerg Med. 2011;57(2):138–40. https://doi.org/10.1016/j.annemergmed.2010.06.006.

Rosen JL, Dumitru JK, Langley EW, Meade Olivier CA. Emergency department death from systemic loxoscelism. Ann Emerg Med. 2012;60(4):439–41.

Rowe AH, Xiao Y, Scales J, Linse KD, Rowe MP, et al. Isolation and characterization of CvIV4: a pain inducing α-scorpion toxin. PLoS One. 2011;6(8):e23520. https://doi.org/10.1371/journal.pone.0023520.

Russell FE, et al. Preparation of a new antivenin by affinity chromatography. Am J Trop Med Hyg. 1985;34(1):141–50. https://doi.org/10.4269/ajtmh.1985.34.141.

Ryan NM, et al. Treatments for Latrodectism—a systematic review on their clinical effectiveness. Toxins. 2017;9(4):148. https://doi.org/10.3390/toxins9040148.

Schioldann E, Mahmood MA, Kyaw MM, Halliday D, Thwin KT, Chit NN, et al. Why snakebite patients in Myanmar seek traditional healers despite availability of biomedical care at hospitals? Community perspectives on reasons. PLoS Negl Trop Dis. 2018;12:e0006299. https://doi.org/10.1371/journal.pntd.0006299.

Seifert SA, et al. Snake envenomation. N Engl J Med. 2022;386(1):68–78. https://doi.org/10.1056/NEJMra2105228.

Severino M, Bonadonna P, Passalacqua G. Large local reactions from stinging insects: from epidemiology to management. Curr Opin Allergy Clin Immunol. 2009;9(4):334–7. https://doi.org/10.1097/ACI.0b013e32832d0668.

Sherman RP, Groll JM, Gonzalez DI, Aerts MA. Black widow spider (Latrodectus mactans) envenomation in a term pregnancy. Curr Surg. 2000;57(4):346–8. https://doi.org/10.1016/s0149-7944(00)00276-2.

Silva A, et al. Neurotoxicity in Russell's viper (*Daboia russelii*) envenoming in Sri Lanka: a clinical and neurophysiological study. Clin Toxicol (Phila). 2016;54(5):411–9. https://doi.org/10.3109/15563650.2016.1143556.

Silva A, et al. Antivenom for neuromuscular paralysis resulting from snake envenoming. Toxins. 2017;9(4):143. https://doi.org/10.3390/toxins9040143.

Smith C, Mackessy S. The effects of hybridization on divergent venom phenotypes: characterization of venom from Crotalus scutulatus scutulatus × Crotalus oreganus helleri hybrids. Toxicon. 2016;120:110–23. https://doi.org/10.1016/j.toxicon.2016.08.001.

Sofer S, Shalev H, Weizman Z, Shahak E, Gueron M. Acute pancreatitis in children following envenomation by the yellow scorpion Leiurus quinquestriatus. Toxicon. 1991;29(1):125–8. https://doi.org/10.1016/0041-0101(91)90045-s.

Steinhorst J, Aglanu LM, Ravensbergen SJ, Dari CD, Abass KM, Mireku SO, Adu Poku JK, Enuameh YAK, Blessmann J, Harrison RA, Amuasi JH, Stienstra Y. 'The medicine is not for sale': practices of traditional healers in snakebite envenoming in Ghana. PLoS Negl Trop Dis. 2021;15(4):e0009298. PMID: 33861735; PMCID: PMC8081335. https://doi.org/10.1371/journal.pntd.0009298.

Stoecker WV, Vetter RS, Dyer JA. NOT RECLUSE-A mnemonic device to avoid false diagnoses of Brown recluse spider bites. JAMA Dermatol. 2017;153(5):377–8.

Sutherland SK, Coulter AR, Harris RD. Rationalisation of first-aid measures for elapid snakebite. Lancet. 1979;313:183–6. https://doi.org/10.1016/S0140-6736(79)90580-4.

Tednes M, Slesinger TL. Evaluation and treatment of snake envenomations. In: StatPearls [Internet]. Treasure Island, FL: StatPearls; 2023. https://www.ncbi.nlm.nih.gov/books/NBK553151/. Accessed 19 Oct 2022.

Toschlog EA, et al. Surgical considerations in the management of pit viper snake envenomation. J Am Coll Surg. 2013;217(4):726–35. https://doi.org/10.1016/j.jamcollsurg.2013.05.004.

Vetter RS, Visscher PK, Camazine S. Mass envenomations by honey bees and wasps. West J Med. 1999;170(4):223–7. PMID: 10344177; PMCID: PMC1305553.

Vital Brazil O, Vieira RJ. Neostigmine in the treatment of snake accidents caused by Micrurus frontalis: report of two cases (1). Rev Inst Med Trop SP. 1996;38(1):61–7. https://doi.org/10.1590/s0036-46651996000100012.

Wagener M, et al. Wound infection secondary to snakebite. S Afr Med J. 2017;107(4):315–9. https://doi.org/10.7196/SAMJ.2017.v107i4.12084.

Ward MJ, Ellsworth SA, Nystrom GS. A global accounting of medically significant scorpions: epidemiology, major toxins, and comparative resources in harmless counterparts. Toxicon. 2018;151:137–55. Epub 2018 Jul 17. https://doi.org/10.1016/j.toxicon.2018.07.007.

Ward-Smith H, Arbuckle K, Naude A, Wüster W. Fangs for the memories? A survey of pain in snakebite patients does not support a strong role for defense in the evolution of snake venom composition. Toxins. 2020;12:201. https://doi.org/10.3390/toxins12030201.

Warrell DA, Williams DJ. Clinical aspects of snakebite envenoming and its treatment in low-resource settings. Lancet. 2023;401(10385):1382–98. Epub 2023 Mar 14. https://doi.org/10.1016/S0140-6736(23)00002-8.

Watt CH Jr. Treatment of poisonous snakebite with emphasis on digit dermotomy. South Med J. 1985;78(6):694–9. https://doi.org/10.1097/00007611-198506000-00020.

Watt G, Padre L, Tuazon ML, Theakston RD, Laughlin LW. Tourniquet application after cobra bite: delay in the onset of neurotoxicity and the dangers of sudden release. Am J Trop Med Hyg. 1988;38:618–22. https://doi.org/10.4269/ajtmh.1988.38.618.

Weinstein SA, Warrell DA, Keyler DE. "Venomous" bites from "Non-Venomous" snakes. Amsterdam: Elsevier; 2022.

White J. Elapid snakes. In: Dart RC, editor. Medical toxicology. 3rd ed. Philadelphia, PA: Lippincott Williams & Wilkins; 2003. p. 1566–78.

White J. A comprehensive approach to managing a neglected, neglected tropical disease; the Myanmar snakebite project (MSP). Toxicon X. 2018;1:100001. https://doi.org/10.1016/j.toxcx.2018.100001.

Willhite LA, et al. Death after bite from severed snake head. Clin Toxicol. 2018;56(9):864–5. https://doi.org/10.1080/15563650.2018.1439951.

World Health Organization. Guidelines for the prevention and clinical management of snakebite in Africa. Brazzaville: WHO; 2010a. https://www.who.int/snakebites/resources/9789290231684/en/.

World Health Organization. Guidelines for the production, control and regulation of snake antivenom immunoglobulins. Geneva: World Health Organization; 2010b. http://www.who.int/bloodproducts/snake_antivenoms/en.

World Health Organization. Guidelines for the management of snakebites. 2nd ed. Geneva: World Health Organization; 2016. https://apps.who.int/iris/handle/10665/249547.

World Health Organization. Snakebite envenoming: a strategy for prevention and control. Geneva: World Health Organization; 2019. https://doi.org/10.1016/S0140-6736(18)32745-4.

Zeng L, et al. Effectiveness of clotting factor replacement therapy after antivenom treatment on coagulopathic envenomation following green pit viper bites: a retrospective observational study. BMC Emerg Med. 2022;22(1):9. https://doi.org/10.1186/s12873-022-00569.

Poisonous Plants and Mushrooms 19

Ricky L. Langley

Mushrooms

There are more than 10,000 species of mushrooms worldwide of which 50–100 are known to be toxic and only 200–300 are known to be safely edible (Pajouhi 2018). Several of the more toxic mushrooms have ominous common/local names such as Death cap, Destroying angel, Deadly skullcap, Fool's funnel, Deadly webcap, Fly agaric, Deadly dapperling, Panther cap, Devil's bolete, and Jack O'lantern.

A recent study of US mushroom exposures as reported to national poison control centers from 1999 to 2016 found that over 18 years, 133,700 cases (7428/year) of mushroom exposure, mostly by ingestion, have been reported (Brandenburg and Ward 2018). Cases were most frequently unintentional (83%, $P < 0.001$); caused no or only minor harm (86%, $P < 0.001$); and most occurred in children <6 years old (62%, $P < 0.001$). Approximately 704 (39/year) exposures resulted in major harm. Fifty-two (2.9/year) fatalities were reported, mostly from cyclopeptide (68–89%)-producing mushrooms ingested by older adults unintentionally. The vast majority of reported ingestions resulted in no or minor harm, although some groups of mushroom toxins or irritants, such as cyclopeptides, ibotenic acid, and monomethylhydrazine, have been deadly. Misidentification of edible mushroom species appears to be the most common cause and may be preventable through proper training.

The mechanism of mushroom toxicity varies by the genus and species of the mushroom, and the amount of toxin varies considerably even among members of the same species depending on local geography and weather conditions. In 75 to 95% of cases, the exact species of mushroom ingested is not identified (Trestrail 1991) by health care workers. Thus, one must rely upon the presenting signs and symptoms to aid in the clinical diagnosis and to guide treatment recommendations.

Mushroom Toxins

There are numerous mushroom toxins and many syndromes have been associated with certain toxins. Goldfrank (2015) has a clinical classification based on 14 different toxic components.

Toxins found in various mushrooms and which are associated with different toxidromes include amatoxins, momomethylhydrazine, muscarine, coprine, ibotenic acid and mucimol, allenic norleucine, orellanine, psilocybin and psilocin, acromelic acids, Lycoperdon spores, polyporic acid, an immune-mediated response to involutin, and unidentified toxins (Goldfrank 2015; Pajouhi 2018).

R. L. Langley (✉)
Department of Biological Sciences,
North Carolina State University, Raleigh, NC, USA
e-mail: rllangley@ncsu.edu

W. J. Meggs, R. L. Langley (eds.), *Farm Toxicology*, https://doi.org/10.1007/978-3-031-80441-0_19

The cyclopeptide-containing mushrooms includes many of the most dangerous mushroom toxins including amatoxins. Other cyclopeptide toxins include phallotoxins and virotoxins. Amatoxins, gyromitrins, and orellanine are toxins usually implicated in fatal mushroom poisonings worldwide (Horowitz 2023a). Amatoxins are the most toxic and responsible for liver and kidney damage. Gyromitrins are also hepatotoxic. Several types of mushrooms produce amatoxins, including various species of *Amanita*, *Galerina*, and some *Lepiota* and *Conocybe* (Pajouhi 2018). The amatoxins are very potent toxins with a minimum lethal dose of about 0.1 mg/kg. One *Amanita phalloides* cap may contain a lethal dose of 10–15 mg. In contrast, 15–20 caps of *Galerina*, which contains less toxin, would be a fatal dose in adults (Olson 2018). Most deaths worldwide are associated with ingestion of cyclopeptide-containing mushrooms (Goldfrank 2015).

Orellanine and allenic norleucine are nephrotoxic. Muscarine, psilocybin, muscimol, and ibotenic acid are central nervous system poisons while gyromitrins are also epileptogenic. Coprine causes a disulfiram-like reaction when combined with alcohol.

Evaluation of Suspected Mushroom Poisoning

The diagnosis of mushroom poisoning is dependent upon a history of ingestion, even if symptoms are delayed for 12 or more hours after ingestion. It is important to get a description of the mushroom, where it was harvested, whether eaten raw or cooked, was more than one type of mushroom consumed, how much was eaten, were the mushrooms eaten at more than one meal, time of onset of symptoms after ingestion (symptoms that develop more than 6 h after ingestion indicate poisoning with potentially lethal mushroom toxins such as amatoxin, gyromitrin, or orellanine), are other people ill that may have eaten or not eaten mushrooms, and whether alcohol was ingested after eating the mushrooms (a disulfiram-like reaction can occur from coprine-containing mushrooms from 30 min up to 5 days after ingestion) (Pajouhi 2018). If photos or samples of the mushroom are brought in, obtaining assistance from a botanist, mycologist, horticulturist, or cooperative extension agents may be able to help identify local mushrooms.

Symptomatic patients and any asymptomatic person who might be at risk for life-threatening toxicity (e.g., amatoxin-, gyromitrin-, and orellanine-containing mushrooms) warrant emergent medical evaluation.

Signs and symptoms may point to a specific type of mushroom poisoning. The following clinical findings are from Tran and Juergens (2023):

Acute gastroenteritis: Symptoms of nausea, vomiting, abdominal cramping, and possibly diarrhea associated with ingestion account for the majority of reported mushroom poisonings. It manifests typically within 1–3 h and occurs from a variety of mushroom species.

Hallucinations: Symptoms of altered sensorium and euphoria occur 30 min to 2 h after ingestion and last typically 4–12 h depending on the amount ingested. Caused by psilocybin and psilocin-containing species, which include *Psilocybe*, *Conocybe*, *Gymnopilus*, and *Panaeolus*. These agents act as agonists or partial agonists at 5-hydroxytryptamine (5-HT) subtype receptors.

Cholinergic toxicity: Signs and symptoms include abdominal cramping, diaphoresis, salivation, lacrimation, bronchospasm, bronchorrhea, and bradycardia. Onset is usually within 30 min of ingestion. Cholinergic toxicity is caused by muscarine-containing species in various genera such as *Clitocybe* and *Inocybe*. Though *Amanita muscari* contains small amounts of muscarine, levels are typically not sufficient to cause a cholinergic presentation.

Disulfiram-like reaction: The toxin's metabolites result in aldehyde dehydrogenase inhibition leading to headache, nausea, vomiting, flushing, tachycardia, and rarely hypotension. Symptoms occur if alcohol is ingested hours to days after the consumption of coprine-containing mushrooms such as *Coprinus atramentarius*.

Hepatic toxicity: Amatoxin in species of *Galerina*, and *Lepiota* and especially *Amanita* disrupt RNA polymerase II, leading to protein deficiency at the cellular level. Toxicity characteristically occurs in three distinct phases. Gastrointestinal effects start typically 6–12 h post-ingestion, followed by a quiescent interval of 24–36 h after ingestion with symptomatic improvement. During this phase, however, there may be laboratory signs of hepatotoxicity. After 48 h, hepatic damage intensifies, leading to liver failure and its sequelae. Death may occur within a week in severe cases or may require liver transplantation.

Nephrotoxicity: The typical course includes acute gastroenteritis symptoms progressing to renal injury in 12–24 h. Renal symptoms can be delayed for 1–2 weeks after ingestion. Mushrooms of the *Cortinarius* genus produce orellanine, a nephrotoxic agent. Nephrotoxicity also results from allenic norleucine found most commonly in *Amanita smithiana*, but present in other *Amanita* species. Although some patients will require hemodialysis, most patients have a full recovery with appropriate supportive care.

Seizures: Toxicity is due to a metabolite, monomethylhydrazine, that leads to pyridoxine (Vitamin B6) and ultimately Gamma-aminobutyric acid (GABA) depletion. These seizures may be intractable to anticonvulsant therapy and may require supplemental treatment including pyridoxine. The toxin is gyromitrin present in species of *Gyromitra*, *Paxina*, and *Cyathipodia micropus*, though the latter two are far less common.

Isoxazole syndrome is caused by ingesting mushrooms containing isoxazole derivatives. Symptoms are nausea, vomiting, lethargy or hyperactivity, muscle jerking, hallucinations, delirium, and rarely seizures. Onset is 30 min to 2 h after ingestion and can last up to 12 h. This syndrome can occur after ingesting *Amanita muscaria*, *Amanita pantherina*, and *Amanita gemata*. The syndrome is due to ibotenic acid and muscimol toxins.

Other manifestations: These include but are not limited to headaches, vertigo, somnolence, palpitations, dysrhythmias, rhabdomyolysis (*Tricholoma equestre*), methemoglobinemia, hemolysis (*Paxillus involutus*), erythromelalgia (acromelic acid), dermatitis, and cramping. An allergic bronchoalveolitis may occur after inhalation of spores from puffball mushrooms (*Lycoperdon* sp.).

Time to onset of symptoms may help in the diagnosis of the causative mushroom (Pajouhi 2018). If symptom onset occurs within 6 h, the likely categories of mushrooms include those causing allergic pneumonitis, cholinergic syndrome, GI irritants, hallucinogenic, immunohemolytic (hemolysis), and isoxazole syndrome.

If symptoms occur from 6 to 24 h after ingestion, consider mushrooms containing amatoxins, monomethylhydrazine, and acromelic acids. Symptom onset after 24 h post-ingestion suggests poisoning by orellanines that cause kidney damage and mushrooms that cause rhabdomyolysis or delayed Central Nervous System (CNS) toxicity.

Findings on physical examination may offer some clues as to the type of mushroom involved:

Fever may be observed with psilocybin and muscimol poisonings.

Tachycardia is nonspecific, may be seen with any of the mushrooms, or may be a manifestation of hypoxia or hypovolemia from any cause.

Cyanosis due to methemoglobinemia may occur with gyromitrin poisoning.

Facial flushing may be a manifestation of anticholinergic poisoning and may also be noted in a patient experiencing a coprine-related disulfiram-like reaction.

Profuse sweating and facial flushing are prominent features of muscarinic poisoning. Bradycardia may be a manifestation of muscarine poisoning; reflex tachycardia has also been observed in this setting.

Mydriasis is commonly observed with the ingestion of mushrooms that contain psilocybin and muscimol (because they also contain anticholinergic substances).

Miosis is observed with toxicity caused by muscarine-containing mushrooms.

Jaundice may be observed in patients with liver failure due to gyromitrin and amatoxin poisoning.

Jaundice may also be a manifestation of hemolysis, rarely seen with *Paxillus* ingestion.

Laboratory Test

Lab testing in patients with mushroom exposures is guided by the clinical presentation: Asymptomatic individuals with ingestions that are unlikely to be toxic (the mushroom has been identified) may be observed without any testing.

Symptomatic patients and asymptomatic patients with ingestion of potentially lethal mushrooms should undergo baseline assessment. Abdominal pain, vomiting, and diarrhea, are nonspecific and occur commonly in patients with mushroom poisoning and may cause electrolyte abnormalities.

Useful lab studies include complete blood count (CBC), electrolytes, glucose, bilirubin, liver and renal panels, PT/INR/PTT, and creatine kinase. While detection of the toxin may be available at certain clinical labs, this is often not the case in rural settings.

If physical examination or laboratory testing suggests liver failure, altered mental status, cyanosis, or hypoxia, additional tests should be considered:

- Liver failure—Blood gas determination, serum lactate, blood ammonia, and serum lactate dehydrogenase (LDH).
- Altered mental status—Blood gas determination, and, if hepatic encephalopathy is suspected or the patient shows signs of increased intracranial pressure, neuroimaging (e.g., computed tomography/MRI of the brain) to assess for cerebral edema.
- Cyanosis—If not responsive to oxygen therapy or ingestion of mushrooms containing gyromitrin toxin, then check a methemoglobin level.
- Hypoxia or respiratory distress—Blood gas determination, pulse oximetry, and chest radiography.

Hepatic studies are typically normal in most acute mushroom exposures. However, ingestion of any of the following mushrooms containing amatoxin or gyromitrin toxins (*Gyromitra esculenta*) can cause elevation of liver enzymes and patients should have reassessment approximately 24 to 36 h after ingestion.

Amatoxins can be found among various genera of mushrooms including Amanita, Lepiota, and Galerina.

The Amanita group includes the following species:

- *Amanita phalloides*
- *Amanita virosa*
- *Amanita verna*
- *Amanita ocreata*
- *Amanita bisporigera*
- *Amanita suballiacea*
- *Amanita magniverrucata*
- *Amanita muscaria*

The Lepiota group includes the following species:

- *Lepiota helveola*
- *Lepiota chlorophyllum*
- *Lepiota josserandi*
- *Lepiota fulvella*
- *Lepiota subincarnata*
- *Lepiota brunneoincarnata*
- *Lepiota brunneolilacea*

The Galerina group includes the following species:

- *Galerina autumnalis*
- *Galerina sulcipes*
- *Galerina marginata*

Thrombocytopenia, coagulopathy, hyperbilirubinemia, or hyperammonemia with encephalopathy indicates progressive toxicity in such patients and may be associated with gastrointestinal bleeding. Acidosis, hypoglycemia, and renal failure signifying hepatorenal syndrome are markers for poor prognosis. The mortality rate from amatoxin ingestion is 6–10% with intensive supportive care (Olson 2018; Olano et al. 2021; Horowitz 2023b).

In a retrospective study of 144 amatoxin-poisoned patients seen between 1996 and 2009, Trabulus and Altiparmak (2011) reported a mortality of 9.7% (14 patients). Factors associated with a greater likelihood of death included the following: low mean arterial pressure, encephalopathy, mucosal hemorrhage, oliguria-anuria, hypoglycemia, and thrombocytopenia during the hospitalization. Low sodium values and high urea, AST, ALT, total bilirubin, LDH, prothrombin time, international normalized ratio, and activated partial thromboplastin time values were associated with an increased likelihood of mortality.

Acutely, renal insufficiency may occur as a nonspecific result of hypovolemic shock due to vomiting and diarrhea or may indicate ingestion of allenic norleucine toxin (*Amanita smithiana* and *Amanita proxima*). Renal insufficiency occurring days to weeks after mushroom ingestion is characteristic of orellanine toxicity (*Cortinarius* mushroom species). Although orellanine poisoning is rare in the United States, mushrooms containing orellanine account for the most mushroom fatalities in some areas of Europe. A shorter time course between ingestion and toxicity portends a worse prognosis. Mild renal insufficiency may resolve a few months after the ingestion. Some patients may develop chronic renal failure (Goldfrank 2015). In a study of long-term effects of orellanine poisoning, the outcomes of 28 patients who ingested mushrooms of the *Cortinarius* species in the period from 1979 to 2012 were reviewed (Hedman et al. 2017). The researchers reported 22 patients (78%) developed acute kidney injury requiring dialysis of which 15 received a kidney transplantation.

Abnormal findings on the CBC/urinalysis may indicate hemolysis as noted by anemia, red blood cell fragments on blood smear, and hemoglobinuria. This may indicate an immune-mediated hemolytic anemia caused by *Paxillus involutus*, and possibly *Clitocybe claviceps* and *Boletus luridis*.

Gyromitrin-containing mushrooms such as *Gyromitra esculenta* may cause cyanosis due to methemoglobinemia. Most patients recover from gyromitrin poisoning. In the United States, death from this event is rare, but in some areas of Europe, mushrooms containing gyromitrin accounts for the most mushroom fatalities (Horowitz 2023b).

Rhabdomyolysis as noted by an elevated creatine kinase level occurring 1–3 days after mushroom ingestion suggests ingestion of *Tricholoma equestre* or Russula species (e.g., *Russula emetica*). Other mushrooms implicated in less severe forms of rhabdomyolysis are *Russula subnigricans*, *Boletus edulis*, *Leccinium versipelle*, and *Albatrellus ovinus* (Horowitz 2023b).

Respiratory symptoms in association with bilateral reticulonodular infiltrates (allergic bronchoalveolitis) seen on chest radiographs can occur from inhalational of spores of puffballs from various species of *Lycoperdon*.

The prognosis for muscarine poisonings is excellent and fatalities are very rare. Many patients who ingest muscarine-containing mushrooms have minor or no symptoms; when symptoms do occur, they tend to be temporary, and self-limited, lasting 6–24 h. Most patients recover without drug therapy (Horowitz 2023b).

Treatment

It is recommended that in all cases of suspected mushroom poisoning, the rural practitioner should consult with a medical toxicologist or call the Poison Center (1-800-222-1222) for guidance. Treatment of the vast array of possible symptoms primarily consists of supportive care. Early volume resuscitation is important if liver and kidney toxidromes are suspected.

Depending on the timing of ingestion, activated charcoal may provide some benefit by binding to some mycotoxins undergoing enterohepatic circulation (Horowitz 2023b; Olson 2018; Pajouhi 2018). For poisoning from amatoxin-containing mushrooms, additional treatments may be available or used in other countries that are not used in the United States. There may be a role of whole bowel irrigation for amatoxins if given within the first hour after ingestion (Horowitz 2023b). Acute gastrointestinal effects may benefit from rehydration and antiemetics in addition to correction of any electrolyte derangements.

Administration of specific drugs and antidotes (Horowitz 2023b) such as anticonvulsants, antiemetics, activated charcoal, polyethylene glycol, N-acetylcysteine, pyridoxine, methylene blue, penicillin G, atropine, ipatropium and glycopyrrolate, fomepizole, benzodiazepines, cimetidine, and silibinin should be per toxicologist recommendations. There are ongoing studies in animals evaluating experimental therapeutics for amatoxin poisoning (Wang et al. 2023).

It is important to follow-up patients after mushroom poisoning to make sure they do not develop delayed effects such as kidney or liver damage. Severe hepatic damage may require a liver transplant. Dialysis, or even renal transplant, may be required if patients develop renal failure. If amatoxin-containing mushroom ingestion is suspected, other consultations to consider include a transplants surgeon, nephrologists, and possibly a psychiatrist if ingestion may have been a suicide attempt.

Poisonous Plants

Hundreds of various plant species are poisonous and thousands may cause skin irritation or allergic skin reactions. Plant poisoning is one of the top 20 causes of poisoning in the United States with approximately 54,000 calls to US poison centers in 2021 (Gummin et al. 2022). Common plant poisonings reported by US poison centers included American pokeweed, cherry and cherry pits, Elephant's Ear, Poison Ivy, various species of *Ilex*, and various species of lilies. Many exposures were to unknown plants or berries (Gummin et al. 2022).

Poisonous plant ingestions occur frequently in children, but fortunately, serious toxicity is rare as indicated by the following studies:

- Of approximately 500,000 toxic plant ingestions in children ≤5 years of age reported to the United States poison control centers over 10 years, more than 90% of children had minimal or no effects, and only one child died as a result of ingestion (Krenzelok and Mrvos 2011).
- Of almost 60,000 potentially toxic plant ingestions in children under 15 years of age reported to German poison information centers, 90% had no effects at the time of the call, 9% had minimal effects, and less than 1% had moderate or major effects (Pietsch et al. 2008).

On farms, plant poisonings are responsible for millions of dollars of loss from livestock poisonings each year. Various factors affect plant toxicity on farms, including adverse climatic conditions, agricultural practices, and animal management practices (Osweiler 1996). Under certain conditions, plants may become poisonous as a result of the accumulation of toxic inorganic minerals such as copper, lead, cadmium, fluorine, manganese, nitrates, or selenium that may be naturally present in the soil or contained in biosolids or fertilizers that have been applied to the fields.

Many ornamental house plants are poisonous and grow as native plants in other countries, especially in tropical and subtropical areas, and cause poisonings worldwide. Some have been cultivated in the United States and escaped into surrounding areas such as the balsam pear. However, this chapter is focused on plants in the United States and Canada that are collected in the wild (foraging) for human consumption. Unfortunately, many people believe that plants and berries are edible because birds or wildlife eat them without adverse effects. Many of the most toxic plants in the United States foragers collect are mistaken for wild carrots, wild onions/garlic, or parsnip.

Poisonous plants may be classified according to the chemical nature of their toxic components, their phylogenetic relationship, or their botanical characteristics. The following classification, which is based on their toxic effects, is often utilized: (1) plants that are poisonous to eat, (2) plants that are poisonous upon contact, (3) plants that produce photosensitization, and (4) plants that produce airborne allergens (Klaassen et al. 2024).

Plant Toxins

Plant poisons vary widely in their chemical properties and structure and many toxins with similar chemical properties occur across a variety of genera and species. Toxicity of the plant varies depending on the part of the plant (leaves, stem, root, seeds, or flowers), geography, season of the year, growing environment, the age of the plant (whether freshly harvested or pre-dried), the method of preparation (for homeopathic remedies—syrups, tinctures, and lotions), and the exposure route (dermal, oral, or via inhalation).

Plant poisons, or phytotoxins, include a wide range of biologically active chemical compounds (Osweiler 1996). Classification of plant toxins varies by different authors (Goralka and Albertson 2018; Nelson and Goldfrank 2015). One common classification scheme categorizes plant toxins into primary groups (Nelson and Goldfrank 2015):

1. Alkaloids—Alkaloid characteristics include the presence of nitrogen and their ability to combine with acids to form salts. They are usually bitter in taste. It has been estimated that about 10% of the plant species contain some type of alkaloid. Typically they cause a strong physiological reaction when administered to an animal.
2. Glycosides—which are compounds that yield one or more sugars (glycones) and one or more other compounds—aglycones (nonsugars)—when hydrolyzed, are extremely toxic to animals. Toxicity resides in the aglycone component or a part of it.
3. Terpenes and resins—Assemblages of 5-carbon units with many types of attached functional groups. Most essential oils are mixtures of monoterpenes. Resins differ widely in chemical properties but have certain similar physical properties. Some resins are physiologically very active, causing irritation to nervous and muscle tissue.
4. Proteins, peptides, and lectins—Proteins are composed of amino acid units with various side chains. Peptides consist of linkages of amino acids. Lectins are glycoproteins. Toxalbumins are highly toxic lectins. Ricin, a toxalbumin from the castor bean (*Ricinus communis*), is one of the most toxic substances known.
5. Phenols and phenylpropanoids—Phenols contain phenyl rings with one or more hydroxyl attached groups. Phenyl ring attached to a propane side chain is a phenylpropanoid molecule. Among these plant toxins are coumarins, capsaicin, flavonoids, lignans, and tannins.
6. Carboxylic acids—Aristolochic acids, oxalic acid, and oxalate raphides. Consumption of aristolochic acids may cause nephropathy while calcium oxalates in certain plants may cause painful irritation to the skin or mucus membranes upon contact.
7. Alcohols—Cicutoxin, a diacetylene diol, is found in various species of hemlock plants and ingestion of these plants can be lethal. Absorption of cicutoxin can also occur through the skin.
8. Unidentified toxins—Many plants contain toxins that have not been well characterized.

Toxidromes

Another classification system developed by Diaz (2016) utilizes a toxidromic classification of plant poisonings to assist in rapid identification of poisonous plant–induced toxidromes. The four specific toxidromes of plant poisonings identified are stratified as cardiotoxic, neurotoxic, cytotoxic, and gastrointestinal/hepatotoxic poisonings, all of which have resulted in deaths after both intentional and unintentional ingestions.

The cardiotoxic toxidrome includes an assortment of digitalis toxicity–like symptoms and signs, including nausea, vomiting, bradycardia, hyperkalemia, atrioventricular conduction blocks, and ventricular arrhythmias.

The neurotoxic toxidrome includes a variety of neurological symptoms and signs ranging from predominantly anticholinergic manifestations (mydriasis, facial flushing, dry skin, tachycardia, mental status changes, combative behavior, and hallucinations) to nicotinic and neuromuscular manifestations (ataxia, tachycardia, hypertension, seizures, weakness, paralysis, and respiratory failure).

The cytotoxic toxidrome includes a constellation of abdominal pain, nausea, vomiting, watery-to-bloody diarrhea, weakness, dehydration, hypotension, metabolic acidosis, elevated serum creatinine, and multiorgan failure.

The gastrointestinal/hepatotoxic toxidrome includes a cluster of manifestations ranging from upper gastrointestinal signs of drooling and dysphagia to abdominal pain with increasing hepatic enzyme levels and later jaundice.

Table 19.1 is a partial list of plants (by commonly known names) that may be collected and often misidentified while foraging and which can cause poisoning if ingested. (Nelson and Goldfrank 2015; Diaz 2016; Nelson and Balick 2020). It should be noted that many plants contain a variety of poisons and may cause signs/symptoms in more than one organ system.

Approach to the Patient with Plant Ingestion

If the plant is known, then its toxicity can be looked up in modern medical databases or by calling poison control (1-800-222-1222). If the plant is unknown, seeking assistance from local botanists, extension agents, horticulturists, or the local poison center in identification may be useful. Photographs should be taken which can help in the identification. Fortunately, most exposures do not cause serious effects.

Evaluation of exposed persons by health care practitioners involves obtaining an accurate history to determine extent of exposure and subsequent risk of illness. The following items may provide important information:

- Name of plant (note that common names vary considerably by region).

Table 19.1 Plants associated with different toxidromes

GI/Hepatotoxic	Cardiotoxic	Neurotoxic	Cytotoxic
Baneberry	Angel's trumpet	Ackee tree	Autumn crocus
Black locust	Azalea	Balsam apple Balsam pear	Elderberry (except ripe, cooked berries are edible)
Black nightshade	Deadly nightshade	Blue cohosh	Hydrangea
Buttercup	Death camas	Bloodroot	May apple
English ivy	False hellebore	Jequirty pea	Pits of various fruits such as apple, cherry, crab apple, plum, and peach
Horse chestnut	Fetterbush	Blue lobelia	Periwinkle
Jack-in-the-pulpit	Foxglove	Morning glory	Ragwort
Lilies (most)	Jimson weed	Myrtle-leaved sumac	Seaside heliotrope
Pokeweed (especially berries)	Lily of the Valley	Peyote	
Skunk cabbage	Monkshood	Pinkroot	
Virginia creeper	Mountain laurel	Poison hemlock	
Wisteria	Oleander	Southern mistletoe	
	Rhododendron	Tobacco	
	Yew	Water hemlock	
		Wild indigo	

- Actual plant (if available, allows for detailed description of features).
- Part of the plant ingested, in general, roots and stems, have higher concentrations of toxins than flowers or berries.
- Amount ingested or exposed.
- Duration of time since exposure occurred.
- Initial symptoms and time between exposure and symptom onset.
- Past medical history, current medication, and allergies (these may alter host response and risk).
- Prominent symptoms—See toxidromes above.

Physical Examination

Many patients will be asymptomatic with a normal physical examination after ingestion of a potentially toxic plant.

Among symptomatic patients, potential physical findings include:

- Swelling of the oral mucosa, excessive oral secretions.
- Bradycardia or tachycardia.
- Hypotension.
- Skin may appear flushed, warm, or cherry-red.
- Hyperthermia or diaphoresis.
- Dilated pupils or constricted pupils.
- Seizures, muscle weakness, or fasciculations.
- Decreased bowel sounds.

Laboratory Tests

Although specific plant toxins can be identified, these analytic methods are neither usually available in most hospital laboratories nor timely enough to aid in acute management. Thus, the diagnosis usually relies upon clinical findings and identification of the plant.

Asymptomatic individuals with ingestions that are unlikely to be toxic may be observed without any testing. Ancillary studies in symptomatic patients with potentially toxic plant ingestions are guided by the clinical presentation and, when possible, plant identification:

- Patients presenting with an altered mental status (delirium lethargy and coma) or seizures:
  - Rapid blood glucose.
  - Arterial or venous blood gas.
  - Complete blood count (CBC, especially if hematemesis or hematochezia).
  - Serum electrolytes, blood urea nitrogen (BUN), and serum creatinine.
  - Creatine kinase, urine for myoglobin (especially patients with seizures, anticholinergic poisoning, or nicotinic findings).
- Patients who have ingested plants that may cause cardiac arrhythmias:
  - Electrolytes—Hyperkalemia suggests ingestion of plants that contain cardiac glycosides.
  - Serum digoxin level—Some plant cardiac glycosides can cross-react with digoxin. A detectable level is strongly suggestive of acute exposure, however, the absence of a detectable level cannot exclude exposure. However, the level obtained is not a useful prognostic indicator and cannot be used to dose digoxin antibody (Fab) fragments.
  - 12-lead electrocardiogram and continuous cardiac monitoring.
- Patients with findings suggestive of cyanide poisoning:
  - Cyanide level.
  - Serum lactate, which is often markedly elevated.

Treatment

In general, management of poisonings by unknown plants should be supportive and based on the four presenting toxidromes (Diaz 2016). A regional Poison Center should be contacted to discuss likely plant species ingested based upon clinical findings, identification of any plant parts available for analysis, and advice on treatment of specific toxic effects.

Activated charcoal administration may be indicated if the poisoned patient is conscious, alert, and cooperative, and presents within 60 min of potentially dangerous or lethal plant ingestions. Whole bowel irrigation may be considered for patients who have ingested significant amounts of poisonous plant matter that will release toxins slowly over time in the gastrointestinal tract such as apple, cherry, or apricot pits containing cyanogenic glycosides or oleander seeds containing cardiotoxic glycosides (Diaz 2016). However, there are few effective antidotes for most plant toxins. Digoxin-specific Fab antibodies (Digibind, DigiFab) to inactivate ingested plant-derived cardiac glycosides and physostigmine to reverse plant toxin-induced central anticholinergic syndromes may be effective for some plant poisonings. Severe poisonings with cardiotoxic plants, toxalbumins, and colchicine may result in cardiovascular collapse and multiorgan failure, and require intensive care monitoring and treatment.

Irritant and Allergic Contact Dermatitis from Plants

Dermatitis caused by plant exposure is due to mechanical injury (thorns, briars, and spikes), chemical injury (the plant may contain calcium oxalate crystals and proteolytic enzymes causing bradykinin and histamine release), allergic contact dermatitis, contact urticaria, and phytophotodermatitis (Shih and Goldfrank 1998). Many plants can cause a nonallergic, inflammatory skin reaction. Known plant chemical irritants include calcium oxalate, protoanemonin, isothiocyanates, bromelain, diterpene esters, alkaloids, and other chemical irritants such as naphthoquinone and acids (Modi et al. 2009). Some examples of plant irritants include calcium oxalate (agave, daffodil, daisy, and hyacinth), thiocyanates (radish, wasabi, and horseradish), and diterpene esters (castor bean plant, croton, and poinsettia). An increasing number of cases of dermatitis, often severe, are being recognized from exposure to the giant hogweed plant. The toxic component appears to be furocoumarins in this plant.

The most commonly seen plant caused allergic contact dermatitis is Toxicodendron dermatitis due to urushiol oils in poison ivy, poison oak, and poison sumac plants. Many plant families other than *Toxicodendron* can cause allergic contact dermatitis in sensitized individuals. Examples include Asteraceae or Compositae (*Achillea millefolium*, *Chrysanthemum*, *Matricaria chamomilla*, and *Taraxacum officinale*), Alliaceae (*Allium sativum* [garlic], *Allium cepa* [onion]), and Myrtaceae (*Melaleuca alternifolia* [tea tree]).

Approximately 50 to 75% of the United States adult population is sensitized to poison ivy, oak, and sumac (Kim et al. 2019). Poison ivy and poison oak are often identified by three leaflets with flowering branches arising on a single stem (See Fig. 19.1). Poison sumac more often forms leaflets of five, seven, or more that angle upward toward the top of the stem.

Poison ivy, oak, and sumac dermatitis are classic type IV hypersensitivity (cell-mediated) allergic reactions.

Toxicodendron dermatitis usually will present as an acute, intensely itchy skin eruption with erythematous papules or plaques, vesicles, and bullae, often arranged in characteristic, linear or streak-like configurations where a portion of a plant has touched the skin. The so-called "black spot" poison ivy dermatitis occurs when urushiol is left on the skin and oxidizes, appearing as black spots that cannot be washed off (Kurlan and Lucky 2001). Involvement of the face and genitals may cause significant edema. Airborne exposure from burning these plants may cause facial dermatitis and respiratory injury from inhalation of the urushiol oil resin.

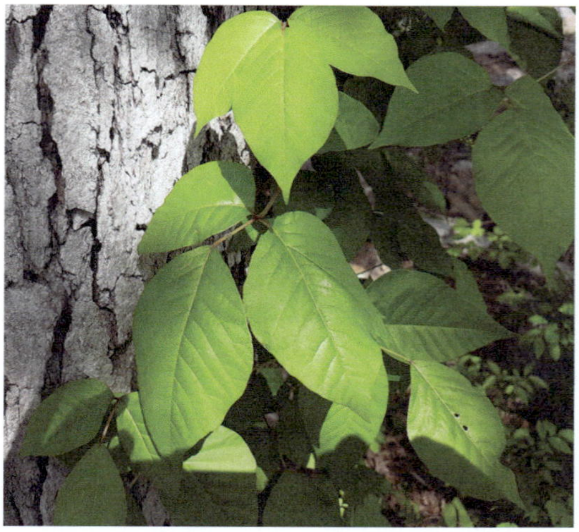

Fig. 19.1 Poison Ivy (*Toxicodendron radicans*)

Symptoms of Toxicodendron dermatitis in sensitized individuals generally develop within 4 to 96 h after exposure and peak between 1 and 14 days after exposure (Kim et al. 2019). Depending on the amount of urushiol present on the skin and the thickness of the stratum corneum layer of the epidermis at the areas of contact, lesions may present in different locations at different times after exposure. Left untreated, the dermatitis usually resolves in 7–21 days.

Complications are uncommon and include postinflammtory hyperpigmentation and secondary bacterial infection (Fisher 1996).

First Aid

After a known exposure, patients should remove any contaminated clothing and wash the whole body with mild soap or dish soap on a damp washcloth under very warm or hot running water as soon as possible. One study found that after approximately 10 min on the skin, 50% of the urushiol can be removed. This number falls to 10% after 30 min and 0% after 1 h (McGovern and Barkley 1998). If washing is not possible within 30 min, it may still be worthwhile to wash at the first opportunity to avoid any continued exposure from contaminated clothing. Some clinicians suggest washing the entire body three times while always wiping in one direction, not back and forth; this seems to reduce irritation and help remove the oils (Neill et al. 2019). If there is no rapid access to dishwashing liquid, plain water can be used to wipe the skin in the same fashion. This will at least remove some of the resin. There are some over-the-counter preparations that may help reduce symptoms if applied soon after exposure including Tecnu, Zanfel, Goop, and Dial ultra dishwashing soap (Gladman 2006).

Barrier creams are topical preparations that are applied prior to exposure to a contact allergen in an attempt to prevent the development of dermatitis The effectiveness of barrier creams to prevent contact dermatitis is controversial but may be effective (Gladman 2006).

Clothing, tools, or other items that may be contaminated with urushiol resin should also be washed with warm, soapy water prior to reuse.

Treatment of Dermatitis

Symptomatic treatment of dermatitis from plant exposure includes soothing measures, such as oatmeal baths and cool, wet compresses. Topical treatment with calamine lotion may also provide symptomatic relief. Topical astringents such as aluminum acetate (Burow's solution) or aluminum sulfate calcium acetate used under occlusion may be useful to dry weeping lesions. Topical agents with known allergenic potential, including topical anesthetics containing benzocaine, topical antihistamines, and topical antibiotics containing neomycin or bacitracin, should be avoided.

The approach to pharmacologic treatment is based on dermatitis severity (Butt et al. 2022). Because allergic contact dermatitis (ACD) is a type IV hypersensitivity reaction, both topical and/or oral corticosteroids have been used with previous success to inhibit the inflammatory and immunologic response and alleviate symptoms associated with ACD. For mild cases of ACD, midpotency topical corticosteroids (such as triamcinolone) can be used as primary treatment with escalation to high-potency topical corticosteroids (such as clobetasol) should the patient's symptoms persist or worsen. Topical corticosteroids can cause skin pigmentation so should be avoided on the face. Treatment of moderate cases should begin with higher-potency topical corticosteroids and escalate to a 14- to 20-day tapered course of oral prednisone. Severe cases of ACD should use a 14- to 20-day tapered course of oral prednisone as the primary treatment along with high-potency topical corticosteroids. The duration of 14 to 20 days also provides enough coverage to prevent possible rebound dermatitis, which can occur when clinical and physical symptoms of ACD return with insufficient duration of oral corticosteroids. In cases of severe ACD, optional treatments can include administering 40 to 80 mg of intramuscular (IM) triamcinolone.

First-generation, sedating H1 antihistamines given at bedtime may be beneficial for patients who experience exacerbations of pruritus at night. Sedating antihistamines may increase daytime sleepiness and should be used with caution.

Phytophotodermatitis

Topical exposure to plant-derived substances may also cause a phototoxic reaction termed phytophotodermatitis (Baugh 2021). Phytophotodermatitis is a phototoxic reaction entirely independent of the immune system and prior sensitization or an intact immune system is not required. The most common plants that cause phytophotodermatitis in agricultural workers include celery, wild parsnip, and parsley, as well as lemons, limes, and giant hogweed (Fig. 19.2). The sap of certain trees such as fig trees is additional inducer of phytophotodermatitis.

The majority of these plants contain furocoumarins, of which psoralens and angelicins are the most notable. The furocoumarins alone are inactive, but, following exposure to long-wave ultraviolet A (UV-A, 320–380 nm) radiation they may induce a photosensitivity reaction.

The clinical findings appear approximately 24 h after sun exposure and patients will typically present with erythema, edema, and bullae in linear or bizarre configurations on sun-exposed skin that reflect the manner in which they have come in contact with the plant. Lesions are not pruritic but may be painful (burning). The phototoxic result may be intensified by wet skin, sweating, and heat. Once the rash does occur, it may take weeks to resolve. Hyperpigmentation may develop after the acute eruption clears and may take months to years to disappear. It should be noted that often the preceding skin redness may be inapparent and only the hyperpigmentation is observed.

Cool wet compresses may be used for acute lesions. Topical steroids may be used if the eruption is severe and edematous. Low-to-high potency topical steroids may be applied to affected areas to reduce local inflammation induced by the photoactivated psoralens. They may help to relieve the burning sensation associated with phytophotodermatitis as well as to reduce the associated postinflammatory hyperpigmentation. Over-the-counter nonsteroidal anti-inflammatory drugs (NSAIDs) may help reduce pain and swelling. If a severe case evolves or greater than 30% of the body is affected, then it is recommended for the patient to be admitted to a burn unit for local wound care (Baugh 2021).

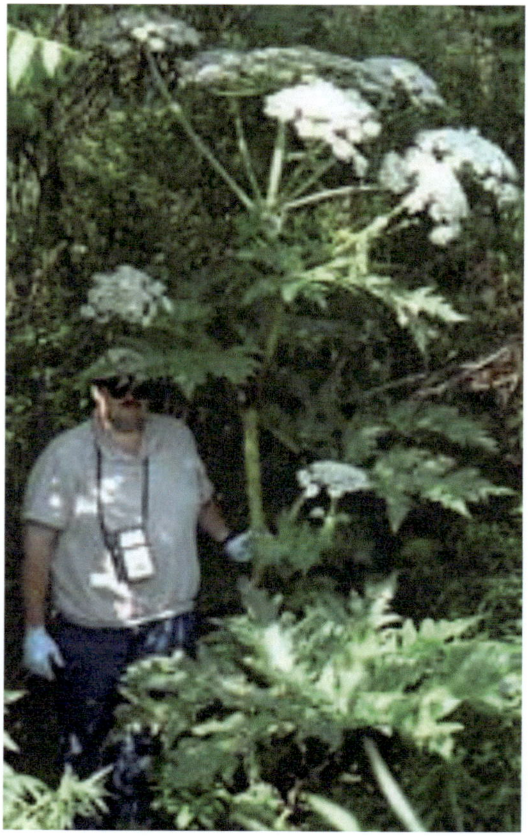

Fig. 19.2 Giant Hogweed (*Heracleum mantegazzianum*). (Photo © USDA APHIS PPQ Archive, USDA APHIS PPQ, Bugwood.org)

Regular use of UV-A–blocking sunscreens may help to diminish the cutaneous effects of phytophotodermatitis if contact with plant psoralens occurs.

References

Baugh WP. Phytophotodermatitis. Medscape Updated: Nov 04, 2021. https://emedicine.medscape.com/article/1119566-overview. Accessed 25 Apr 2024.

Brandenburg WE, Ward KJ. Mushroom poisoning epidemiology in the United States. Mycologia. 2018;110(4):637–41.

Butt M, Marks JG Jr, Flamm A. Establishing consensus on the treatment of toxicodendron dermatitis. Dermatitis. 2022;33(3):220–6. https://doi.org/10.1097/DER.0000000000000894.

Diaz JH. Poisoning by herbs and plants: rapid toxidromic classification and diagnosis. Wilderness Environ Med. 2016;27(1):136–52. https://doi.org/10.1016/j.wem.2015.11.006.

Fisher AA. Poison ivy/oak/sumac. Part II: specific features. Cutis. 1996;58(1):22.

Gladman AC. Toxicodendron dermatitis: poison ivy, oak, and sumac. Wilderness Environ Med. 2006;17(2):120–8. https://doi.org/10.1580/PR31-05.1.

Goldfrank LR. Mushrooms. In: Hoffman RS, Howland MA, Lewin NA, Nelson LS, Goldfrank LR, editors. Goldfrank's toxicologic emergencies. 10th ed. McGraw Hill Education: New York; 2015. p. 1500–14.

Goralka JM, Albertson TE. Plants. In: Olson K, editor. Poisoning & drug overdose. 7th ed. McGraw Hill Education: New York; 2018. p. 375–93.

Gummin DD, Mowry JB, Beuhler MC, Spyker DA, Rivers LJ, Feldman R, Brown K, Pham Nathaniel PT, Bronstein AC, Weber JA. 2021 Annual report of the National Poison Data System© (NPDS) from America's poison centers: 39th annual report. Clin Toxicol. 2022;60(12):1381–643. https://doi.org/10.1080/15563650.2022.2132768.

Hedman H, Holmdahl J, Mölne J, Ebefors K, Haraldsson B, Nyström J. Long-term clinical outcome for patients poisoned by the fungal nephrotoxin orellanine. BMC Nephrol. 2017;18:121. https://doi.org/10.1186/s12882-017-0533-6.

Horowitz BZ. Mushroom toxicity. Medscape. Updated April 26, 2023a. https://emedicine.medscape.com/article/167398-overview#a3. Accessed 24 Apr 2024.

Horowitz BZ. Mushroom toxicity treatment & management. Medscape. Updated April 26, 2023b. https://emedicine.medscape.com/article/167398-treatment?form=fpf. Accessed 24 Apr 2024.

Kim Y, Flamm A, ElSohly MA, Kaplan DH, Hage RH Jr, Hamann CP, Marks JG Jr. Poison ivy, oak, and sumac dermatitis: what is known and what is new? Dermatitis. 2019;30(3):183–90. https://doi.org/10.1097/DER.0000000000000472.

Klaassen CD, Wong KL, Halstead BW. Poisons. 2024. https://www.britannica.com/science/poison-biochemistry/Plant-poisons-phytotoxins#:~:text=Plant%20poisons%20(phytotoxins). Accessed 12 Apr 2024.

Krenzelok EP, Mrvos R. Friends and foes in the plant world: a profile of plant ingestions and fatalities. Clin Toxicol (Phila). 2011;49:142.

Kurlan JG, Lucky AW. Black spot poison ivy: a report of 5 cases and a review of the literature. J Am Acad Dermatol. 2001;45(2):246.

McGovern TW, Barkley TM. Botanical dermatology. Int J Dermatol. 1998;37(5):321.

Modi GM, Doherty CB, Katta R, Orengo IF. Irritant contact dermatitis from plants. Dermatitis. 2009;20(2):63.

Neill BC, Neill JA, Brauker J, Rajpara A, Aires DJ. Postexposure prevention of toxicodendron dermatitis by early forceful unidirectional washing with liquid dishwashing soap. J Am Acad Dermatol. 2019;81(2):e25. https://doi.org/10.1016/j.jaad.2017.12.081.

Nelson LS, Goldfrank LR. Plants. In: Hoffman RS, Howland MA, Lewin NA, Nelson LS, Goldfrank LR, editors. Goldfrank's toxicologic emergencies. 10th ed. New York: McGraw Hill Education; 2015. p. 1517–36.

Nelson LS, Balick MJ. Handbook of Poisonous and Injurious Plants. Third edition. Springer, New York, NY. 2020.

Olano JD, Wang JJ, Villeneuve E, Gosselin S, Biary R, Su MK, Hoffman RS. Current fatality rate of suspected cyclopeptide mushroom poisoning in the United States. Clin Toxicol (Phila). 2021;59(1):24–7.

Olson K. Mushrooms, Amatoxin-type. In: Olson K, editor. Poisoning and drug overdose. New York: McGraw-Hill Education; 2018. p. 333–5.

Osweiler GD. Plant-related toxicosis. In: Toxicology. The National Veterinary Medical Series. Philadelphia: William & Wilkins; 1996. p. 361–408.

Pajouhi A. Mushrooms. In: Olson K, editor. Poisoning and drug overdose. New York: McGraw-Hill Education; 2018. p. 330–3.

Pietsch J, Koch I, Hermanns-Clausen M, et al. Pediatric plant exposures in Germany, 1998–2004. Clin Toxicol (Phila). 2008;46:686.

Shih RD, Goldfrank LH. Plants. In: Goldfrank LR, Flomenbaum NE, Lewin NA, Weisman RS, Howland MA, Hoffman RS, editors. Goldfrank's toxicologic emergencies. 6th ed. Norwalk, CT: Appleton & Lange; 1998. p. 1243–60.

Trabulus S, Altiparmak MR. Clinical features and outcome of patients with amatoxin-containing mushroom poisoning. Clin Toxicol (Phila). 2011;49(4):303–10.

Tran HH, Juergens AL. Mushroom toxicity. In: StatPearls [internet]. Treasure Island, FL: StatPearls; 2023.

Trestrail JH. Mushroom poisoning in the United States-an analysis of 1989 United States poison center data. J Toxicol Clin Toxicol. 1991;29(4):459–65. https://doi.org/10.3109/15563659109025741.

Wang B, Wan AH, Xu Y, Zhang RX, Zhao BC, Zhao XY, Shi YC, Zhang X, Xue Y, Luo Y, Deng Y, Neely GG, Wan G, Wang OP. Identification of indocyanine green as a STT3B inhibitor against mushroom α-amanitin cytotoxicity. Nat Commun. 2023;14:2241. https://doi.org/10.1038/s41467-023-37714-3.

Miscellaneous Farm Toxicological and Environmental Hazards

20

Ricky L. Langley

Air Quality

Indoor Air Quality

For any building, the four basic factors that affect indoor environmental quality (IEQ) are indoor pollutant sources; heating, ventilation, and air-conditioning (HVAC) systems; pollutant pathways; and occupants and their activities or practices. On farms the indoor air quality will often differ depending on the structure (home, barn, shed, warehouse), the residing population (humans, animals), or the purpose of the building (equipment repair, crop storage, animal housing). Factors adversely affecting IEQ are tightly sealed buildings to reduce energy costs, the use of synthetic building materials and furnishings, increased use of chemical products such as pesticides, housekeeping supplies, and personal care products (N.C. DHHS 2019b).

Confined animal farm operations (CAFOs) often house hundreds to thousands of animals inside a structure and generate both gases and particulate matter that may be harmful for humans working and animals living within such facilities. These indoor pollutants may arise from feed for the animals (inorganic and organic grain dusts, endotoxins, mycotoxins, glucans, tannins, plicatic acid), from the animals themselves (feces and urine and bacterial degradation of these waste products), chemical agents used to clean, sanitize or disinfect the facilities, and equipment used in the facilities (fossil fuel burning heaters). Ammonia, hydrogen sulfide, and methane arise from the decomposition of animal waste; carbon dioxide and carbon monoxide (CO) are produced from fossil fuel combustion and gasoline-powered pressure washers; and carbon dioxide generated from animal respiration are the primary agents of concern. Ammonia is the most common noxious gas in animal quarters and is a mucus membrane and respiratory irritant. In addition, up to 200 different chemical compounds can be produced from animal waste decomposition and contribute to odors emitted from CAFOs (Donham and Thelin 2016a).

Individuals working in CAFOs are at risk of developing various respiratory illnesses. The most common respiratory symptoms reported in 1/3rd to 2/3rd of workers include cough, sputum production, scratchy throat, runny nose, burning or watery eyes, chest tightness, shortness of breath, and wheezing. Headaches and muscle aches and pains are also reported in approximately 1/4th to 1/3rd of workers (Donham 1993).

Respiratory illnesses in confinement housing and dairy barn workers include acute and chronic bronchitis, allergic asthma, nonallergic asthma-like condition (nonallergic occupational asthma or reactive airways disease), mucus membrane

R. L. Langley (✉)
Department of Biological Sciences,
North Carolina State University, Raleigh, NC, USA
e-mail: rllangley@ncsu.edu

W. J. Meggs, R. L. Langley (eds.), *Farm Toxicology*, https://doi.org/10.1007/978-3-031-80441-0_20

irritation, Monday morning syndrome, organic dust toxic syndrome, and hypersensitivity pneumonitis (Murphy 1992; Donham and Thelin 2016a). These conditions arise from agricultural dust exposure. Often dust and gas exposure occur simultaneously and the resulting health effects may be additive or synergistic.

In situations where the ventilation system in a CAFO is not working properly or the heaters are malfunctioning, levels of carbon monoxide and carbon dioxide may increase to asphyxiating levels and become hazardous to both humans and animals in the facility. Deaths have also occurred from hydrogen sulfide exposure when manure in pits (often located under the building) is being agitated for emptying. During agitation, lethal levels of hydrogen sulfide may occur within seconds. Workers have also died from entering a pit to repair equipment or damage to the pit, clean out solids, or remove animals or tools that may have fallen into the pit. In several cases, other family members and even first responders have also died trying to rescue the initial victim(s) due to not wearing proper respiratory protective equipment.

Other structures on farms such as machine shops, machine sheds, garages, and controlled atmosphere storage facilities present a risk to workers in these facilities. There are usually various solvents and machine fluids (such as hydraulic fluid, brake fluid, chainsaw oils, etc.) used to clean or maintain farm equipment in these shops and garages. Gasoline, diesel fuel, kerosene, or propane is often used to power the equipment and these diverse fuels and solvents present risks from dermal and inhalational exposures. In addition, activities such as welding often occur on farms and overexposure to welding fumes may result in metal fume fever. Large quantities of fruits and vegetables are often placed in controlled atmosphere storage where the temperature within the facility is lowered, oxygen concentration is lowered, and carbon dioxide concentrations are raised in order to retard metabolic processes in these harvested crops to retard perishable quality. Fossil fueled generators are often used to initially establish the low oxygen atmosphere and may result in high carbon monoxide levels in these structures (Murphy 1992). Hydrocarbon powered forklifts may be used to load or unload these structures and may generate carbon monoxide and carbon dioxide at very high levels so proper ventilation is required to prevent worker overexposure to these gases (Hirsch et al. 2016).

Carbon monoxide (CO) results from incomplete combustion of hydrocarbons used on farms such as gasoline, diesel fuel, propane, kerosene. Proper ventilation is required wherever these products are used. Carbon monoxide is colorless, odorless, tasteless, and nonirritating and has an affinity for hemoglobin 200–250 times that of oxygen. Exposure to CO results in a decrease in blood oxygen-carrying capacity. The oxyhemoglobin dissociation curve is shifted to the left impairing oxygen delivery to the tissues. The consequence of this is cellular hypoxia and ischemia. CO also disrupts oxygen utilization and respiration at the cellular level. Overexposure can result in fatalities. Symptoms of overexposure are predominantly in organs with high oxygen consumption. Most patients complain of headaches, dizziness, and nausea. Persons with coronary artery disease may complain of angina symptoms or even develop myocardial infarction. Symptoms of severe CO poisoning include malaise, shortness of breath, headache, nausea, chest pain, irritability, ataxia, altered mental status, other neurologic symptoms, loss of consciousness, coma, and death; signs include tachycardia, tachypnea, hypotension, various neurologic findings including impaired memory, cognitive and sensory disturbances, metabolic acidosis, arrhythmias, myocardial ischemia or infarction, and noncardiogenic pulmonary edema, although any organ system might be involved (CDC 2020). Survivors of serious poisoning may experience long-term neurologic deficits from the hypoxic-ischemic insult including personality and memory disorders to Parkinsonism to a persistent vegetative state. Exposure during pregnancy may result in fetal death. In animal confinement facilities, an increased number of abortions in animals may be a warning of high CO levels. Also see Chap. 14 Toxic Gases for additional information.

An elevated carboxyhemoglobin (CO-Hgb) level of $\geq 2\%$ for nonsmokers and $>9\%$ CO-Hgb level for smokers strongly supports a diagnosis of CO poisoning. While blood CO-Hgb levels may not reliably correlate with the severity of the poisoning, levels greater than 25% are considered significant and greater than 40–50% are usually associated with obvious signs and symptoms (Olson 2018). If there is any suspicion that carbon monoxide overexposure may have occurred, obtain a specific CO-Hgb level by co-oximetry with arterial or venous blood. Note that routine arterial blood gas instrumentation and conventional pulse oximetry are unreliable in detecting carbon monoxide intoxication. Treatment of carbon monoxide poisoning begins with the administration of 100% oxygen which speeds the rate of elimination of CO from hemoglobin from about 6 h in room air to 1 h. Depending on symptoms and CO-Hgb level, the exposed victim may benefit from hyperbaric oxygen. Contact the Poison Control Center (1-800-222-1222) for guidance. Also be aware that if the victim had smoke exposure, then consider the possibility of cyanide poisoning, methemoglobinemia, and irritant gas injury.

Within human residential structures, air quality issues are a fairly common concern. Examples of concerns/complaints that may indicate an air quality problem include stale (stuffy) air, lingering disagreeable odors, mold or mildew growth/odors, mucus membrane irritation, relative humidity levels below 30% or above 60%, tobacco smoke, and excessive dust or pet dander (AIHA 2023). While most indoor air problems may cause discomfort, in general most usually do not cause serious health issues. However serious illness may result from exposure to carbon monoxide from appliances that burn natural gas, propane, fuel oil, or wood such as stoves, space heaters, fireplaces, water heaters, and clothes dryers. These appliances need routine inspection and cleaning to make sure they are properly operating. In addition, carbon monoxide detectors should be installed along with fire detectors. Long-term exposure to environmental tobacco smoke and radon may increase the risk of developing lung cancer.

In addition, numerous products within the residential home may release chemicals into the air which can cause headaches and mucus membrane irritation. Off-gassing of various chemicals (volatile organic compounds) can occur from paints, paint strippers, moth balls, new carpets, new furniture, foam insulation, plywood, and particle board in the home. Formaldehyde-based resins are often used in press board products and urea foam insulation. Formaldehyde can cause mucus membrane and eye irritation and some individuals can become sensitized to it and develop lower respiratory symptoms such as asthma or dermatologic symptoms such as rash and urticaria. Formaldehyde is also recognized as a human carcinogen (ACS 2022).

In addition to carbon monoxide, combustion products include nitrogen dioxide and particulates. Nitrogen dioxide is a reddish-brown odorless gas that irritates the mucus membranes and may contribute to respiratory diseases. Nitrogen dioxide can decrease the lungs' defenses against bacteria making them more susceptible to infections. It can also aggravate asthma. There is also evidence from animal studies that repeated exposures to elevated nitrogen dioxide levels may lead or contribute to the development of lung diseases such as emphysema. People at particular risk from exposure to nitrogen dioxide include children and individuals with asthma and other respiratory diseases. Particulates can contribute to cardiovascular and respiratory disease, and cancer-causing pollutants such as radon and benzo (a) pyrene can attach to these particles and be transported to the lungs if inhaled (U.S. EPA 2023f).

If there is a history of roof leaks or the home has been affected by flooding (either due to plumbing issues or natural causes) then persistent moisture problems indoors can result in the growth or amplification of biological and microbial organisms like mold, mildew, dust mites, and bacteria. In addition to disagreeable odors from volatile organic compounds (mold and mildew smell), exposure to these organisms can increase the risk of allergic illness, trigger asthma attacks, cause respiratory infections, or have other adverse health effects such as mucus membrane irritation and skin rash. To remedy the problem, the source of excess moisture must be found and fixed, and contaminated materials must be removed and discarded if they cannot be thoroughly cleaned. Proper cleaning and building maintenance, especially moisture control, are essential in controlling mold and other biological agents (N.C. DHHS 2023b).

Outdoor Air Quality

The outdoor air quality changes daily just as the weather does. While outdoor air in rural areas may be cleaner than in urban areas, air pollution from cities can drift to rural areas. In addition, smoke from wildfires may contribute to unhealthy air quality. Because poor air quality may adversely affect health, in the United States, the U.S. Environmental Protection Agency (U.S. EPA) has developed the Air Quality Index (AQI) for reporting air quality (U.S. EPA 2003b). Rural practitioners must know what the AQI means and how to advise their patients.

The U.S. EPA establishes AQI for five major air pollutants regulated by the Clean Air Act. Each pollutant has a national air quality standard set by U.S. EPA to protect public health. The five pollutants include ground-level ozone; particulate matter including PM 2.5 and PM 10; carbon monoxide; sulfur dioxide; and nitrogen dioxide. Ozone and particulates are the major sources of unhealthy air quality 99% of the time in the United States according to the U.S. EPA.

The AQI runs from 0 to 500 with the higher the AQI value the greater the health concern. AQI values at or below 100 are generally thought of as satisfactory and levels above 100 are unhealthy (at first for sensitive groups, then for everyone as AQI values get higher). The AQI is divided into six categories and each category is color-coded. Each category corresponds to a different level of health concern. Knowing the AQI in your area can provide information to protect the health of outdoor workers (Table 20.1).

Certain groups of individuals with heart or lung disease or certain age groups may be more sensitive to the effects of a certain pollutant when the AQI is greater than 100 for the pollutant:

Ozone: People with lung disease, children, older adults, people who are active outdoors (including outdoor workers).

PM 2.5: People with heart or lung disease, older adults, children, lower socioeconomic status.

PM 10: People with heart or lung disease, older adults, children, lower socioeconomic status.

CO: People with heart disease.

NO_2: People with asthma, children, and older adults.

SO_2: People with asthma, children, and older adults.

Table 20.1 U.S. EPA Air Quality Index

Daily AQI color	Levels of concern	Value of index	Description of air quality
Green	Good	0–50	Air quality is satisfactory and air pollution poses little to no risk
Yellow	Moderate	51–100	Air quality is acceptable. However, there may be a risk to some people, particularly those unusually sensitive to air pollution
Orange	Unhealthy for sensitive groups	101–150	Members of sensitive groups may experience health effects. The general public is less likely to be affected
Red	Unhealthy	151–200	Some members of the general public may experience health effects, and members of more sensitive group s may experience more serious health effects
Purple	Very unlikely	201–300	Health alert. The risk of health effects is increased for everyone
Maroon	Hazardous	301 or higher	Health warning of emergency conditions: everyone is more likely to be affected

In Table 20.2, the U.S. EPA provides the following information for these sensitive groups (U.S. EPA 2018b).

Metropolitan areas with a population of more than 350,000 are required to report the daily AQI. Many more areas report it as a public service. The U.S. EPA has partnered with the National Oceanic and Atmospheric Administration (NOAA), National Park Service, NASA, Centers for Disease Control, and tribal, state, and local air quality agencies to develop a one-stop source for air quality data called AirNow (airnow.gov). You can find the daily AQI on AirNow (airnow.gov) and on state and local agency websites. The U.S. EPA uses two algorithms, called "NowCasts," to relate hourly readings from air quality monitors to the AQI for ozone and the AQI for particle pollution. AQI reporting is required for all criteria pollutants when they have an index value of 50 or above. Most cities forecast for ozone and particle pollution as these pollutants are the major sources of unhealthy air quality around 99% of the time. However, several cities forecast for all five pollutants. EPA requires ozone monitoring during the time of year when weather conditions are most favorable for ozone formation. This season varies by state. In some states with warmer climates, monitoring is required year-round. In states where the climate is colder, ozone monitoring is required for as little as 5 months during the summertime. AirNow should be checked before embarking in outdoor activities. You can find forecasts for your area on AirNow, on state, local and tribal air agency websites, in your local news media, and through some national media outlets.

Table 20.2 Pollutant-specific sub-indices and cautionary statements for guidance on the Air Quality Index (AQI) from U.S. EPA

AQI categories (index values)	Ozone (ppm)		Particulate matter (μg/m³) C		Carbon monoxide (ppm) (8-h)	Sulfur dioxide (ppb) (1-h)	Nitrogen dioxide (ppb) (1-h)
	(8-h)	(1-h)	PM 2.5 (24-h)	PM 10 (24-h)			
Good (up to 50)	0–0.054 None		0–12.0 None	0–54 None	0–4.4 None	0–35 None	0–53 None
Moderate (51–100)	0.055–0.070 Unusually sensitive people should consider reducing prolonged or heavy outdoor exertion		12.1–35.4 Unusually sensitive people should consider reducing prolonged or heavy exertion	55–154 Unusually sensitive people should consider reducing prolonged or heavy exertion	4.5–9.4 None	36–75 None	54–100 Unusually sensitive individuals should consider limiting prolonged exertion especially near busy roads
Unhealthy for sensitive groups (101–150)	0.071–0.085	0.125–0.164	35.5–55.4	155–254	9.5–12.4	76–185	101–360

(continued)

AQI categories (index values)	Ozone (ppm)		Particulate matter (µg/m³) C		Carbon monoxide (ppm) (8-h)	Sulfur dioxide (ppb) (1-h)	Nitrogen dioxide (ppb) (1-h)
	(8-h)	(1-h)	PM 2.5 (24-h)	PM 10 (24-h)			
	People with lung disease (such as asthma), children, older adults, people who are active outdoors (including outdoor workers), people with certain genetic variants, and people with diets limited in certain nutrients should reduce prolonged or heavy outdoor exertion		People with heart or lung disease, older adults, children, and people of lower socioeconomic status should reduce prolonged or heavy exertion		People with heart disease, such as angina, should limit heavy exertion and avoid sources of CO, such as heavy traffic	People with asthma should consider limiting outdoor exertion	People with asthma, children and older adults should limit prolonged exertion especially near busy roads
Unhealthy (151–200)	0.086–0.105	0.165–0.204	55.5–150.4	255–354	12.5–15.4	186–304	361–649
	People with lung disease (such as asthma), children, older adults, people who are active outdoors (including outdoor workers), people with certain genetic variants, and people with diets limited in certain nutrients should avoid prolonged or heavy outdoor exertion; everyone else should reduce prolonged or heavy outdoor exertion		People with heart or lung disease, older adults, children, and people of lower socioeconomic status should avoid prolonged or heavy exertion; everyone else should reduce prolonged or heavy exertion		People with heart disease, such as angina, should limit moderate exertion and avoid sources of CO, such as heavy traffic	Children, people with asthma, or other lung diseases, should limit outdoor exertion	People with asthma, children and older adults should avoid prolonged exertion near roadways; everyone else should limit prolonged exertion especially near busy roads
Very unhealthy (201–300)	0.106–0.200	0.205–0.404	150.5–250.4	355–424	15.5–30.4	305–604 (24-h)	650–1249
	People with lung disease (such as asthma), children, older adults, people who are active outdoors (including outdoor workers), people with certain genetic variants, and people with diets limited in certain nutrients should avoid all outdoor exertion; everyone else should reduce outdoor exertion.		People with heart or lung disease, older adults, children, and people of lower socioeconomic status should avoid all physical activity outdoors. Everyone else should avoid prolonged or heavy exertion		People with heart disease, such as angina, should avoid exertion and sources of CO, such as heavy traffic	Children, people with asthma, or other lung diseases should avoid outdoor exertion; everyone else should reduce outdoor exertion	People with asthma, children, and older adults should avoid all outdoor exertion; everyone else should avoid prolonged exertion, especially near busy roads
Hazardous (301–500)	–	0.405–0.604	250.5–500.4	425–604	30.5–50.4	605–1004 (24-h)	1250–2049

(continued)

Table 20.2 (continued)

AQI categories (index values)	Ozone (ppm)		Particulate matter (μg/m³) C		Carbon monoxide (ppm) (8-h)	Sulfur dioxide (ppb) (1-h)	Nitrogen dioxide (ppb) (1-h)
	(8-h)	(1-h)	PM 2.5 (24-h)	PM 10 (24-h)			
	Everyone should avoid all outdoor exertion		Everyone should avoid all physical activity outdoors; people with heart or lung disease, older adults, children, and people of lower socioeconomic status should remain indoors and keep activity levels low		People with heart disease, such as angina, should avoid exertion and sources of CO, such as heavy traffic; everyone else should limit heavy exertion	Children, people with asthma, or other lung diseases, should remain indoors; everyone else should avoid outdoor exertion	People with asthma, children, and older adults should remain indoors; everyone else should avoid all outdoor exertion

Source: U.S. EPA (2018b)

Aquaculture

Aquaculture is one of the fastest growing segments in agriculture and rural practitioners may have patients working in this arena. Aquacultural practices include farming finfish, crustaceans, mollusks, seaweeds, and other aquatic organisms such as eels for human consumption. In addition, aquaculture also includes hatchery production of fish and shellfish for conservation, stock enhancement, recreational angling and bait, ornamental fish, and algae (e.g., kelp) for a variety of uses including cosmetics, fertilizer, fuel, and animal feed (Fry et al. 2019).

Water is the growing environment for aquatic animals so a source of good quality water is vital to their growth. Many aquaculture farms use ozone or ultraviolet lights to lower microbial growth in the water supply. Ultraviolet (UV) radiation exposure can damage the skin and eyes, and ozone gas can injure lung tissue. Oxygen is also routinely used during aquaculture production and transportation of aquaculture products. Oxygen increases the risks of fire and explosions, and liquid oxygen can cause freezing (cryogenic) burns and tissue damage. Workers may also be exposed to high concentrations of radon, occurring naturally in groundwater (depending on local geology) used in aquaculture production.

Finfish and shellfish hatcheries contain chemical, biological, and physical hazards. Chemical hazards in hatcheries can originate from veterinary pharmaceuticals, disinfectants, sterilizers, and other sources. Workers at freshwater operations can be exposed to anesthetics, antibiotics, vaccines, chemical disinfectants, chemical sterilizers, solvents, fuels, oxyacetylene systems, pesticides, herbicides, water-testing chemicals, and chemicals that alter water chemistry (Myers 2010).

Medications approved by the U.S. Food and Drug Administration (FDA) for use in aquaculture to control external bacteria and fungi (Fry et al. 2019) include chloramine-T, formalin, hydrogen peroxide, and oxytetracycline hydrochloride. Tricaine methanesulfonate has been used as an anesthetic and chorionic gonadotrophin for spawning. Fry et al. (2019) provide a list of potential adverse human health effects from these agents.

Antibiotic-medicated feed includes florfenicol, oxytetracycline dehydrate, and sulfadimethoxine/ormetoprim. Localized skin reactions, respiratory problems, development of allergies, and even anaphylactic reactions may occur with repeated contact with these antibiotics. In addition, misuse of antibiotics may lead to development of antibiotic resistance in the water microbes, some of which may be pathogenic to humans (Durborow 1999).

Fish vaccines are typically delivered by injection, and accidental needle sticks to the worker injecting the fish can occur resulting in localized tissue damage, fever, muscle aches, malaise, edema, lymphangitis, dizziness, rash, and potential anaphylactic shock. Even amputation of injected digits from vaccines containing a mineral oil adjuvant has been reported (Durborow 1999).

A variety of other chemicals are used in various aspects of aquacultural practice including aquatic herbicides, algaecides, disinfectants, and chemicals to maintain water quality. Some of the chemicals utilized include the following: formalin, ethanol, copper sulfate, potassium chloride, potassium permanganate, iodine, silicone-based defoaming agents (food grade emulsions), quaternary ammonia, bleach (chlorine), carbon dioxide, sodium thiosulfate, diquat, rodeo aquatic herbicide, malachite green, and sulfuric acid. Again (Fry et al. 2019) provide a list of health effects from these agents.

Preservatives such as sodium metabisulfite (sometimes called "shrimp dip") may be used. In sulfite-sensitive individuals, bronchospasm and urticaria/angioedema may result from exposure to this chemical. If sodium metabisulfite mixes with acid and water, then sulfur dioxide may be generated and may have been responsible for deaths in shrimp trawler fishermen (Durborow 1999).

Arsenic

Arsenic is a naturally occurring metal found in the earth's crust. It occurs in various forms: elemental (metallic) arsenic; combined with other elements such as oxygen, chlorine, and sulfur (inorganic arsenic), or combined with carbon and hydrogen (organic arsenic). Inorganic arsenicals are generally more toxic than organic forms. Inorganic arsenic compounds are found in soils, sediments, and groundwater. These compounds occur naturally or as a result of mining, ore smelting, and industrial use of arsenic. In the past, inorganic forms of arsenic were used in pesticides, paint pigments, and wood preservatives, and may persist for decades in the soil. In the United States, usage of arsenic-containing pesticides and wood preservatives (chromated copper arsenate) is mostly restricted. Inorganic arsenic and arsenic compounds are considered to be cancer-causing chemicals. Most of the arsenic in fish/shellfish is in the organic form which is the less harmful form. Some seaweed may contain arsenic in inorganic forms that may be more harmful (CDC 2009; N.C. DHHS 2019c).

People are exposed to elevated levels of inorganic arsenic through drinking contaminated water, using contaminated water in food preparation and irrigation of food crops, eating contaminated food, smoking tobacco, and from occupational exposure to industrial processes using arsenic compounds. Inorganic arsenic is naturally present at high levels in the groundwater of a number of countries, including Argentina, Bangladesh, Cambodia, Chile, China, India, Mexico, Pakistan, the United States, and Vietnam. People are exposed to organic arsenic primarily by consuming seafood.

Arsenic-treated wood should never be burned in open fires, in stoves, residential boilers, or fire places, and should not be composted or used as mulch.

The U.S. EPA has set a limit of arsenic in drinking water at 10 ppb (parts per billion) (U.S. EPA 2023a). The most important action in affected communities is the prevention of further exposure to arsenic by the provision of a safe water supply for drinking, food preparation, and irrigation of food crops. There are a number of options to reduce levels of arsenic in drinking water (WHO 2022).

- Substitute high-arsenic sources, such as groundwater, with low-arsenic, microbiologically safe sources such as rainwater and treated surface water. Low-arsenic water can be used for drinking, cooking, and irrigation purposes, whereas high-arsenic water can be used for other purposes such as bathing and washing clothes.

- Blend low-arsenic water with higher-arsenic water to achieve an acceptable arsenic concentration level.
- Install arsenic removal systems —either centralized or domestic —and ensure the appropriate disposal of the removed arsenic. Technologies for arsenic removal include oxidation, coagulation-precipitation, absorption, ion exchange, and reverse osmosis techniques. Exposure can also be reduced by using bottled water or connecting to a public water supply, if possible.

Ingestion of inorganic arsenic, depending on dose, can cause acute symptoms ranging from nausea, vomiting, and diarrhea to dehydration. These are followed by numbness and tingling of the extremities, muscle cramping, shock, and death in extreme cases. Long-term exposure to inorganic arsenic in drinking water has been associated with skin disorders such as hyperpigmentation and hypo-pigmentation, and increased risks for diabetes, high blood pressure, peripheral neuropathy, peripheral vascular disease, and several types of cancer including skin cancer, bladder, and lung cancer. Forms of organic arsenic (e.g., arsenobetaine) found in seafood are not known to be toxic to humans (WHO 2022).

Laboratory tests can measure arsenic in your blood, urine, hair, or fingernails, and these tests are often helpful in determining if you have been exposed to above-average levels of arsenic in the past. If arsenic is detected, then your physician may recommend treatment (depending on your symptoms and the level detected). If arsenic is detected, ask the laboratory to speciate the forms of arsenic as organic arsenics (such as arsenobetaine) are much less toxic than inorganic forms. Contact the Poison Control Centers for guidance on treatment including possible chelation and subsequent monitoring.

Asbestos

Asbestos is a generic term for fibrous silicate minerals that are heat, corrosion, and acid resistant with high tensile strength, and some varieties are also flexible. There are two morphological types of silicates: amphibole and serpentine fibers. Amphibole fibers are straight, rigid, needlelike fibers while serpentines are curly, pliable fibers. The major types of amphiboles are crocidolite (blue asbestos), amosite (brown asbestos), tremolite, anthophyllite, and actinolite. Amphiboles account for about 10% of asbestos in use. Serpentine accounts for about 90% of asbestos products in use. Chrysotile (white asbestos) is the primary serpentine of commercial use. All forms of asbestos appear to cause cancer and nonmalignant diseases (ATS 2004).

While many uses of asbestos have been banned by the U.S. EPA, there are still numerous potential sources of asbestos on farms and in farm houses. Asbestos may even occur naturally in soils in some areas (ATSDR 2007) or as a contaminant in soil enhancement products such as vermiculite.

Many farms in the United States are likely to contain asbestos-containing materials. Many residential structures built before the mid-1970s may contain asbestos. These would include steam pipes, boilers and furnace ducts, resilient floor tiles and adhesives for installing the tiles, insulation used around furnaces and wood stoves, door gaskets in furnaces and wood stoves, sound proofing or decorative materials sprayed on walls and ceilings, artificial ashes and embers for use in gas-fired fireplaces, and older household products such as fireproofing gloves, stove top pads, ironing board covers and some hairdryers.

People seeking reclaimed wood from barns and farmhouses should be aware of the potential for asbestos contamination. The wood may contain traces of asbestos insulation, and it could bear asbestos-containing paint or varnish. Other sources of asbestos in farm buildings may include asbestos roofing cement, shingles, siding, roofing sheets, building partitions, wall boards, insulation materials, gutters, and exhaust pipes (Whitmer 2023).

If asbestos-containing material is in good shape, it should be left alone because the material will not release asbestos fibers. Regular inspection for signs of damage such as tears, abrasions, or water damage should be done as damaged material may release fibers. If damage is suspected then limit access to the area and do not touch or disturb it. Contact your local or state health department to find out about proper handling and disposal procedures (U.S. CPSC 2019).

Asbestos friction materials such as brakes, clutches, gaskets, insulation, and heat panels were used in farming equipment because asbestos made these products heat-resistant. When repairing equipment that may potentially contain asbestos, wet methods are recommended to limit exposure and use asbestos-free replacement parts.

Farmers may also be exposed to asbestos in the soil of their fields. Asbestos in soil may occur naturally, or it may have been added to the soil as a vermiculite-based fertilizer or conditioning agent (ATSDR 2007). Farmers who unknowingly work on lands contaminated with asbestos fibers may face a moderate to high risk of exposure during activities that generate dust. ATSDR has recommendations to decrease exposure to workers that may disturb soil with naturally occurring asbestos present (ATSDR 2005).

Vermiculite is a natural mineral that is like asbestos in that it is heat-resistant and a good insulator. Vermiculite is the mineralogical name given to hydrated laminar magnesium-aluminum-iron silicate that resembles mica in appearance. All vermiculite ores contain a range of other minerals that were formed along with the vermiculite in the rock. Vermiculite ores from some sources have been found to contain asbestos minerals but asbestos is not intrinsic to vermiculite and only a few ore bodies have been found to contain more than trace amounts (U.S. EPA 2023d). Vermiculite has been used in a variety of products such as brake linings, fireproofing materials, potting soils, and soil conditioners. Some of the farming purposes for vermiculite include:

- Animal feed.
- Fertilizer.
- Pesticides.
- Seed encapsulation.
- Soil conditioner.
- Potting mix.
- Root cuttings.
- Seed germination.
- Sowing composts.

If using vermiculite, the U.S. EPA recommends using it outdoors, keeping it damp to reduce dust and avoid bringing dusty clothing into the home.

Asbestos exposure may cause both malignant and nonmalignant disease. Inhalation of asbestos fibers induces alveolitis and inflammation in the surrounding interstitium that can result in fibrosis in the respiratory bronchioles that extends into adjacent alveolar tissue. Asbestos inhalation can also result in pleural inflammation (ATS 2004).

Diseases of the pleura that may occur include pleural effusions which may occur within 10–20 years even after minimal exposure. Diffuse pleural thickening is a complication that may result from multiple benign associated pleural effusions. Pleural plaques usually develop about 20 years after exposure. Plaques and effusions may develop at lower levels of exposure than that which causes asbestosis (Norbert et al. 2015).

Asbestosis (a form of parenchymal fibrosis) is commonly associated with prolonged exposure to high concentrations of asbestos usually over 10–20 years. However, asbestosis would be unusual in farmers given exposures are usually not at high levels for prolonged periods of time. Cigarette smoking increases the risk of developing asbestosis presumably due to decreased clearance of asbestos fibers in the lung.

Asbestos exposure has been associated with several forms of cancer including lung cancer, mesothelioma, laryngeal cancer, and ovarian cancer. Some studies have also suggested that workplace asbestos exposure may be linked to other cancers, including cancers of the pharynx (throat), stomach, colon, and rectum and gastrointestinal cancer (ACS 2023). Cigarette smoking acts synergistically with asbestos to increase the risk of lung cancer as compared to nonsmokers exposed to asbestos.

Detergents, Disinfectants, and Cleaning Agents

A variety of cleaning agents are used on farms, especially farms with livestock. Soaps and detergents are among the most commonly used. Soaps and detergents are surfactant agents that lower the surface tension of water to enable it to wet surfaces more efficiently and help to remove dirt, soil, fats, and greases. Soaps are generally low in toxicity; however soaps made with alkali (homemade soap or laundry soaps) may potentially be a corrosive hazard.

Detergents are non-soap surfactants in combination with inorganic ingredients such as carbonates, phosphates, and silicates (Kore and Kiesche-Nesselrodt 1990). Detergents can be further classified as nonionic surfactants, anionic surfactants, and cationic surfactants according to their charge in solution.

Nonionic detergents are uncharged in aqueous solutions at neutral pH. Examples of nonionic detergents include alkyl ethoxylate, alkyl phenoxy polyethoxy ethanols, and polyethylene glycol stearate. Most nonionic detergents have a low order of irritation and toxicity (Kore and Kiesche-Nesselrodt 1990).

Anionic surfactants are primarily sulfonated or phosphorylated straight-chain hydrocarbons. Examples include alkyl sodium sulfates, alkyl sodium sulfonates, dioctyl sodium sulfosuccinate, sodium lauryl sulfate, tetrapropylene benzene sulfonate, and linear alkyl sulfonates. Most anionic detergents are slightly to moderately toxic although some may have high alkalinity and be more corrosive (Kore and Kiesche-Nesselrodt 1990).

Cationic detergents are often quaternary ammonium compounds with aryl or alkyl substituent groups often with a long-chain hydrophobic carbon chain and a halogen attached. Depending on the concentration of the cationic detergent, signs and symptoms range from mucus membrane irritation to corrosive burns that may occur from contact with these agents. Ingestion of these compounds may cause adverse systemic effects. In animals, signs may mimic organophosphate poisoning.

Disinfectants are usually applied in animal facilities to destroy microorganisms or inhibit their growth. They are often applied as a high-pressure spray of active biocides including chlorine, quaternary ammonia compounds, organic iodines, phenolic compounds, pine oil disinfectants, cresol-based compounds, formaldehyde, and glutaraldehyde. Exposure to these products can result in acute and chronic problems including throat and nose irritation, nosebleeds, eye irritation, skin rashes, and even asthma (Hill 1999; Kore and Kiesche-Nesselrodt 1990; Meggs 1999; Popendorf and Reynolds 1997). Formaldehyde is considered a human carcinogen (ACS 2022).

Wearing appropriate personal protective equipment (PPE) is mandatory when handling these products. It should also be remembered that certain PPE may also contain a sensitizer such as latex and should be considered in the differential diagnosis of a farm worker with skin rash or asthma.

Depending on the route of exposure treatment may include dilution with milk or water and rinsing eyes with copious amounts of water. Call the Poison Center (800-222-1222) for guidance.

Drugs of Abuse

While not traditionally considered farm chemicals, the farmer and his/her family are not immune from the toxic and addictive effects of illicit drugs or intentional abuse/misuse of veterinary medications. A 2017 survey found that 3 of 4 farmers were affected by the opioid epidemic (Morning Consult 2017).

With more than 100,000 deaths occurring yearly in the United States (CDC 2023a) from substance abuse (not including alcohol and tobacco smoking), the rural practitioner needs to be able to recognize signs and symptoms of abuse and overdose. For example, a migrant worker collapses in a field. Could this be from heat exposure, pesticide exposure, or an illicit drug overdose? A quick assessment by the emergency responder/rural practitioner may offer clues to the condition leading to collapse. Were the pupils dilated suggesting possible stimulant overdose such as from methamphetamine or were they constricted which can occur in organophosphate pesticide poisoning or opiate overdose? Was the skin hot and dry which may suggest heat stroke? This section will briefly describe signs and symptoms from the major classes of illicit drug use including narcotics, sedative-hypnotics, stimulants, hallucinogens, and inhalants. Also, see the Veterinary Pharmaceutical section for veterinary medications that are being abused. A useful reference source for street names of drugs of abuse has been compiled by the Drug Enforcement Agency (DEA 2017). Table 20.3 is a quick overview of physical signs useful in the differential diagnosis of various substances often abused. Consider referral to an addiction specialist to help manage patients with drug abuse problems.

Narcotics

In the United States, opiates are responsible for most fatal overdoses, and fentanyl and its analogs are increasingly being detected in overdoses. Additionally, many drug overdoses involve a mixture of various classes of substances. There are many potential reasons why the farming community has been affected by the opioid epidemic. Farming and jobs in agriculture are high-risk jobs with a strong likelihood of being injured at work on the farm. Treatment often includes prescribing (or over-prescribing) an opiate for pain management. Another explanation for opioid misuse in the agricultural community could be due to the stressful nature of the occupation. Farmers often work long hours and are faced with challenges like the weather, commodity prices, input costs, and government regulations. Illicit drug or alcohol use is sometimes used as a coping strategy (Meadowcroft et al. 2023).

Narcotics include naturally derived compounds such as opium from poppy plants (the opium poppy is the key source for many narcotics including morphine, codeine, and heroin) to synthetically produced compounds (fentanyl and its scores of analogs). Opiates bind to receptors (primarily mu-opioid receptors) in various body regions.

Table 20.3 Physical signs of drug use/overdose

Drugs	Temp.	HR and BP	RR	Pupils	Bowel sounds	Skin moisture
Opioid Morphine, codeine, meperidine, heroin, fentanyl, hydromorphone, methadone, oxycodone, propoxyphene, tramadol	↓	↓	↓	Pinpoint	↓	Dry
Sympathomimetic (stimulants) Caffeine, cocaine, amphetamines, methamphetamines, Ritalin, theophylline, MDMA	↑	↑	↑	Dilated	↑	Wet
Sedative-hypnotic Anti-anxiety agents, muscle relaxants, antiepileptics, and pre-anesthetic medications-barbiturates-benzodiazepines	↓	↓	↓	No Δ	↓	Dry
Cholinergic Organophosphorous compounds, carbamates, arecoline, pilocarpine, urecholine, carbachol, choline, methacholine, mushrooms	No Δ	No Δ	No Δ	Pinpoint	↑	Wet
Anticholinergic Anticholinergics-atropine, scopolamine, glycopyrrolate, benztropine, trihexyphenidyl Antihistamines-cyproheptadine, chlorpheneramine, doxylamine, hydroxyzine, diphenhydramine, dimenhydrinate, meclizine, promethazine	↑	↑	No Δ	Dilated	↓	Dry
Hallucinogens LSD, mescaline, psilocybin, morning glory, nutmeg	No Δ or ↑	↑	↑	Dilated	↑	Wet

With mild or moderate overdose lethargy is common. The pupils are constricted (miosis). Blood pressure and pulse rate decreased, bowel sounds diminished and the muscles are usually flaccid. With higher doses respiratory depression and coma are seen. Apnea may result in sudden death. Noncardiogenic pulmonary edema may occur. Seizures are not common but may occur and cardiotoxicity may occur.

If an opiate overdose is suspected, the victim should be given nalaxone (an opiate antagonist) and the dose can be repeated every 2–3 min if no response. The duration of action of naloxone is 1–2 h and may be shorter than that of many opiates (methadone has a long half-life). Therefore, do not release a patient who has awakened after naloxone treatment until 3–4 h have passed since the last dose of naloxone and consider observation for 6–12 h if naloxone was required to reverse opioid-induced coma (Albertson 2018). Nalmefene is an opioid antagonist with a longer duration of action (3–5 h) than naloxone.

Symptoms suggestive of opiate withdrawal include watery eyes, runny nose, loss of appetite, nausea, vomiting, irritability, tremors, panic, chills and sweating, and cramps.

Sedative-Hypnotics

Sedative-hypnotics are widely used for the treatment of insomnia and anxiety and as muscle relaxants. These agents lower the arousal levels and reduce nervous system excitability by a range of pharmacological mechanisms; the most prominent are the facilitation of gamma-aminobutyric acid (GABA) receptors, opioid receptors, or an inhibition of glutamatergic or catecholaminergic activity. Common agents used as sedative-hypnotics include barbiturates, benzodiazepines, and non-benzodiazepines that act on the same GABA receptors as benzodiazepines, and gamma-hydroxybutyric acid (GHB), and carisoprodol (skeletal muscle relaxant).

Physical signs of overdose include shallow respiration, clammy skin, dilated pupils, nystagmus, weak and rapid pulse, slurred speech, loss of motor coordination, blurred vision, nausea and vomiting, low blood pressure, and coma. Hypothermia may be seen (Weimer 2019).

Withdrawal symptoms include anxiety, insomnia, tremors, delirium, and convulsions.

Stimulants

Stimulants enhance the activity of the central and peripheral nervous system. Effects vary depending on the stimulant. Examples of stimulants include cocaine, amphetamines, methamphetamines, and synthetic cathinones (bath salts), and gabapentinoids (Weimer 2019).

Signs of stimulant overdose include increased alertness, agitation, hallucinations, hyperthermia, tremors, headache, seizures, flushed skin, chest pain and palpitations, hypertension, excessive sweating, dry mouth, vomiting, abdominal cramps, dilated pupils (mydriasis). Myocardial infarction and cerebral hemorrhage/edema may develop. Renal failure secondary to rhabdomyolysis may develop.

Withdrawal symptoms may include apathy, irritability, mood swings, sleep disturbance, depression, exhaustion, depression, anxiety, and drug craving.

Hallucinogens

Hallucinogens are drugs that cause hallucinations in which the user sees or hears things that are not actually present. Rather than hallucinations, most street hallucinogens produce distorted perceptions and are often referred to as illusionogens. In this category are drugs that include lysergic acid diethylamide (LSD), MDMA, phencyclidine (PCP), mescaline, psilocybin, ketamine, morning glory and nutmeg, and jimson weed. The mechanism of toxicity is thought to be an alteration of serotonin and dopamine in the brain. Central and peripheral sympathetic stimulation may account for some of the side effects (Weimer 2019).

Signs of overdose may include illusions and hallucinations, poor perception of time and distance, and paranoid or bizarre reasoning. Sympathomimetic side effects (similar to stimulant overdose) may include tachycardia, hyperthermia, hypertension, dilated pupils, diaphoresis, bruxism, tremor, and hyperreflexia in mild to moderate intoxication. Life-threatening toxicity from intense sympathomimetic stimulation can include seizures, severe hyperthermia, hypertension, intracranial hemorrhage, and cardiac arrhythmias.

Hallucinogen addiction is rare and most hallucinogens are not considered addictive, although some do produce tolerance, cravings, and withdrawal symptoms. Not all hallucinogens produce withdrawal symptoms, but some drugs like PCP or ketamine do. Some people may become physically dependent on these drugs and experience withdrawal symptoms when they try to stop.

Common hallucinogen withdrawal symptoms include stiff muscles, depressed breathing, convulsions, rapid heart rate, extreme changes in body temperature, cravings, headaches, sweating, seizures, and flashbacks.

Inhalants

Many individuals are intentionally inhaling volatile substances often referred to as huffing, sniffing, and bagging. Substances often inhaled include typewriter correction fluid, glue, felt-tipped marking pens, paint, paint stripper, and gasoline. Chemicals that may be present in these products include freons, benzene, 1,1,1-trichloroethane, trichloroethylene, carbon tetrachloride, methylene chloride, toluene, and miscellaneous hydrocarbons.

Adverse effects from inhalants include altered mental status, slurred speech, incoherence, poor coordination, ataxia, abdominal pain, nausea vomiting, cough, shortness of breath, dysrhythmia, and asystole. Two (or more) of the following signs often develop during, or shortly after, inhalant use or exposure: dizziness, nystagmus, incoordination, slurred speech, unsteady gait, lethargy, depressed reflexes, psychomotor retardation, tremor, generalized muscle weakness, blurred vision or diplopia, stupor or coma, or euphoria. Chronic users may suffer damage to the heart (cardiomyopathy), lungs, kidneys (renal tubular acidosis), liver (hepatotoxicity), and bone marrow (anemia) (Anderson and Loomis 2003).

Tolerance to inhalants can develop with frequent use. A withdrawal syndrome has been described, although it occurs infrequently. Symptoms can include sleep disturbance, irritability, jitteriness, diaphoresis, nausea, vomiting, tachycardia, and, occasionally, hallucinations or delusions. Withdrawal can last one month or longer, and relapse rates are high.

Fertilizers and Lime

Fertilizers are used to supply plants with nutrients for growth and usually consist of a combination of nitrogen, phosphorous (phosphates), and potassium (potash). Trace metals may also be added for plant nutrition. There are two basic types of fertilizers-chemical fertilizers and animal manures. Chemical fertilizers are available in solid (dry), liquid, and gaseous forms. Most commonly it is in granular form and spread on the soil.

Dry fertilizer is hygroscopic-it attracts moisture. It may cause minor skin burns and irritation of the eyes and mucus membranes. Much more serious injuries can occur from the use of anhydrous ammonia. It is a colorless gas at room temperature but can be changed to a liquid under pressure and is usually transported, stored, and handled as a liquid. Anhydrous ammonia is a strong alkali.

Direct exposure to anhydrous ammonia can result in freezing skin burns and eye injuries due to the vaporization if contact is made with the liquid as it escapes from its container. In addition, anhydrous ammonia is very water soluble and forms a strongly alkaline solution (ammonium hydroxide) that can produce severe skin, eye, and mucus membrane burns. Liquefacient necrosis of tissues may result. Ocular exposure can be serious and requires referral to an ophthalmologist due to the severity of corneal burns (Shaver and Tong 1991; U.S. DOL 1994). Also see Chap. 14 Toxic Gases.

Inhalation of gaseous anhydrous ammonia can result in laryngospasm and bronchospasm with coughing and wheezing, acute pulmonary edema, adult respiratory distress syndrome (ARDS), bronchiolitis obliterans, and chronic bronchiectasis. Fatalities may occur from airways obstruction and survivors may develop pulmonary fibrosis or obstructive airways impairment.

After an initial lung injury from inhalation of anhydrous ammonia, an exacerbation may occur 2–3 weeks later. Gradual deterioration in pulmonary function can continue for 2–6 months followed by a slight improvement. Therefore, close monitoring after an inhalation injury is necessary.

Aqueous (aqua) ammonia is a frequently used fertilizer. It is similar to household ammonia but more concentrated and is not usually stored under pressure as is anhydrous ammonia. However, in hot weather conditions, it can build up pressure and vaporize in the supply tank and lines. Hazards are similar to anhydrous ammonia (Bittner et al. 1987).

Agricultural lime, also called aglime, agricultural limestone, and garden lime is a soil additive made from pulverized limestone or chalk. The primary active component is calcium carbonate. Additional chemicals vary depending on the mineral source and may include calcium oxide (Wikipedia 2023). Lime is also frequently applied to fields to increase productivity by the following actions:

- It increases the pH of acidic soil, reducing soil acidity and increasing alkalinity.
- It provides a source of calcium for plants.
- It improves water penetration for acidic soils.
- It improves the uptake of major plant nutrients (nitrogen, phosphorus, and potassium) of plants growing on acid soils.

Lime is an alkaline substance (calcium hydroxide forms when calcium oxide contacts water) and can result in skin irritation/burns and ocular burns if it gets in the eyes. Mild to severe mucus membrane and throat/lung irritation may also occur from inhalation. Oral exposure may cause gastrointestinal irritation/erosions.

Green Tobacco Sickness

Green tobacco sickness (GTS) is a condition associated with the planting, cultivating, or harvesting of tobacco plants. Workers new to handling and harvesting tobacco are at increased risk for GTS. Green tobacco sickness is a type of nicotine poisoning. Risk of nicotine poisoning increases when the nicotine contained in the tobacco leaves mixes with rain, morning dew, or sweat, allowing nicotine to get onto the skin and pass into the bloodstream more easily. GTS symptoms may occur while at work or several hours after the workday ends.

Symptoms of GTS include weakness, headache, nausea, vomiting, dizziness, abdominal cramps, breathing difficulty, abnormal temperature, pallor, diarrhea, chills, fluctuations in blood pressure or heart rate, and increased perspiration and salivation. The onset of the illness is three to 17 h after exposure and the duration of illness ranges from 1 to 3 days (CDC 2015; McBride et al. 1998).

Workers with GTS have also noted difficulty sleeping or eating. Symptoms usually resolve within 24 h once exposure ceases. Tobacco workers suffering from Green Tobacco Sickness are at greater risk for heat illness. Symptoms of GTS may be similar to those of heat illness and pesticide poisoning, which can make it difficult to diagnose. Clinical diagnosis of GTS is based on the presence of symptoms consistent with the condition and on a history of working with tobacco plants. The diagnosis of GTS may be achieved by a test for urinary or serum nicotine (half-life = 3–4 h) or, in the case of nontobacco users, cotinine (a nicotine metabolite with a half-life of 36 h) may be useful diagnostically.

Treatment may include intravenous rehydration, anti-emetics, dimenhydrinate (Trade name Dramamine), and supportive care (Reddy and Ashok 2019). Gloves, long-sleeved shirts, long pants, and water-resistant clothing are recommended to prevent exposure to nicotine from tobacco leaves. Washing with soap and water immediately after working is recommended to reduce exposure to nicotine.

Lead

Lead (Pb) is a naturally occurring metal found in small quantities in rock and soil. Lead has been used industrially in the production of gasoline, ceramic products, paints, metal alloys, batteries, and solder. While lead arising from the combustion of leaded gasoline was a major source of exposure in past decades, today deteriorated lead-based paint and resulting dust and soil contamination are the primary sources of environmental lead exposure for children and occupational and recreational sources are the main exposures among adults.

Residential farm houses and other structures and farm equipment are often decades old and may have been painted with lead-based paint. The federal government banned lead-based paint from housing on February 28, 1978. Older homes may also have lead pipes or used lead solder on the joints in plumbing. Peeling paint may be ingested by infants and young children and cause lead poisoning which may be insidious in onset. Lead may leach from pipes and drinking water may become contaminated leading to elevation in blood lead levels (BLLs). Other sources/activities of lead exposure to farmers or their household members may include remodeling and scraping paint from older homes, welding with lead-based solder or welding on lead-painted equipment, use of glazes in ceramics, recreational activities such as reloading of ammunition and making fishing sinkers, and using imported spices or medicines from other countries (U.S. EPA 1999, 2003a). Mouthing of toy jewelry (often imported) by infants and young children can be a source of lead poisoning.

There is no safe level of lead in humans. Several mechanisms of lead toxicity exist (Kosnett 2018a) including inactivation or alteration of macromolecules and enzymes by binding to carboxyl, sulfhydryl, and phosphate groups. Lead may interact with essential cations such as calcium, iron, and zinc. Alterations in cell and mitochondrial membranes, neurotransmitter synthesis and function, heme synthesis, cellular redox states, and nucleotide metabolism are other toxic mechanisms from lead exposure.

The usual route of lead exposure in nonindustrial jobs is through ingestion, particularly in children less than 6 years of age, who absorb more lead than adults (45–50% vs. 10–15%). Gastrointestinal lead absorption is increased by fasting, iron deficiency, and low dietary calcium. After absorption, lead is distributed by blood to multiple tissues including kidneys, liver, bone marrow, and nervous tissue. Lead in soft tissues causes the majority of symptoms and toxicities. Lead is lastly stored in the bone (95% in adults, 70% in children) where it is incorporated into the hydroxyapatite lattice (Wahl and Friede 2001).

Clearance of lead from the body follows a multicompartmental kinetic model with the “fast” compartments in the blood and soft tissue (half-life about 28–36 days from blood, 40–120 days in soft tissue) and the “slow” compartment in bone (half-life of 15–25 years) (CLN 2023; Moline and Landrigan 2005). Absorbed lead is eliminated primarily in urine and feces by adults. Small amounts are excreted in sweat, saliva, hair, nails, and breast milk. Lead can cross the placental barrier putting fetuses at risk, and infants may be exposed from breast feeding.

Traditionally, clinical symptoms were believed to occur at blood levels of 30–40 μg/dL but more recent scientific studies have shown adverse cognitive effects at levels lower than 5 μg/dL (ATSDR 2023a). Acute symptomatic intoxication is rare after a single exposure but may occur within hours or days after ingestion of gram quantities of soluble compounds (Kosnett 2018a). Symptoms and signs from acute ingestion (gram quantities) include vomiting, abdominal pain, hyperactivity, fatigue, lethargy, ataxia, behavioral changes, seizures, and coma. Laboratory findings may include basophilic stippling, anemia (may be hemolytic), increased urinary coproporyhrins, hemolysis, and toxic hepatitis. Abdominal X-rays may show opacities present. The blood lead level is usually >60 μg/dL in acute symptomatic poisonings.

Subacute or chronic exposure is more common than acute ingestion of large amounts of lead. Lead concentration in the body depends on the level (amount), frequency, and duration of lead exposure. The most common diagnostic test for lead (Pb) in the body is the concentration of Pb in blood (PbB). Blood Pb concentration reflects both ongoing exposure and Pb stores in bone, which can be transferred to blood. Because of the relatively rapid elimination of Pb from blood compared to bone, blood Pb will reflect mainly the exposure history of the previous few months and not necessarily the larger burden of Pb in bone (ATSDR 2020). The signs and symptoms from lead exposure generally become more noticeable as BLLs increase but symptoms may vary by individual. Children, infants, and fetuses are more vulnerable to the effects of lead because the blood-brain barrier is not fully developed in them. Thus, a smaller amount of lead will have a greater effect on children than on adults. In addition, lead absorption can be up to five times greater in children compared to adults (U.S. EPA 2022). A continuum of signs and symptoms can often be seen as shown in Table 20.4 (WHO 2021).

Fortunately, blood lead levels have been decreasing in the United States. In 2017–2018, median blood lead levels by age group were: 0.7 μg/dL for age 1 year; 0.8 μg/dL for age 2 years; 0.6 μg/dL for ages 3 to 5 years; 0.5 μg/dL for ages 6 to 10 years; 0.4 μg/dL for ages 11 to 15 years; and 0.4 μg/dL for ages 16 to 17 years (U.S. EPA 2023i). In 2021, CDC lowered the blood lead reference value (BLRV) from 5 to 3.5 μg/dL. CDC uses a BLRV of 3.5 μg/dL to identify children with blood lead levels that are higher than most children's levels. This level is based on the 97.5th percentile of the blood lead values among U.S. children ages 1–5 years from the 2015–2016 and 2017–2018 National Health and Nutrition Examination Survey (NHANES) cycles. Children with blood lead levels at or above the BLRV represent the top 2.5% with the highest blood lead levels (CDC 2022). If lead is detected in a child's blood, recommendations have been provided by Pediatric Environmental

Table 20.4 Blood lead concentration and signs and symptoms from lead exposure (adapted from WHO 2021)

Blood lead level (μg/dL)	Adults	Children
<5	Reduced fetal growth (based on maternal level)	Decreased IQ, cognitive performance, and academic achievement Increased incidence of behavioral problems Increased diagnosis of ADHD
<10	Reduced synthesis of 5-ALA dehydratase contributing to anemia Decreased cognitive function, altered mood, and behavior Possible increases in cardiovascular-related deaths Hypertension Possible increase in spontaneous abortions Possible increased preterm births	Reduced synthesis of 5-ALA dehydratase contributing to anemia Decreased cognitive function, altered mood, and behavior Delayed puberty
>30	Anemia Reduced fertility Spontaneous abortion Reduced birth weight	
>40	Subclinical peripheral neuropathy Neurobehavioral effects Abdominal colic Nonspecific symptoms such as headache, fatigue, anorexia	
>50	Altered neuromotor and neurosensory function (decreased motor skills)	Altered neuromotor and neurosensory function (decreased motor skills) Abdominal colic
>80	Encephalopathy	Encephalopathy

Health Specialty Units for follow-up and management (PESHU 2021).

If the blood lead level in a child is greater than 45 µg/dL, then chelation therapy should be considered. If the blood lead is >70 µg/dL consider hospitalization plus chelation. For asymptomatic children with elevated blood lead levels, oral succimer (DMSA) is often used, while for symptomatic cases such as severe gastrointestinal toxicity or encephalopathy, parenteral agents such as dimercaprol (BAL) and calcium disodium ethylenediamine tetraacetic acid ($CaNa_2$ EDTA) are used. Symptomatic cases should be hospitalized. Contact your local Poison Center for the latest therapeutic agents and dosages (1-800-222-1222).

Blood lead levels have also been falling in adults. In the 2017–2018 NHANES survey, adults 20 years and older had the highest geometric mean blood lead level (0.855 µg/dL) of all the reported age groups (U.S.EPA 2023i).

Recent recommendations on lead exposure among workers have been developed by the American College of Occupational and Environmental Medicine and recommend that workers maintain a BLL <10 µg/dL and <3.5 µg/dL if pregnant or wanting to become pregnant (Kosnett et al. 2023).

For asymptomatic adults, the usual treatment is removal from exposure and observation. Consider oral succimer for asymptomatic adults with BLL > 80 µg/dL (Young et al. 2020). For symptomatic adults without encephalopathy, consider treating with oral succimer or parenteral $CaNa_2$ EDTA (Kosnett 2018a). For encephalopathy, hospitalize and treat with BAL and $CaNa_2$ EDTA. Contact your local Poison Center for the latest therapeutic agents and dosages.

Mercury

Mercury (Hg) is a naturally occurring element. It can be present in three forms: elemental (metallic) mercury, inorganic mercury, and organic mercury. As mercury is a naturally occurring element, it can be found in the air, water, or soil. It can also be found in the environment due to industrial releases to air and water. Other sources of mercury include batteries; thermometers and other scientific and medical devices; electronic switches and lighting applications; paints and pigments; fungicides and pesticides. Mercury is also present in many types of light bulbs that are used in many homes and farm buildings such as:

- Fluorescent bulbs:
  - Linear, U-tube, and circline fluorescent tubes.
  - Bug zappers.
  - Tanning bulbs.
  - Black lights.
  - Germicidal bulbs.
  - High output bulbs.
  - Cold-cathode fluorescent bulbs.
- High-intensity discharge bulbs:
  - Metal halide.
  - Ceramic metal halide.
  - High-pressure sodium.
  - Mercury vapor.
- Mercury short-arc bulbs.
- Neon bulbs.

Mercury can enter private wells from erosion of rocks underground or from industrial and agricultural activities, such as mining and smelting operations, or from emissions from coal-fired power plants. The improper disposal of household products to soil, such as outdoor paints containing mercury, can also reach well water supplies. Historical mercury-based pesticides used on farms and orchards may leave high levels of mercury residue in the soil, which could transfer to well water since the initial application (often years prior). Some cultures use mercury in traditional medicines or religious practices.

Mercury does not break down in the environment. In the air, mercury may spread far from where it was released. Mercury can be present in drinking water from the erosion of natural deposits, discharges from refineries and factories, and runoff from landfills and croplands. When deposited into water bodies, mercury can be methylated by anaerobic bacteria producing a highly bioaccumulative form of organic mercury (methylmercury) that biomagnifies up the aquatic food web. For this reason, mercury can often be detected at high levels in fish and other aquatic organisms, rice, and other vegetation. Ingestion of plants and fish contaminated by methylmercury may cause adverse health effects including birth defects (Wahl and Finke 2001).

A common exposure to small amounts of mercury in homes occurs from broken light bulbs, thermostats, or thermometers. Inhalation is the primary risk from elemental (metallic) mercury exposure as it tends to readily volatilize once released in the environment. Occasionally a person may be exposed to high amounts of elemental mercury such as from collecting and storing mercury in containers that break. The U.S. EPA provides cleanup guidance when thermometers or mercury-containing light bulbs break in the home (U.S. EPA 2023b).

Mercury reacts with sulfhydryl groups resulting in enzyme inhibition and alteration of cellular membranes. The health effects of exposure to mercury depend on a number of factors including the amount and form of mercury, route and length of exposure, and person's age (Kosnett 2018b).

Signs and symptoms from inhalation of high concentrations of elemental mercury vapor may include cough, dyspnea, chest pain, nausea, vomiting, stomatitis, diarrhea, fever, and a metallic taste in the mouth. The clinician needs to watch for the development of interstitial pneumonitis, necrotizing bronchiolitis, and pulmonary edema after significant exposure. Children less than 30 months of age appear to be at increased risk for pulmonary toxicity. Renal manifestations include proteinuria, acute tubular necrosis, and oliguric renal failure. Conjunctivitis and an erythematous, pruritic rash have been reported with relatively mild exposure to mercury vapor (Kosnett 2018b).

According to ATSDR (2018) chronic mercury exposure primarily affects the central nervous system. Chronic exposure produces a classic triad of tremor, gingivitis, and erethism (insomnia, excessive shyness, and emotional lability). Other neuropsychological findings include headache, short-term memory loss, anorexia, incoordination, impaired vision, impaired learning, memory, and mood changes. Fine tremors in the fingers, eyelids, and lips are early signs of mercury toxicity. Other peripheral nervous system findings include distal paresthesias, motor and sensory nerve conduction delay, and limb weakness. Gingivitis, stomatitis, and excessive salivation may occur. Acrodynia, a nonallergic hypersensitivity reaction, may develop in children exposed to mercury vapors.

Some children born in communities that consumed food with high levels of organic mercury had learning, sensory, and movement problems. Many states have advisory levels on fish consumption due to methylmercury that concentrates in fish tissue. In children exposed to mercury, developmental milestones should be evaluated.

The blood Hg level for the 95th percentile of the U.S. population is below 5 μg/L; a blood concentration of 50 μg/L or greater is considered the threshold for symptoms of toxicity. Mercury has a short half-life in blood (3 days), so blood analysis may be performed during the first 3 days after an acute high-level exposure. After that, urine levels of mercury provide the most appropriate assessment of elemental mercury exposure and are useful for the assessment of acute and chronic exposures (Table 20.5).

Symptomatic patients who have experienced acute high-dose elemental mercury inhalation exposure should receive supportive care and be

Table 20.5 Relationship of urinary mercury concentration with health effects

Urinary mercury concentration (μg/L)	Signs and symptoms
<20	None
20–100	Decreased response on tests for nerve conduction, brain-wave activity, and verbal skills Early indication of tremor on testing
100–500	Irritability, depression, memory loss, minor tremor, other nervous system disturbances
	Early signs of disturbed kidney function
500–1000	Kidney inflammation
	Swollen gums
	Significant tremor and nervous system disturbances

monitored for the development of acute pneumonitis and pulmonary edema in a hospital setting. For severe symptoms and highly elevated levels of elemental mercury chelation treatment (such as DMSA (succimer), DMPS (unithol), BAL, and penicillamine) may be required (ATSDR 2018; Kosnett 2018b). Contact the Poison Center for the latest management guidelines.

If mercury is found in well water, then the installation of a treatment system is effective. Carbon or granular activated carbon (GAC) treatment systems, installed at the point of entry should be used to reduce levels of mercury in the well water. Exposure can also be reduced by using bottled water or connecting to a public water supply, where possible (N.C.DHHS 2022b).

Nitrates/Nitrites

The rural practitioner must be aware of the harmful and potentially fatal effects of nitrates/nitrites contamination of ground water. Pregnant females and infants are especially at risk from consuming nitrates/nitrites. High nitrate levels are usually due to human activities although sometimes they may naturally occur in the water.

Nitrates and nitrites form naturally in soil from the decomposition of soil organic matter, from the application of organic materials like animal manure and application of inorganic nitrogen fertilizers. Poultry and livestock feedlot operations produce large amounts of manure that can be a source of nitrate and nitrite from feedlot runoff or application as a soil amendment or fertilizer. Ground water contamination problems occur when nitrate and nitrite from these sources are over-applied to lawns, gardens, crop land, or pastures. If there is more nitrite and nitrate than plants can use, they can move easily through the soil with excess rainwater and can end up in groundwater. Other causes of well water contamination include improperly constructed or maintained wells that are located close to septic tanks, cesspools, or spray fields.

There are many potential health problems associated with high nitrate and nitrite levels in drinking water (ATSDR 2013). The toxic effects of nitrate are closely related to its conversion to nitrite by bacteria in the alimentary tract. Nitrate and nitrite can react with amines and amides to form N-nitroso compounds (NOC). These effects depend not only on dose but also on the concentration and type of bacteria present in the alimentary tract. The International Agency for Research on Cancer (IARC) noted that the presence of nitrite and some types of amines or amides in the acid environment of the stomach may result in the production of some cancer-causing N-nitroso compounds; under these conditions, IARC determined that ingested nitrate and nitrite is probably carcinogenic to humans (Group 2A) (IARC 2010).

High nitrate and nitrite levels can cause a condition called methemoglobinemia or "blue baby syndrome." Methemoglobinemia (MetHgb) is the primary adverse health effect associated with human exposure to nitrate or nitrite. To cause methemoglobinemia, nitrate must be converted to nitrite. Methemoglobinemia occurs when nitrite oxidizes the Fe^{2+}in hemoglobin to Fe^{3+}, a form that does not allow oxygen transport. Methemoglobinemia can lead to cyanosis (insufficient oxygenation of the blood characterized by bluish skin and lips), headaches, weakness, dizziness, difficulty breathing, and even death at high levels.

Methemoglobinemia in adults is rare. Due to oxidative stress, methemoglobin is continually produced within red blood cells, but its levels are kept low (0.5% to 2.5% of total hemoglobin) by enzymatic pathways that work to reduce methemoglobin. However certain groups of individuals are at higher risk of developing symptomatic methemoglobinemia. Infants under 4–6 months of age who have been fed formula mixed with nitrate-containing well water or food with a high nitrate content or who have diarrhea are at higher risk of developing methemoglobinemia. It should be remembered that boiling drinking water does not remove the nitrates/nitrites but instead may increase the concentration.

Other groups at higher risk of developing methemoglobinemia include pregnant females and individuals with hemoglobin variants or certain enzyme deficiencies, which are described later (ATSDR 2013).

Infants

Infants are at highest risk of developing methemoglobinemia due to a number of factors including the following:

- Infant Gut pH
  The high pH of the infant gastrointestinal system favors the growth of nitrate-reducing bacteria particularly in the stomach and especially after ingestion of contaminated waters. The stomach of adults is typically too acidic to allow for significant bacterial growth and the resulting conversion of nitrate to nitrite.
- HgbF
  A large proportion of hemoglobin in young infants is in the form of fetal hemoglobin. Fetal hemoglobin (Hgb F) is more readily oxidized to MetHb by nitrites than is adult hemoglobin. Over the first year of life, the adult forms of hemoglobin (Hgb A) gradually increase and Hgb F decreases. Infants with a higher proportion of fetal hemoglobin may have severely reduced oxygenation before cyanosis appears clinically. Therefore, infants, especially premature ones, are particularly susceptible.
- Impaired Reduction of MetHgb
  At birth, NADH-dependent methemoglobin reductase (also called cytochrome-b5 reductase), the major enzyme responsible for the reduction of induced methemoglobin back to normal hemoglobin, has only about half the activity it has in adults. The level of cytochrome-b5 reductase does not reach adult levels until at least 4 months of age.
- Other Factors
  Infection and inflammatory reactions can increase the endogenous synthesis of nitrate in both infants and adults. Gastroenteritis with vomiting and diarrhea can exacerbate nitrite formation in infants. Young infants can develop methemoglobinemia with systemic metabolic acidosis. The systemic metabolic acidosis is often caused by dehydration associated with diarrhea or sepsis, but it can occur with renal disorders.

It is important that the rural practitioner knows the differential diagnosis of cyanosis in the infant so that proper medical therapy can be provided. The differential diagnosis for cyanosis in an infant includes:

- Alveolar hypoventilation.
  - CNS depression (i.e., asphyxia, seizure, meningitis, encephalitis, intraventricular hemorrhage, drug-induced).
  - airway obstruction (i.e., choanal atresia, laryngomalacia),
  - neuromuscular disease (i.e., phrenic nerve injury, myasthenia gravis),
- Decreased oxygen-carrying capacity of blood (less oxygen available at tissue level).
  - Methemoglobinemia (acquired or congenital).
- Decreased peripheral circulation (peripheral cyanosis).
  - Sepsis.
  - Shock (any cause).
  - Polycythemia.
  - Hypothermia.
  - Hypoglycemia.
  - Low cardiac output (i.e., hypocalcemia, cardiomyopathy).
- Impaired oxygen diffusion.
  - Pulmonary edema (i.e., left-sided obstructive cardiac disease as seen with aortic stenosis, cardiomyopathy).
  - Pulmonary fibrosis.
- Right-to-left shunt.
  - Cardiac anomalies (i.e., tetralogy of Fallot, transposition of the great arteries, truncus arteriosus, total anomalous pulmonary venous return, tricuspid atresia, pulmonary atresia, hypoplastic left heart).
  - Persistent pulmonary hypertension of the newborn.
  - Pulmonary anomalies (i.e., pulmonary arteriovenous malformation).
- Ventilation/perfusion mismatch.
  - Airway disease (i.e., transient tachypnea of the newborn (TTN), respiratory distress syndrome (RDS), pneumonia, aspiration,

atelectasis, diaphragmatic hernia, pulmonary hypoplasia, pulmonary hemorrhage).
 - Extrinsic compression of the lungs (i.e., pneumothorax, pleural effusion, hemothorax).

In an infant with no known cardiopulmonary disease, cyanosis that is unresponsive to oxygen therapy is most likely due to methemoglobinemia.

Pregnancy

The pregnant woman and her fetus represent another high-risk group. Pregnancy is a high oxygen-demand physiologic state. An increase in intake and utilization of oxygen and increased levels of oxidative stress occurs. The hematologic changes of pregnancy include a 40–50% expansion of blood volume (plasma greater than RBC mass) at around 30 weeks. With plasma volume increasing more than the RBC mass, the maternal hematocrit falls reaching a nadir at 30 to 34 weeks resulting in a "physiologic anemia of pregnancy". The high oxygen demand and increased levels of oxidative stress of pregnancy may overwhelm the body's ability to reconvert methemoglobin back to hemoglobin, resulting in increased methemoglobin levels.

Exposure to nitrates also increases oxidative stress and depletes antioxidant reserves so that pregnant women may be more sensitive to the induction of clinical methemoglobinemia by nitrites or nitrates at or near the 30th week of pregnancy when oxidative stress peaks. Maternal exposure to environmental nitrates and nitrites may increase the risk of pregnancy complications, such as:

- Anemia.
- Threatened abortion/premature labor.
- Preeclampsia.

There are some reproductive outcome studies of high nitrate levels in the water supply that show some evidence of placental transfer of nitrate and nitrite. Recent epidemiologic data have suggested an association between developmental effects in offspring and the maternal ingestion of nitrate from drinking water, such as:

- Spontaneous abortions.
- Intrauterine growth restriction.
- Various birth defects.

Other Groups at Risk

An increased risk of developing methemoglobinemia from exposure to oxidizing agents has been reported in individuals with coexisting conditions including:

- Anemia, cardiovascular disease, lung disease, sepsis.
- Glucose-6-phosphate deficiency (more common in individuals of African, Asian, or Mediterranean descent).
- Metabolic problems with pyruvate kinase and RBC methemoglobin reductase.
- Presence of other abnormal hemoglobin species (structural abnormalities of the hemoglobin molecule itself) including carboxyhemoglobin, sulfhemoglobin, sickle hemoglobin (Hgb S).

The most useful diagnostic test for nitrate toxicity is a blood MetHgb level. This can accurately be determined using arterial blood gas measurements with co-oximetry. MetHgb levels are typically reported as a percentage of hemoglobin, symptoms may vary depending on the total hemoglobin level. Due to the large excess capacity of the blood to carry oxygen, levels of MetHgb up to 10% typically do not cause significant clinical signs in an otherwise healthy individual. A chocolate-brown or slate-gray central cyanosis—involving the trunk and proximal portions of the limbs, as well as the distal extremities, mucous membranes, and lips—is one of the hallmarks of methemoglobinemia and can become noticeable at a concentration of 10%–15% of total hemoglobin. As an easy- to- remember guideline, the treatment action level is often considered to be 20% MetHgb in symptomatic patients and 30% in asymptomatic patients. Patients that have significant concurrent problems that compromise oxygen delivery such as heart disease, lung disease, carbon monoxide poisoning, or anemia may need antidotal treatment at MetHgb levels as low as 10% (ATSDR 2023b). Signs and symptoms found in individuals with methemoglobinemia are noted in Table 20.6.

Treatment decisions must be made immediately once methemoglobinemia is recognized and confirmed. General principles of supportive care, with attention to removal of the cause, will suffice for most identified cases of methemoglobinemia. Proper fluid, electrolyte, and pH balance is vital, especially in infant methemoglobinemia complicated or caused by serious illness. Not all patients require specific antidotal therapy. Methylene blue is an effective antidote for most patients with methemoglobinemia (should be used with caution in patients with G6PD deficiency). Call the Poison Center for the latest advice on managing cases of methemoglobinemia.

The U.S. EPA has developed recommendations for exposure to nitrates/nitrites in drinking water. The Maximum Contaminant Level (MCL) for drinking water for nitrate is 10 mg/L, and nitrite is 1 mg/L. Both are based on the potential health effects of shortness of breath and blue baby syndrome in infants (U.S. EPA 2023l).

Table 20.6 Signs and symptoms of methemoglobinemia

Methemoglobin concentration (%)	Clinical findings
10–20	• Central cyanosis of limbs/trunk; often asymptomatic but may have weakness, tachycardia
20–35	• Central nervous system depression (headache, dizziness, fatigue) • Dyspnea • Nausea
35–55	• Lethargy • Syncope • Coma • Arrhythmias • Shock • Convulsions
>70	• High risk of mortality

From ATSDR (2023b)

There are several steps that can be taken if well tests high in nitrate (UGAE 2022).

- Determine the source of contamination and try to eliminate it. For example, apply only the amount of fertilizer or manure that plants can use.
- Make sure the wellhead is adequately protected.
- Install a point-of-use water treatment system such as an anion exchange resin, reverse osmosis, or a distillation system.
- Use bottled water for drinking and cooking.
- Switch to a public water supply.
- Retest to see if corrective actions or treatment systems are working.

Per- and Polyfluoroalkyl Substances (PFAS)

Per- and polyfluoroalkyl substances (PFAS) are a group of man-made chemicals that have been used in industry and consumer products since the 1940s because of their useful properties such as oil and water repellency, friction reduction, temperature resistance, and stain resistance. These compounds go by the moniker "forever chemicals." There are over 10,000 different PFAS. PFAS are characterized by a fully or partially fluorinated carbon chain, some with a hydrophilic tail. Some are characterized as long-chain compounds, and some are characterized as short-chain compounds. The carbon-fluorine bond is very strong which makes it persistent in the environment.

Of the thousands of PFAS compounds few have been studied as to their health and environmental effects. Perfluorooctanoic acid (PFOA) and Perfluorooctane sulfonate (PFOS) are two of the most widely used and studied chemicals in the PFAS group. The next most commonly studied are perfluorohexane sulfonic acid (PFHxS) and perfluorononanoic acid (PFNA). PFOA and PFOS are being replaced in the United States with other PFAS compounds. GenX chemicals are considered a replacement for PFOA, and perfluorobutane sulfonate

(PFBS) is considered a replacement for PFOS. One common characteristic of concern of PFAS is that many break down very slowly and can build up in people, animals, and the environment over time. Because of their widespread use and their persistence in the environment, PFAS are found in the blood of people and animals all over the world and are present at low levels in a variety of food products and in the environment. The United States Geological Survey (USGS) has found at least one PFAS could be detected in about 45% of U.S. drinking water samples (Smalling et al. 2023).

PFAS can be present in our water, soil, air, and food as well as in materials found in our homes or workplaces. Sources of PFAS compounds include:

- Biosolids —for example, fertilizer from wastewater treatment plants that is used on agricultural lands can affect ground and surface water and animals that graze on the land.
- Drinking water —in public drinking water systems and private drinking water wells.
- Fire extinguishing foam —in aqueous film-forming foams (AFFFs) used to extinguish flammable liquid-based fires. Such foams are used in training and emergency response events at airports, shipyards, military bases, firefighting training facilities, chemical plants, and refineries.
- Food —for example, in fish caught from water contaminated by PFAS and dairy products from livestock exposed to PFAS.
- Food packaging —for example in grease-resistant paper, fast food containers/wrappers, microwave popcorn bags, pizza boxes, and candy wrappers.
- Household products and dust —for example, in stain and water-repellent used on carpets, upholstery, clothing, and other fabrics; cleaning products; nonstick cookware; paints, varnishes, and sealants.
- Manufacturing or chemical production facilities that produce or use PFAS— for example, at chrome plating, electronics, and certain textile and paper manufacturers.
- Personal care products— for example, in certain shampoos, dental floss, and cosmetics.
- Soil and water at or near waste sites —at landfills, disposal sites, and hazardous waste sites such as those that fall under the federal Superfund and Resource Conservation and Recovery Act programs.

Most people in the United States and in other industrialized countries have measurable amounts of protein-bound and free PFAS in their blood. Some PFAS remain in the body for a long time. Most PFAS are not metabolized by the body. Biological half-life varies by chemical species. A few examples are: 2,3,4,5,6 PFBA—72 to 81 h; PFOA—2.1 to 10.1 years; PFOS—3.3 to 27 years; PFHxS—4.7 to 35 years. PFAS compounds like perfluorobutanoic acid (PFBA) with shorter carbon chains may have a shorter half-life. PFOS and PFOA are slowly eliminated through menstruation, breast milk, and feces but are primarily excreted in urine.

Environmental risks differ among PFAS based on their potential toxicity, mobility, and bioaccumulation. The risk of adverse effects in humans and wildlife depends on several factors, including the exposure dose, the frequency of exposure, the route and duration of exposure, and the time of exposure during the lifecycle (e.g., fetal development, early childhood).

Current peer-reviewed scientific studies have shown that exposure to certain levels of PFAS may lead to many adverse effects (ATSDR 2022; NAS 2022; U.S. EPA 2023e):

- Reproductive effects such as decreased fertility.
- Developmental effects or delays in children, including low birth weight, accelerated puberty, bone variations, or behavioral changes.
- Increased risk of some cancers, including prostate, kidney, and testicular cancers.
- Reduced ability of the body's immune system to fight infections, including reduced vaccine response.
- Interference with the body's natural hormones such as thyroid hormone.
- Increased cholesterol levels and/or risk of obesity.

- Decreased vaccine response in children.
- Changes in liver enzymes.
- Increased risk of high blood pressure or pre-eclampsia in pregnant women.
- Small decreases in infant birth weights.

Additional health effects noted include ulcerative colitis and thyroid toxicity (NAS 2022). Note many of these findings are associations and do not necessarily indicate causation.

There are certain groups of individuals that may be at increased risk of exposure and/or health risk from PFAS exposure. Industrial workers who are involved in making or processing PFAS or PFAS-containing materials, or fire fighters who use fire fighting foam, or people who live or recreate near PFAS-producing facilities or areas where PFAS contamination may have occurred such as farms where sewage sludge may have been applied, commercial airports, military bases, wastewater treatment plants, landfills, or incinerators that have received PFAS-containing waste. Pregnant and lactating women tend to drink more water per pound of body weight than the average person and as a result, they may have higher PFAS exposure compared to other people if it is present in their drinking water. Because children are still developing, they may be more sensitive to the harmful effects of chemicals such as PFAS. They can also be exposed more than adults because children drink more water, eat more food, and breathe more air per pound of body weight than adults, which can increase their exposure to PFAS. Young children crawl on floors and put things in their mouths which lead to a higher risk of exposure to PFAS in carpets, household dust, toys, and cleaning products.

Breast milk from mothers with PFAS in their blood and baby formula made with water containing PFAS can expose infants to PFAS, and it may also be possible for children to be exposed in-utero during pregnancy. Scientists continue to do research in this area. Based on current science, the benefits of breastfeeding appear to outweigh the risks for infants exposed to PFAS in breast milk (AAP 2019). To weigh the risks and benefits of breastfeeding, mothers should discuss them with their health care practitioner.

According to the recommendations from a recent panel of experts (NAS 2022), clinicians should offer PFAS testing to patients likely to have a history of elevated exposure. In all discussions of PFAS testing, clinicians should describe the potential benefits and harms of the testing and the potential clinical consequences (such as additional follow-up), related social implications, and limitations of the testing so that patient and clinician can make a shared, informed decision. Clinicians should use serum or plasma concentrations of the sum of PFAS (simple additive sum of MeFOSAA, PFHxS, PFOA (linear and branched isomers), PFDA, PFUnDA, PFOS (linear and branched isomers), and PFNA in serum or plasma). In case the laboratory does not include all these analytes, the sum of PFAS should include PFOA, PFOS, PFHxS, and PFNA as these four analytes are most commonly detected in the United States.

To inform clinical care of exposed patients, use the following guidelines/recommendations for interpretation (NAS 2022):

- Adverse health effects related to PFAS exposure are not expected at less than 2 ng/mL.
- There is a potential for adverse effects, especially in sensitive populations, between 2 and 20 ng/mL.
- There is an increased risk of adverse effects above 20 ng/mL.

Recommendation 1: Clinicians should treat patients with serum PFAS concentration below 2 ng/mL with the usual standard of care.

Recommendation 2: For patients with serum PFAS concentration of 2 ng/mL or higher and less than 20 ng/mL, clinicians should encourage PFAS exposure reduction if a source of exposure is identified, especially for pregnant persons. Within the usual standard of care, clinicians should:

- Prioritize screening for dyslipidemia with a lipid panel (once between 9 and 11 years of

age, and once every 4 to 6 years over age 20) as recommended by the American Academy of Pediatrics (AAP) and the American Heart Association (AHA).
- Screen for hypertensive disorders of pregnancy at all prenatal visits per the American College of Obstetricians and Gynecologists (ACOG).
- Screen for breast cancer based on clinical practice guidelines based on age and other risk factors such as those recommended by the U.S. Preventive Services Task Force (USPSTF).

Recommendation 3: For patients with serum PFAS concentration of 20 ng/mL or higher, clinicians should encourage PFAS exposure reduction if a source of exposure is identified, especially for pregnant persons. In addition to the usual standard of care, clinicians should:

- Prioritize screening for dyslipidemia with a lipid panel (for patients over age 2) following American Academy of Pediatrics (AAP) guidelines for high-risk children and American Heart Association (AHA) guidance for high-risk adults.
- At all well visits, conduct thyroid function testing (for patients over age 18) with serum thyroid stimulating hormone (TSH), assess for signs and symptoms of kidney cancer (for patients over 45), including with urinalysis, and for patients over 15, assess for signs and symptoms of testicular cancer and ulcerative colitis.

Because certain PFAS are known to cause risks to human health, the most important step you and your family can take to protect your health is to understand how to limit your exposure to PFAS (U.S. EPA 2023e). There are methods to reduce one's exposure to PFAS. The primary route to PFAS in nonoccupational settings is likely ingestion, which may include drinking contaminated water; eating seafood from contaminated water; or consuming other contaminated foods, such as vegetables, game, or dairy products.

If you get your water from a public drinking water system:

- Find out if PFAS are in your drinking water**:** If you get your water from a public drinking water system, reach out to your local water utility to learn about how they may be addressing PFAS as well as ask them to test the water for PFAS or to share information with you if they have already tested the water. Compare your results to your state's standards for safe levels of PFAS in drinking water. If your state does not have standards, compare your levels to EPA's Health Advisory levels for certain PFAS.
- If you remain concerned about the level of PFAS in your drinking water, you can:
  - Contact your state environmental protection agency or health department and your local water utility to find out what actions they recommend.
  - Consider installing in-home water treatment (e.g., filters) that is certified to lower the levels of PFAS in your water (N.C. DHHS 2022a; U.S. EPA 2018a).

If you get your water from a home drinking water well:

- Conduct regular well testing—for information on the overall quality of the water and whether it contains PFAS.
- Compare your results to your state standards for safe levels of PFAS in drinking water**.** If your state does not have standards, compare your levels to EPA's Health Advisory levels for PFOA and PFOS.
- If you remain concerned about the level of PFAS in your drinking water:
  - Contact your state environmental protection agency or health department and your local water utility to find out what actions they recommend.
  - If possible, consider using an alternate water source for drinking, preparing food, cooking, brushing teeth, preparing baby formula, and any other activity when your family might swallow water. Boiling water

does not remove PFAS. Studies have shown that only a small amount of PFAS can get into your body through your skin. Therefore, showering, bathing, and washing dishes in water containing PFAS are unlikely to significantly increase your risk.

- Consider installing an in-home water treatment (e.g., filters) that is certified to lower the levels of PFAS in your water (N.C. DHHS (2022c; U.S. EPA 2018a).

Steps You Can Take to Reduce Risk from Consuming Fish or Wildlife Contaminated with PFAS

Avoid eating fish from waterways impacted by PFAS. Check with your local or state health, environmental, or wildlife agencies for food/fish/wildlife consumption advisories in your area.

Steps You Can Take to Reduce Risk from Consumer Products Containing PFAS

Even though recent efforts to remove certain PFAS from commerce have reduced the likelihood of exposure, some household products and indoor air or dust may still contain PFAS. People can reduce the use of products containing PFAS, including packaged foods, products with nonstick or stain and water-resistant coatings, and some personal care products. Information about consumer products that have been identified as PFAS-free can be found at PFAS Central (https://pfascentral.org/pfas-free-products/) or Environmental Working Group (https://www.ewg.org/withoutintentionallyaddedpfaspfc). If you have questions about the products you use in your home, contact the Consumer Product Safety Commission at (800) 638-2772. The Federal Food and Drug Administration also has a testing program on PFAS and has the authority to recall products if levels of health concern are detected (U.S. FDA 2023).

Radon

Radon is a radioactive gas that forms naturally when uranium, thorium, or radium (which are radioactive metals) break down in rocks, soil, and groundwater. People can be exposed to radon primarily from breathing radon in air that typically moves up through the soil to the air above and into your home through cracks and other holes in the foundation. Your home traps radon inside, where it can build up. Sometimes radon enters the home through well water. In a small number of homes, the building materials can give off radon. However, building materials rarely cause radon problems by themselves (U.S. EPA 2023h).

Radon concentrations are measured in picocuries/liter (pCi/L). The average indoor radon level is about 1.3 picocuries per liter (pCi/L) in the air in the United States. The average outdoor level is about 0.4 pCi/L. In 2005, the U.S. Surgeon General issued a Health Advisory warning Americans about the health risks from exposure to radon in indoor air. The Surgeon General urged Americans to test their homes to find out how much radon they might be breathing and also stressed the need to remedy the problem as soon as possible when the radon level is 4 pCi/L or more (U.S. DHHS 2005).

The U.S. EPA recommends homes be fixed if the radon level is ≥4 pCi/L. Because there is no known safe level of exposure to radon, EPA also recommends that Americans consider fixing their home for radon levels between 2 pCi/L and 4 pCi/L. Elevated radon levels are found in 1 in 15 homes in the United States. While certain areas of the country have higher radon levels due to local geology, without measurement you cannot know the actual level of radon in your home/building. The level in an individual's home may be elevated while his neighbors' level is within acceptable limits. Therefore, it is important that homes are tested for radon.

Radon is a carcinogen and is the second leading cause of lung cancer behind tobacco smoking. It is estimated that 21,000 cases of lung cancer in the United States are due to radon (about 12–13% of lung cancers in the United States). Additionally, a few cancers of stomach cancer may be due to ingestion of radon in ground water.

For smokers the risk of lung cancer is significant due to the synergistic effects of radon and smoking. For this population about 62 people in a

Table 20.7 Radon risk of lung cancer in smokers[a]

Radon level	If 1000 people who smoked are exposed to this level over a lifetime
20 pCi/L	About 260 people could get lung cancer
10 pCi/L	About 150 people could get lung cancer
8 pCi/L	About 120 people could get lung cancer
4 pCi/L	About 62 people could get lung cancer
2 pCi/L	About 32 people could get lung cancer
1.3 pCi/L	About 20 people could get lung cancer
0.4 pCi/l	About 3 people could get lung cancer
0 pCi/L	Calculated absence of risk

Note: If you are a former smoker, your risk could be lower
[a]Lifetime risk of lung cancer deaths from EPA Assessment of Risks from Radon in Homes (EPA 402-R-03-003)

Table 20.8 Radon risk of lung cancer in nonsmokers[a]

Radon level	If 1000 people who did not smoke were exposed to this level over a lifetime…[a]
20 pCi/L	About 36 persons could get lung cancer
10 pCi/L	About 18 persons could get lung cancer
8 pCi/L	About 15 persons could get lung cancer
4 pCi/L	About 7 persons could get lung cancer
2 pCi/L	About 4 persons could get lung cancer
1.3 pCi/L	About 2 persons could get lung cancer
0.4 pCi/L	On average, fewer than 1 person (0.7) could get lung cancer
0 pCi/L	Calculated absence of risk

Note: If you are a former smoker, your risk may be higher
[a]Lifetime risk of lung cancer deaths from EPA Assessment of Risks from Radon in Homes (EPA 402-R-03-00)

Table 20.9 Treatment methods to remove radionuclide contaminants in well water

Treatment	Uranium	Radium	Radon	Gross alpha	Gross beta
Ion exchange[a]	X	X			X
Reverse osmosis	X	X		X	X
Surface and decay storage			X		
Aeration system			X		
Granular activated carbon			X		

Source: N.C. DHHS (2022c)
[a]The type of ion exchange depends on contaminants detected and location of treatment system (point of entry or point of use)

1000 will die of lung cancer, compared to 7.3 people in a 1000 for never smokers. The following Tables 20.7 and 20.8 show the lifetime risk of lung cancer in smokers and nonsmokers exposed to different levels of radon in their home (U.S. EPA 2012).

Testing for radon is relatively easy and can be done by the home occupant. Most radon tests last between 2 and 7 days. Many local home improvement or hardware stores sell test kits. Test kits can also be ordered online. The state radon office may offer testing kits (varies by state). You also can hire a qualified tester to do a radon test for you. Kansas State University, under a cooperative agreement with EPA, provides national radon program services, including selling radon test kits and answering toll-free radon hotlines. For more information about radon testing call 1–800-SOS-RADON (1-800-767-7236) or visit www.epa.gov/radon/find-radon-test-kit-or-measurement-andmitigation-professional.

There are several proven methods to reduce radon in homes/buildings. One frequently used method is a vent pipe system and fan, which pulls radon from beneath the house and vents it to the outside. Sealing foundation cracks and other openings makes this kind of system more effective and cost-efficient. If planning a structural renovation, such as converting an unfinished basement area into a living space, it is especially important to test the area for radon before beginning the renovation and after the work is completed (U.S. EPA 2000).

If radon or other radionuclides are detected at elevated levels in well water, there are water treatment methods to remove these contaminants as noted in Table 20.9 (N.C. DHHS 2022c).

Lowering high radon levels requires technical knowledge and special skills. It may be difficult to lower levels below 2 pCi/L. Check with your state radon office for names of qualified or state-certified radon contractors in your area. You can also contact private radon proficiency programs for lists of privately certified radon professionals in your area. A good source of information that the rural practitioner can provide to his/her patients available from the U.S. EPA is the "Consumer's Guide to Radon Reduction" (U.S. EPA 2016).

Silica

In general, agricultural dusts may be divided into those of organic and inorganic origin. Organic dusts originate from plant and animal sources and are commonly the source of allergic diseases such as asthma. Inorganic dusts originate predominantly from the soil and tend to result in nonallergic reactions in the lung (Schenker 2000). The composition of inorganic dust in agriculture generally reflects the soil composition. The mineral fraction of most soils is dominated by silicates. Soils of very arid climates are exceptions; there the inorganic fraction may be dominated by calcium carbonate and more soluble salts (evaporites). Very highly weathered soils of warm, humid climates, where oxides and hydroxides of iron (goethite and hematite) and aluminum (gibbsite) predominate, are also exceptions.

Silicate is a generic term for compounds that contain silicon, oxygen, and one or more metals. Naturally occurring silicate minerals make up nearly 90% of the earth's crust. Silicates are classified on the basis of how extensively the silica is polymerized. Generally, the more highly polymerized the structure, the more resistant to chemical weathering. Silica refers to a specific chemical compound, silicon dioxide, with the chemical formula SiO_2. Quartz is a naturally occurring crystalline mineral that primarily consists of silica but contains some impurities. Quartz is the main form in which silica is found in nature. Respirable quartz is found in soil dust. In some agricultural environments crystalline silica may represent up to 20% of the soil composition, and human exposures to these dusts represent a risk for interstitial fibrosis. Other silicates (up to 80% of soil samples) may also cause or contribute to pulmonary fibrosis (mixed-dust pneumoconiosis), although they are less fibrogenic than crystalline silica. Weathering and chemical reactions may make silica in soil less fibrogenic than freshly fractured quartz in other occupations such as mining, quarrying, and sandblasting (Schenker 2000).

Occupational exposure to respirable crystalline silica (RCS) is regulated by most countries by the time-weighted average (TWA). The TWA is the average concentration of an airborne substance encountered over an average work week of 40 h. Generally, the accepted exposure limit of RCS is between 0.05 mg/m^3 and 0.1 mg/m^3. However, even at exposure levels equal to a TWA of 0.05 mg/m^3 over a working career of 40 to 45 years, workers still had a significant risk of at least 1 in 100 developing radiographic silicotic lung disease. Clinically significant exposures to inorganic dusts may occur in agriculture. Such exposures are most common in so-called dry-climate farming, i.e., areas where rainfall occurs for only a few months of the year and agriculture is watered by man-made irrigation. Tractors pulling soil preparation implements may generate tremendous dust clouds. In such locations farming activities that perturb the soil (e.g., plowing, tilling) commonly result in exposures to farm operators of 1–5 mg/m^3 respirable dust, and total dust exposures of 20 mg/m^3 or more are commonly observed, but exposures in an open cab can range up to 80 to more than 100 mg/m^3. These exposure concentrations have been observed to cause chronic bronchitis in other industrial settings and are likely to explain in part the increase in chronic bronchitis observed in agriculture, particularly in areas of dry-climate farming.

The respirable form of silica is small enough to reach the terminal bronchioles and alveoli of the respiratory system. Typical immune mechanisms cannot clear these particles from the lung, initiating a pathologic cycle of inflammation and parenchymal damage that ultimately leads to silicosis. Occupational exposure to crystalline silica has been linked to silicosis, some forms of cancer, kidney disease, and certain autoimmune diseases. Silicosis and silica dust-associated tuberculosis (TB), in particular, are the two diseases that remain high on the list of occupational health priorities in low-income countries and that still occur in some high-income countries (Rees and Murray 2007). Three types of silicosis are described, namely, chronic or ordinary simple silicosis, accelerated silicosis, and acute silicosis (Peters 1986, Redlich and Balmes 1995).

Chronic silicosis, the most commonly encountered form of silicosis, is also known as classic silicosis and may be simple or complicated. Chronic silicosis occurs from exposure to low concentrations of silica dust after 10 to 30 years of exposure. Chest X-ray (CXR) findings usually are first noted at 20 years after initial exposure to <30% silica in dust. Fibrotic nodules located near respiratory bronchioles and hilar lymphadenopathy are noted. Radiographic findings differentiate between simple and complicated chronic silicosis. Simple chronic silicosis is also called nodular silicosis, characterized by pulmonary nodules less than 10 mm in diameter. Patients with simple chronic silicosis are frequently asymptomatic but may present with a dry cough or dyspnea on exertion. Simple silicosis may transition to complicated silicosis as the nodules progress. Complicated chronic silicosis is also known as pulmonary massive fibrosis (PMF). PMF develops when the pulmonary nodules expand and fuse to form conglomerate masses with a diameter of greater than 10 mm. PMF is usually located in the upper lung zones. Chronic silicosis is usually asymptomatic and diagnosed by CXR. Pulmonary function tests (PFT) can be normal or demonstrate mild restriction and or mild obstruction. Chronic complicated silicosis (PMF) may present with significant dyspnea on exertion, malaise, anorexia, and weight loss. Reduced lung volumes and diffusing capacity, arterial desaturation with exercise, pulmonary hypertension, and cor pulmonale may result due to the profound destruction of lung tissue (Baum and Arnold 2023).

Accelerated silicosis occurs 4–8 years after exposure to moderately high dust concentrations. The usual exposure duration is 5–15 years and the percent silica in dust is usually 47–84%. Fibrotic nodules are smaller than those in classical silicosis. Progressive massive fibrosis is more rapid in progression, occurs more frequently, and is found in the mid-zones of the lungs.

Acute silicosis is rare and occurs in workers exposed to very high concentrations of silica. Concentrations of silica in the dust may be as high as 90–100%. CXR changes may be noted 1–3 years after first exposure. On pathology, diffuse interstitial fibrosis and alveolar lipoproteinosis occur. Patients present with marked dyspnea, fever, cough, and weight loss. Usually, rapid progression to respiratory failure occurs.

Although studies show that farming activities in sandy soils can produce respirable silica levels well above generally accepted safe levels, silica-associated diseases are rarely reported in agricultural workers. The paucity of cases may be because silica potency is reduced by other soil components such as iron oxides and clay silicates. In addition, silica in soils is likely to be aged, with most farming activities producing little freshly fractured material. Under-diagnosis is also a possible explanation. While fibrosis has been observed in case reports of agricultural workers, the prevalence and clinical severity of these cases are unknown.

There is no cure for silicosis. Most interventions are supportive and consist of supplemental oxygen in those with hypoxia, recommended vaccinations, prompt treatment of infection, and pulmonary rehabilitation. Cigarette smoking adds to the lung damage caused by silicosis. Quitting smoking is an important part of managing the disease. The primary modality for the treatment of end-stage silicosis is a lung transplant (Baum and Arnold 2023).

Veterinary Medications

Veterinarians, veterinary technicians, animal handlers, livestock producers, farmers, and farm workers use a variety of veterinary medications daily to treat animals either at the veterinary clinic or on-site where the animal is housed and raised. There are over 5000 approved prescription and over-the-counter medications, as well as vaccines, with labeled indications for veterinary patients (Lust et al. 2011). Many veterinary products can be purchased by the lay person without a veterinarian prescription. This often results in the use of veterinary products under little or no professional supervision/control, increasing the risk that the medication, many of which are harmful to humans, to be inappropriately used, including for self-treatment, especially with analgesics and anti-inflammatory agents, antibiotics (systemic and topical), and topical corticosteroids (Erramouspe et al. 2002). There is also concern that these pharmaceutical agents which are excreted in urine and feces and subsequently applied to fields (manure fertilizer) may run off into surface waters and support the development of antibiotic-resistant organisms.

Persons working with and treating animals may be exposed to hazardous drugs when they handle drug vials; compound, administer, or dispose of hazardous drugs; clean up spills; touch surfaces that are contaminated with these drugs; or clean bedding, cages, kennels, or waste of treated animals. Skin absorption, inhalation, and ingestion are the most likely ways these workers may be exposed. Needlestick or sharp injuries pose a risk of exposure in veterinary health care and in farm settings (NIOSH 2010). Many hazardous drugs and their metabolites can be excreted in urine and feces for up to 72 h or more or may be present in vomitus for several hours. There are several products that have significant adverse human health effects upon accidental or intentional exposure or ingestion, such as carfentanil, clenbuterol (Trade name Ventipulmin), ketamine, tilmicosin (Trade name Micotil), testosterone/estradiol (Trade names Component E-H and Synovex H), dinoprost (Trade name Lutalyse/Prostamate), and cloprostenol (Trade name Estromate/EstroPlan), and are explained in more detail later (Lust et al. 2011). The hazards range from mild to life-threatening in terms of severity, and include bronchospasm, central nervous system stimulation, induction of miscarriage, and sudden death. In 2021 the American Association of Poison Control Centers reported 7825 calls from exposure to veterinary drugs without a human equivalent with 463 people treated in a health care facility and 92 of these having moderate to severe adverse effects (Gummin et al. 2022).

Many veterinary agents are used to enhance the immunity to infectious diseases (Donham and Thelin 2016b). These agents are often referred to as biologicals and include antisera, bacterins, vaccines, adjuvants, toxoids, and antitoxins. Most are delivered by inoculation although some may be delivered by aerosol (e.g., Newcastle poultry vaccine). Accidental needle sticks from these biologicals may result in infection (e.g., live vaccines for Contagious ecthyma, Erysipelas, Brucellosis), inflammation from the product (many adjuvants are highly inflammatory and contain mineral oils or mycobacterial cell components used in the adjuvant), or cause a hyperimmune response to which the person has previously been exposed (e.g., person had previous Brucella infection and subsequently exposed to Brucella vaccine). As the same needles are often used to treat multiple animals, they also may be contaminated by bacteria on the animals' hide and accidentally injected leading to infection in the person performing the vaccination.

A variety of antibiotics are used on the farm. These are not only used to treat infection in the animal but may be used to prevent infection in herds and flocks and as an animal growth promotor. Potential adverse effects to humans from antibiotic exposure include direct toxicity from the antibiotic, allergic reaction to the antibiotic, and development of antibiotic-resistant organisms and infections (Donham and Thelin 2016b). Some of the common antibiotics used as growth promoters in animal feed include penicillin, tetracycline, sulfamethazine, and virginiamycin. Dermal and respiratory exposure can occur when feed containing antibiotics is ground, mixed, and handled. Cases of allergic contact dermatitis or asthma may occur (Donham and Thelin 2016b).

One of the more dangerous veterinary medications to humans is the antibiotic tilmicosin (Trade name Micotil 300). This is a prescription injectable antibiotic used to treat respiratory infections in cattle and sheep. It was approved for use in the United States in 1992 and has resulted in over 2200 adverse event reports and 25 deaths in humans (U.S. FDA 2017). Routes of exposure include accidental injection or exposure to the mouth, eyes, or skin to the liquid preparation. Eye pain, burning sensations of the mouth, bad taste, pain, and swelling at the site of injection are symptoms that have been reported. Injection injuries have resulted in severe cardiovascular toxicity due to its calcium channel-blocking effects including tachycardia, decreased heart contractility, and abnormal electrocardiograms, which may lead to death. There is no antidote although most people fully recover. If an exposure by any route has occurred, immediately contact the local/ regional Poison Center for advice (1-800-222-1222). The National Institute for Occupational Safety and Health (NIOSH) has developed recommendations to prevent human exposure to the use of this product (NIOSH 2007).

Reproductive hazards common in the veterinary workplace can be categorized as chemical, biological, and physical hazards. Working with animals (either in the clinic or on the farm) may present a special risk to females, especially if they are pregnant. Chemical hazards include contact with antineoplastic drugs, hormones, pesticides, and anesthetic gases; biological hazards include zoonotic and other infectious agents; and physical hazards include animal-related injuries, radiation exposure, demanding work conditions, and physical work load, needle sticks, and psychosocial hazards from workplace stress, long work hours, and other factors that affect mental well-being (Meggs 1999; Meyer 1999; Scheftel et al. 2017).

Antineoplastic pharmaceuticals, primarily used to treat cancer in dogs and cats, are important reproductive hazards found in the veterinary setting. Many antineoplastic drugs have been reported to be carcinogenic, mutagenic, or teratogenic and have been associated with reduced fertility, spontaneous abortion, and fetal loss (Smith et al. 2018). While there have not been many studies on veterinarians specifically, health care workers (e.g., pharmacy employees, nurses) handling chemotherapeutics (including preparation, administration, and clean up) have been found to have variably increased chromosomal aberrations compared to the general population, as well as urinary excretion of these drugs or their metabolites, which could lead to similar reproductive complications found in cancer patients treated with cytotoxic drugs. Chromosome changes appear to be exposure- and drug-dependent, with high-volume practice and alkylators being associated with the most abnormalities. Some studies have shown an incremental increased risk of infertility and early pregnancy loss with occupational exposure to chemotherapeutics. Additionally, the chance of developing some cancers might be increased. The addition of protective measures such as biologic safety cabinets (BSCs), closed system transfer devices (CSTDs), and personal protective equipment (PPE) markedly decreases, but does not always eliminate, evidence of drug contamination. Smith et al. (2018) provide guidelines on ways veterinary offices can decrease risks of exposure to chemotherapeutic agents.

Beginning in the 1960s and 1970s, there was substantial concern about the effects of inhaled anesthetic gases on reproduction in health care workers. The waste anesthetic gases and vapors of concern are nitrous oxide and halogenated agents (vapors) such as halothane, enflurane, isoflurane, and desflurane (Meyer 1999). Some potential effects of exposure to waste anesthetic gases are nausea, dizziness, headaches, fatigue, and irritability, as well as sterility, miscarriages, birth defects, cancer, and liver and kidney disease, among operating room staff or their spouses (in the case of miscarriages and birth defects). At the present time, owing to the almost universal adoption of scavenging systems, the reproductive risk from occupational exposure to inhalation anesthetics in veterinary personnel appears to be low. Nevertheless, it remains prudent to recommend control measures that reduce occupational exposure. Occupational Safety and Health Administration (OSHA) and NIOSH published recommendations for reducing exposure and risk (NIOSH 2007; OSHA 2000).

Hormones are often used for growth promotion or estrous synchronization in livestock, especially cattle. Hormones used may include estrogens, progesterone, androgens/testosterones, growth hormones, and anabolic steroids. Reproductive hormones used in contemporary veterinary practice are especially hazardous to pregnant women. Oxytocin causes uterine contractions and milk "let down" from mammary glands and is most commonly used in swine and cattle that are having difficulty delivering. Prostaglandins such as dinoprost tromethamine (Trade name Lutalyse) and cloprostenol (Trade name Estromate/EstroPlan) are used in cattle and swine to terminate early pregnancy, to induce parturition in later stages of pregnancy, and to induce an animal "cycle" (estrus). Exposure of pregnant humans to these agents may lead to an abortion/miscarriage. Prostaglandins may also cause difficulty breathing, chest tightness, and respiratory irritation with coughing, wheezing, and sputum production, and may cause eye irritation and can be absorbed through the skin. Prolonged skin contact may cause temporary irritation (Zoetis 2017; MSD 2023). Misoprostol (Trade name Cytotec) is a synthetic prostaglandin has been used in equine reproduction and to treat or reduce risk of ulcers in dogs, cats, and horses taking nonsteroidal anti-inflammatory agents. It is an abortifacient and can cause birth defects, premature births, and miscarriage (Krugh and Maani 2023). Prostaglandins exposure is a risk to individuals with asthma (Donham and Thelin 2016b). Use of these reproductive hormones requires meticulous care and training.

Contact with chemical and biological agents can cause skin dermatitis (irritant or allergic contact dermatitis) or even infections (from live vaccines or zoonotic agents). Many feed additives may contain trace metals and antibiotics used as growth promoters. Table 20.10 shows veterinary pharmaceuticals and feed additives that can cause dermatitis in humans (Meggs 1999). An unexplained rash or dermatitis should be referred to an allergist or dermatologist for evaluation and possibly patch testing. Contact dermatitis can be prevented or reduced by the use of personal protective equipment such as gloves (preferably non-latex), and protective clothing. These should be changed if visibly contaminated. Washing hands and exposed skin with soap and water, (if possible, immediately after handling any pharmaceutical or animal feed), and washing hands before eating and at the end of the work day should be routinely practiced. Wash work clothing separately to protect other family members from residues that may be on work clothing.

Unfortunately, several veterinary medications are now being illicitly used. Some of the more common agents recently detected in human overdoses and which are briefly described include xylazine, ketamine, levamisole, clenbuterol, and fentanyl/carfentanil.

Xylazine (also called "tranq" or "tranq dope") is a non-opioid sedative or tranquilizer. Although not a controlled substance in the United States, xylazine is not approved for use in people. Adulteration of heroin and fentanyl with xylazine is increasingly occurring (D'Orazio et al. 2023).

Table 20.10 Veterinary pharmaceuticals and animal feed additives that cause dermatitis in humans

Bacitracin	Furazolidone	Phenothiazines
Benzocaine	Hydroquinone	Piperazine
Bronopol	Halquinol	Procaine
Carbamate pesticides	Latex	Quindoxin
Dinitolmide	Mercaptobenzothiazole	Quinoxaline
Chlorpromazine	Merthiolate	Spiramycin
Chromate	Neomycin	Sulfacetamide
3,5 Dinitro-o-toluamide	Nitrofurazone	Sulfamethazine
Ethoxyquin	Olaquindox	Thiobendazole
Ethylene diamine	Oxytetracycline	Tylosin
Ethylenediamine dihydroiodine	Penethamate	Virginiamycin
Formalin		

Source: Meggs (1999)

When used in people, xylazine can cause sedation, difficulty breathing, dangerously low blood pressure, slowed heart rate, wounds that can become infected, severe withdrawal symptoms, and death (CDC 2023b).

Fentanyl is an opiate narcotic used to treat moderate to severe pain in humans and animals. Fentanyl and fentanyl analogs are increasingly involved in opioid overdose deaths, and new fentanyl analogs continue to be identified. Carfentanil, ("elephant tranquilizer") the most potent fentanyl analog detected in the United States, is intended for sedation of large animals and is estimated to have 10,000 times the potency of morphine. It has recently been reported in an alarming number of deaths in some states, primarily from illegal import and adulteration of heroin (O'Donnell et al. 2018). It is no longer FDA-approved for animal use in the United States. Alternatives used by wildlife veterinarians include thiafentanil and etorphine, both 3000–5000 times more potent than morphine and pose a potential hazard to persons who work with them (McReynolds 2023).

Ketamine "Special K" is an injectable anesthetic used for general anesthesia as a primary anesthetic and for introducing inhalant anesthesia in veterinary medicine and human medicine. It is also being researched as a treatment for depression. According to the Drug Enforcement Administration ketamine is a dissociative anesthetic that has some hallucinogenic effects. It distorts perceptions of sight and sound and makes the user feel disconnected and not in control. It is referred to as a "dissociative anesthetic" because it makes patients feel detached from their pain and environment. Ketamine can induce a state of sedation (feeling calm and relaxed), immobility, relief from pain, and amnesia (no memory of events while under the influence of the drug). It is abused for its ability to produce dissociative sensations and hallucinations. Ketamine has also been used to facilitate sexual assault (DEA 2020).

Levamisole, a product used to treat parasite infections in animals, has been found as an adulterant in fentanyl and cocaine. There are several reasons as to why levamisole is used to adulterate cocaine. It likely has a cocaine-potentiating effect through inhibition of catecholamine breakdown. By affecting catechol-*O*-methyltransferase and monoamine oxidase, levamisole is believed to potentiate the euphoric effects of cocaine due to increased dopamine activity. A metabolite of levamisole, aminorex, also has amphetamine-like stimulant properties. Levamisole toxicity presents clinically with nonspecific flu-like symptoms, leukopenia, and vasculitis with organ damage to the kidneys or lungs, and potentially serious skin manifestations, ranging from macular cutaneous eruptions to extensive necrosis (Cherlopalle et al. 2016; Vagi et al. 2013).

Some veterinary products are being used illicitly by body builders to build muscle mass. Clenbuterol "clen" (Trade name Ventipulmin) is a beta-2 adrenergic receptor agonist with a rapid onset and long duration of action and used to treat airway obstruction in animals. Most adverse health effects are related to its stimulation of beta-2 adrenergic receptors and clinical manifestations, including hypokalemia, hyperglycemia, hyperlactemia, agitation, tachycardia, and hypotension. Recently cases have been described of poisoning from clenbuterol associated with reported heroin use (CDC 2005; Wingert et al. 2008). The anabolic steroid Trenbelone (also known as trienolone or trienbolone) has been used illicitly in humans to build muscle and metabolize fat and so have the compounds testosterone/estradiol (Trade names Component E-H and Synovex H) (Lust et al. 2011).

Well Water Contamination

Many rural areas and farms rely on ground water from private wells for their personal use and to provide water for the crops and animals. If the well is not properly constructed and maintained, it is at risk of contamination from both chemicals (e.g., fertilizers and pesticides) as well as microbial agents (animal waste runoff). Some contaminants may be especially dangerous for certain high-risk populations such as small children, pregnant women, the elderly, or individuals with compromised immune systems such as people on chemotherapy or with a chronic infection. The rural practitioner may be presented with a patient's well test results and asked for help interpreting them. An understanding of some of the basic well water terminology/testing is provided later.

Groundwater contaminants can come from natural sources and processes (e.g., radionuclides, arsenic) as well as human (e.g., fertilizers, pesticides, gasoline) and animal sources (manure). Groundwater flow is subject to change, which means the distribution and concentration of contaminants in an area may change as well. While the presence of some contaminants can be detected because they change the taste, smell, or appearance of the water, others may only be detected by laboratory testing.

The degree of risk from contact with a contaminant in drinking water depends upon how you are exposed, the length of time that you are in contact with the contaminant, and the amount of the contaminant to which you are exposed, as well as individual susceptibility. The presence of chemical or microbial agents in well water may increase the risk of an adverse outcome. Some contaminants, such as *Escherichia coli* bacteria, may cause short-term illnesses such as gastrointestinal upset with nausea, vomiting, and diarrhea. Whereas long-term exposure to elevated levels of chemical contaminants in drinking water may increase the risk of chronic diseases such as anemia, high blood pressure, and in some cases, cancer.

The U.S. EPA regulates public water supplies. National Primary Drinking Water Regulations NPDWRs (or primary standards) are legally enforceable standards that apply to public water systems. Primary standards protect public health by limiting the levels of contaminants in drinking water. NSDWRs (or secondary standards) are non-enforceable guidelines regulating contaminants that may cause cosmetic effects (such as skin or tooth discoloration) or aesthetic effects (such as taste, odor, or color) in drinking water. The U.S. EPA recommends secondary standards to water systems but does not require systems to comply with the standard. However, states may choose to adopt them as enforceable standards.

The U.S. EPA estimates that more than 23 million households rely on private wells for drinking water in the United States (U.S. EPA 2023k). The U.S. EPA does not regulate private wells nor does it provide recommended criteria or standards for individual wells but offers information regarding the importance of testing private wells and guidance on technologies that may be used to treat or remove any contaminants (U.S. EPA 2023a). Levels established for public water supplies may serve as guidance for health care practitioners if asked to evaluate a patient's well results.

Wells can be tested for a variety of chemicals and microbial contamination. Some of the routine well water tests include pH, alkalinity, water hardness, total dissolved solids (TDS) and total coliform bacteria. In rural areas and or farms, occasionally wells are tested for nitrates/nitrites and pesticides.

pH is classified as a secondary contaminant by the U.S. EPA with a suggested range of 6.5 to 8.5. pH is a measurement of the concentration of hydrogen ions or the acidity of water. Alkalinity is the ability of the water to neutralize or buffer changes in acidity. pH levels and total alkalinity depend on the amount of minerals like carbonate, bicarbonate, and hydroxide in groundwater. pH values below 6.5 may indicate corrosive water which can mobilize metals from pipes. For pH values below 6.5, consider a corrosivity test and/or a test for metals (especially lead and copper) in the water. High alkalinity may lead to scaling in pipes and water heaters. This can shorten the life of water heaters and cause troublesome buildup on fixtures and appliances. Water softening is a common household treatment technique to address scaling issues.

High and low levels of pH can cause gastrointestinal problems. pH less than 4 can cause skin and eye irritation and pH > 10 can cause hair damage.

TDS is basically the sum of all minerals, metals, and salts dissolved in the water and is a good general indicator of water quality. TDS is classified as a secondary contaminant by the U.S. Environmental Protection Agency and a suggested maximum for drinking water is

500 mg/L. This secondary standard is set because elevated TDS can give water a murky appearance and detract from the taste quality of the water. People not accustomed to water with high TDS may experience gastrointestinal irritation from drinking the water.

Total hardness is a measurement of dissolved minerals in the water. Hard water has high levels of calcium, magnesium, and other metals (these elements occur naturally in underground rocks). Total hardness is the sum of the calcium and magnesium concentrations, both expressed as calcium carbonate, in milligrams per liter (mg/L.) (N.C. DHHS 2019a). The degree of water hardness can be ranges from soft to very hard.

General guidelines for classification of water hardness are (USGS 2018):

0 to 60 mg/L as soft
61 to 120 mg/L as moderately hard
121 to 180 mg/L as hard
>180 mg/L as very hard.

Hard water may cause dry skin and itchy scalp. Individuals with medical conditions such as milk-alkali syndrome and hypercalcemia may be affected by drinking water with high calcium content. In addition, persons with kidney disease may be affected by drinking water with high magnesium as it may cause diarrhea or have laxative effects (N.C. DHHS 2019a). Cation exchange (water softener) treatment systems can be used to reduce the levels of total hardness, calcium and magnesium in well water.

Coliform bacteria are found in soil and surface water. Total coliform bacteria water test measures all coliform bacteria in water including fecal coliforms. *E. coli* is a type of fecal coliform that can cause illness in humans and animals. There are several strains of this bacteria. Coliform bacteria can enter the well water if the well is poorly constructed, cracked or unsealed or during times of flooding that may inundate the well. Total coliforms and *E. coli* are used as indicators for the presence of disease-causing organisms that may be present in well water including other bacteria, helminths (roundworms, tapeworms), viruses (polio, hepatitis), and protozoa (*Entamoeba histolytica*).

If the well is contaminated with microbial organisms, shock chlorination is often used to treat the well. If contamination persist ultraviolet filtration systems can be installed to reduce microbial contamination. Local and State environmental health officials can assist you in evaluating and treating well water.

If your patient is complaining about their drinking water, a quick list of potential reasons is provided in Table 20.11 (U.S. EPA 2002).

Table 20.12 lists common conditions or nearby activities that well owners should be aware of and the substance(s) that you should consider testing to ensure your well is safe. Not all of the substances listed pose an immediate or long-term health problem, some impact quality of life only

Table 20.11 Quick reference list of noticeable problems with your water

1. Visible issues
Scale or scum from calcium or magnesium salts in water
Unclear/turbid water from dirt/clay salts, silt, or rust in water
Green stains on sink or faucets caused by high acidity
Brown-red stains on sink, dishwasher, or clothes in wash suggest dissolved iron in water
Cloudy water that clears upon standing may have bubbles from poorly working pump or filter problem
2. Taste issues
Salty or brackish taste from high sodium content in water
Alkali/soapy taste from dissolved alkaline minerals in water
Metallic taste from acidity or high iron content in water
Chemical taste from industrial chemicals or pesticides
3. Smell issues
A rotten egg odor can be from dissolved hydrogen sulfide gas or certain bacteria in the water. If the smell only comes with hot water, it is likely from a part in your hot water heater
A detergent odor and water that foams when drawn could be seepage from septic tanks into your ground water well
A gasoline or oil smell indicates fuel oil or gasoline likely seeping from a tank into the water supply
Methane gas or musty/earthy smell may occur from decaying organic matter in water
A chlorine smell from excess chlorination

Source: U.S. EPA (2002)

Table 20.12 Reasons to test well water based on nearby environmental conditions or activities

Conditions or nearby activities:	Test for:
Recurring gastrointestinal illness	Coliform bacteria
Household plumbing or service lines that contain lead	pH, lead, copper
Radon in indoor air or region is radon rich	Radon
Corrosion of pipes, plumbing	Corrosion, pH, lead
Nearby areas of intensive agriculture	Nitrate, nitrite, pesticides, coliform bacteria
Coal or other mining operations nearby	Metals, pH, corrosion
Gas drilling operations nearby	Chloride, sodium, barium, strontium
Dump, junkyard, landfill, factory, gas station or dry-cleaning operation nearby	Volatile organic compounds, total dissolved solids, pH, sulfate, chloride, metals
Odor of gasoline or fuel oil, and near gas station or buried fuel tanks	Volatile organic compounds
Objectionable taste or smell	Hydrogen sulfide, corrosion, metals
Stained plumbing fixtures, laundry	Iron, copper, manganese
Salty taste and seawater, or a heavily salted roadway nearby	Chloride, total dissolved solids, sodium
Scaly residues, soaps don't lather	Hardness
Rapid wear of water treatment equipment	pH, corrosion
Water softener needed to treat hardness	Manganese, iron
Water appears cloudy, frothy, or colored	Color, detergents

Source: U.S. EPA (2023c)

such as appearance, taste, and odor (U.S. EPA 2023c).

If the water is contaminated there are methods to remove the contaminant(s). Chlorination, distillation, ion exchange, filtration, and reverse osmosis processes are typical methods used to remove contaminants in well water. There are five types of filtration systems and two types of ion exchange systems. The filtration systems include activated charcoal, ultraviolet filter, oxidizing, neutralizing, and sediment filters. The ion exchange systems include cation exchange (water softener) and anion exchange. It may be necessary to use more than one treatment system if multiple contaminants are present (N.C. DHHS 2018).

Table 20.13 shows typical treatment methods utilized to remove specific types of contamination from well water.

The U.S. EPA recommends testing private wells annually for total coliform bacteria, nitrates, total dissolved solids, and pH levels (U.S. EPA 2023k). If other contaminants are suspected, you should test for those also. While recommendations by state may vary, a good source of information on a variety of well contaminants and testing is available from the North Carolina Department of Health and Human Services (N.C. DHHS 2023a).

Wild Fires

A wildfire may be defined as "an unusual or extraordinary free-burning vegetation fire which may be started maliciously, accidently, or through natural means, that negatively influences social, economic, or environmental values" (UNEP 2022). An increasing frequency of wildfires is occurring worldwide. A 2022 United Nations report projected that by 2050, the number of extreme wildfires will rise by up to 30% and by 50% by 2100 (UNEP 2022). That also means more smoke will transcend far beyond country borders and affect health worldwide (Suran 2023). Projected wildfire trends in the United States predict increasing risk of exposure to wildfire smoke because of increases in weather and climate-related factors associated with wildfire risk, including heat, drought, and wind speed (Vargo et al. 2023) Uncontrollable and extreme wildfires can be devastating to people, biodiversity and ecosystems. They also exacerbate climate change, contributing significant greenhouse gases to the atmosphere.

Wildfire smoke produced from combustion of natural biomass contains thousands of individual compounds, including particulate matter, carbon dioxide, water vapor, carbon monoxide, hydro-

Table 20.13 Well treatment methods to remove water contaminants

Contaminant	Filtration	Ion exchange	Distillation	Reverse osmosis	Chlorination
Arsenic	Activated carbon		X	X	
Barium		Cation exchange	X	X	
Cadmium	Activated carbon		X	X	
Calcium		Cation exchange			
Chloride			X	X	
Chromium	Activated carbon	Anion exchange	X	X	
Copper	Activated carbon	Cation exchange	X	X	
Fluoride		Both	X	X	
Iron	Oxidizing	Cation exchange	X	X	
Lead	Activated carbon		X	X	
Magnesium		Cation exchange			
Manganese	Oxidizing	Cation exchange			
Mercury	Activated carbon				
Nitrate/nitrite		Anion exchange	X	X	
Selenium		Anion exchange	X	X	
Silver		Cation exchange			
Sodium			X	X	
Sulfate			X	X	
Thallium		Cation exchange or activated alumina			
VOCs/pesticides	Activated carbon			X	
Zinc	Activated carbon				
pH	Neutralizing				
Total alkalinity	Neutralizing				
Total hardness		Cation exchange			
Turbidity/ sediment	Sedimentation				
E. Coli			X	X	X
Total coliforms			X	X	X

Adapted from NC DHHS (2018)

carbons and other organic chemicals, nitrogen oxides, ozone, polycyclic hydrocarbons, volatile organic compounds, trace minerals, and other harmful air pollutants. Wildfires can move into the wildland– urban interface (WUI), burning homes and structures and thereby consuming man-made materials in addition to natural resources. Residual smoke from wildfires can affect people even if they're far from the burning area. The hotter the fire burns, the greater the chance of larger smoke plumes and the more likely that smoke will rise higher and travel farther. Wildfire smoke can also travel up and destroy the ozone layer.

Wildfire smoke exposure is associated with asthma exacerbations, chronic obstructive pulmonary disease (COPD), respiratory infections, myocardial infarction, ischemic heart disease, heart failure, dysrhythmia, pulmonary embolism, ischemic stroke, transient ischemic attack, out-of-hospital cardiac arrests, and all-cause mortality (U.S. EPA 2023j).

Particulate matter is the principal public health threat from short and longer-term exposure to wildfire smoke (Burke et al. 2023). Fine particulate matter, which is defined as particles that are 2.5 μm or less in diameter, makes up about 90% of wildfire smoke's total particle mass (U.S. EPA 2023j). These particles, referred to as $PM_{2.5}$, can travel deep into the lungs, where they can cause inflammation. They may also enter the bloodstream and travel to other organs. The effects of particulate matter exposure range from eye and respiratory tract irritation to more serious disorders including reduced lung function, bronchitis, exacerbation of asthma, heart failure, and premature death. Short-term exposures (i.e., days to weeks) to fine particles are associated with increased risk of premature mortality and aggravation of pre-existing respiratory and cardiovascular disease. Exposures to fine particles can also affect healthy people, causing respiratory symptoms, transient reductions in lung function, and pulmonary inflammation. Particulate matter may also affect the body's ability to remove inhaled foreign materials, such as pollen and bacteria, from the lungs.

Ground-level ozone, though less of a concern from wildfires than particulate matter, can cause effects such as reductions in lung function, inflammation of the airways, chest pain, coughing, wheezing, and shortness of breath—even in healthy people. These effects can be more serious in people with asthma and other lung diseases. Respiratory effects attributed to ozone exposure can lead to increased use of medication, school absences, respiratory-related hospital admissions, and emergency room visits for asthma and chronic obstructive pulmonary disease (COPD). Although the evidence of ozone's effects on the cardiovascular system (the heart, blood, and blood vessels) is more limited than the evidence of effects on the respiratory system, it indicates that short-term exposure to ozone may cause effects such as changes in heart rate variability and systemic inflammation.

Carbon monoxide is also present in wildfire smoke. Typically, exposures to carbon monoxide from wildfire smoke pose a less significant hazard to the public, except to firefighters and certain at-risk populations. This is because carbon monoxide does not travel far from the point of combustion. Carbon monoxide enters the bloodstream through the lungs and reduces oxygen delivery to the body's organs and tissues. People with cardiovascular disease may experience health effects such as chest pain or cardiac arrhythmias from lower levels of carbon monoxide than healthy people. At higher levels, carbon monoxide exposure can cause headache, weakness, dizziness, confusion, nausea, disorientation, visual impairment, coma, and death, even in otherwise healthy individuals.

Wildfire smoke also contains significant quantities of respiratory irritants that can act in concert to produce eye and respiratory irritation and potentially exacerbate asthma. Additionally, hazardous air pollutants (HAPs) such as acetaldehyde, acrolein, formaldehyde, and benzene are also present in wildfire smoke. These HAPs may lead to adverse health effects in infants, children, pregnant women and their fetuses, elderly persons, those with existing lung, heart, or liver diseases, and persons engaging in physical activity.

Public health recommendations to reduce exposure to wildfire smoke currently include recommendations to stay indoors in places with adequate air filtration, reduce activity during smoke events, reduce other sources of indoor air pollution, use air filters (high-efficiency heating, ventilation, and air-conditioning (HVAC) filters rated MERV 13 or higher). HVAC filtration can help reduce particle concentrations indoors, and those who cannot stay indoors (e.g., agricultural and outdoor workers) should use suitable respiratory protection when outdoors (Stone et al. 2019; U.S. EPA 2023g).

References

AAP (American Academy of Pediatrics, Council on Environmental Health). Breast milk. In: Etzel RA, editor. Pediatric environmental health. 4th ed. Itasca, IL: American Academy of Pediatrics; 2019. p. 238.

ACS (American Cancer Society). Formaldehyde and cancer risk. 2022. https://www.cancer.org/cancer/risk-prevention/chemicals/formaldehyde.html#:~:text=The%20International%20Agency%20for%20Research,cause%20nasopharyngeal%20cancer%20and%20leukemia. Accessed 18 Nov 2023.

ACS. Asbestos and cancer risk. 2023. https://www.cancer.org/cancer/risk-prevention/chemicals/asbestos.html. Accessed 10 Nov 2023.

AIHA (American Industrial Hygiene Association). Indoor air quality 2023. https://www.aiha.org/public--resources/air-quality. Accessed 18 Nov 2023.

Albertson TE. Opiates and opioids. In: Olson KR, editor. Poisoning & drug overdose. 7th ed. New York: McGraw Hill; 2018. p. 350–2.

Anderson CE, Loomis GA. Recognition and prevention of inhalant abuse. Am Fam Physician. 2003;68(5):869–74.

ATS (American Thoracic Society). Diagnosis and initial management of nonmalignant diseases related to asbestos. Am J Respir Crit Care Med. 2004;170:691–715.

ATSDR (Agency for Toxic Substances and Disease Registry). Asbestos. Limiting asbestos exposure while working in areas with naturally occurring asbestos. 2005. https://www.atsdr.cdc.gov/noa/docs/Asbestos-workers.pdf. Accessed 12 Nov 2023.

ATSDR. Naturally occurring Asbestos locations in the contiguous USA and Alaska and the 100 fastest growing U.S. Counties. 2007. https://www.atsdr.cdc.gov/noa/docs/usamap.pdf. Accessed 18 Nov 2023.

ATSDR. ATSDR case studies in environmental medicine: nitrate/nitrite toxicity. 2013. https://www.atsdr.cdc.gov/csem/nitrate_2013/docs/nitrite.pdf. Accessed 31 Oct 2023.

ATSDR. Evaluating mercury exposure: information for health care providers. 2018. https://www.atsdr.cdc.gov/dontmesswithmercury/pdfs/info-for-health-care-providers.pdf. Accessed 14 Oct 2023.

ATSDR. Toxicological profile for lead. 2020. https://www.atsdr.cdc.gov/ToxProfiles/tp13-c1.pdf. Accessed 1 Nov 2023.

ATSDR. What are the health effects of PFAS? 2022. https://www.atsdr.cdc.gov/pfas/health-effects/index.html. Accessed 21 Nov 2023.

ATSDR. What are possible health effects from lead exposure? 2023a. https://www.atsdr.cdc.gov/csem/lead-toxicity/physiological_effects.html. Accessed 2 Nov 2023.

ATSDR. How should patients overexposed to nitrates and nitrites be treated and managed? 2023b. https://www.atsdr.cdc.gov/csem/nitrate-nitrite/patients_exposed.html. Accessed 15 Oct 2023.

Baum L, Arnold TC. Silicosis. StatPearls [Internet]. Treasure Island, FL: StatPearls 2023. https://www.ncbi.nlm.nih.gov/books/NBK594245/. Accessed 2 Dec 2023.

Bittner RH, Childers RE Jr, Doss HJ, Hughes HA, Pickett LK, Wilkinson RH. Chemical equipment. In: Agricultural safety. Moline, IL: Deere & Company Service Training; 1987. p. 196–201.

Burke M, Childs ML, de la Cuesta B, Qiu M, Li J, Gould CF, Heft-Neal S, Wara M. The contribution of wildfire to PM2.5 trends in the USA. Nature. 2023;622(7984):761–6.

CDC (Centers for Disease Control and Prevention). Atypical reactions associated with heroin use—five states, January–April 2005. Morb Mortal Wkly Rep. 2005;54(32):793–6.

CDC. Arsenic. 2009. https://www.epa.gov/sites/default/files/2014-03/documents/arsenic_factsheet_cdc_2013.pdf. Accessed 15 Oct 2023.

CDC. Green Tobacco Sickness. 2015. https://www.cdc.gov/niosh/docs/2015-104/pdfs/2015-104.pdf?id=10.26616/NIOSHPUB2015104. Accessed 15 Oct 2023.

CDC. Clinical guidance for carbon monoxide (CO) poisoning. 2020. https://www.cdc.gov/disasters/co_guidance.html. Accessed 18 Nov 2023.

CDC. Blood lead levels in children. 2022. https://www.cdc.gov/nceh/lead/prevention/blood-lead-levels.htm#:~:text=The%20amount%20of%20lead%20in,higher%20than%20most%20children's%20levels. Accessed 12 Nov 2023.

CDC. Drug overdoses. 2023a. https://www.cdc.gov/nchs/fastats/drug-overdoses.htm. Accessed 10 Nov 2023.

CDC. What you should know about xylazine. 2023b. https://www.cdc.gov/drugoverdose/deaths/other-drugs/xylazine/faq.ht. Accessed 29 Nov 2023.

Cherlopalle S, Enja M, Lippmann M, Lippmann S. Levamisole-adulterated cocaine toxicity: would you recognize it? 2016. https://www.psychiatrist.com/pcc/levamisole-adulterated-cocaine-toxicity/#:~:text=Levamisole%20toxicity%20presents%20clinically%20with,cutaneous%20eruptions%20to%20extensive%20necrosis. Accessed 22 Nov 2023.

CLN (ClinLab Navigator). Leadership 2023. http://www.clinlabnavigator.com/lead.html. Accessed 21 Nov 2023.

DEA (Drug Enforcement Agency). 2017. Drug slang code words. https://www.dea.gov/sites/default/files/2018-07/DIR-020-17%20Drug%20Slang%20Code%20Words.pdf. Accessed 15 Nov 2023.

DEA. Ketamine. 2020. https://www.dea.gov/sites/default/files/2020-06/Ketamine-2020.pdf. Accessed 23 Nov 2023.

D'Orazio J, Nelson L, Perrone J, Wightman R, Haroz R. Xylazine adulteration of heroin-fentanyl drug supply. Ann Intern Med. 2023;176(10):1370–6.

Donham KJ. Respiratory disease hazards to workers in livestock and poultry confinement structures. Semin Respir Infect. 1993;14(1):49–59.

Donham KJ, Thelin A. Agricultural respiratory diseases. In: Agricultural medicine: rural occupational and environmental health, safety, and prevention. 2nd ed. Hoboken, NJ: Wiley; 2016a. p. 95–154.

Donham KJ, Thelin A. Veterinary pharmaceuticals; potential occupational and community health hazards. In: Agricultural medicine: rural occupational and environmental health, safety, and prevention. 2nd ed. Hoboken, NJ: Wiley; 2016b. p. 413–32.

Durborow RM. Health and safety concerns in fisheries and aquaculture. Occup Med. 1999;14(2):373–406.

Erramouspe J, Adamcik BA, Carlson RK. Veterinarian perception of the intentional misuse of veterinary medications in humans: a preliminary survey of Idaho-licensed practitioners. J Rural Health. 2002;18(2):311–8.

Fry JP, Ceryes CA, Voorhees JM, Barnes NA, Love DC, Barnes ME. Occupational safety and health in U.S. Aquaculture: a review. J Agromedicine. 2019;24(4):405–23.

Gummin DD, Mowry JB, Beuhler MC, Spyker DA, Rivers LJ, Feldman R, Brown K, Pham Nathaniel PT, Bronstein AC, Weber JA. 2021 annual report of the National Poison Data System© (NPDS) from America's poison centers: 39th annual report. Clin Toxicol. 2022;60(12):1381–643.

Hill D. Safe handling and disposal of laboratory animal waste. Occup Med. 1999;14(2):449–68.

Hirsch AE, Langley RL, McDaniel JS. Carbon monoxide poisonings from forklift use during produce packing operations. J Agromedicine. 2016;21(2):132–5.

IARC (International Agency for Research on Cancer). Ingested nitrate and nitrite, and cyanobacterial peptide toxins. IARC Monogr Eval Carcinog Risks Hum. 2010;94:v–vii, 1–412.

Kore AM, Kiesche-Nesselrodt A. Toxicology of household cleaning products and disinfectants. Vet Clin N Am Small Anim Pract. 1990;29(2):525–37.

Kosnett MJ. Lead. In: Olson KR, editor. Poisoning & Drug Overdose. 7th ed. New York: McGraw Hill; 2018a. p. 286–91.

Kosnett MJ. Mercury. In: Olson KR, editor. Poisoning & drug overdose. 7th ed. New York: McGraw Hill; 2018b. p. 305–10.

Kosnett MJ, Berenji M, Burton A, Durand-Moreau Q, Esty E, Fischman M, Hudson TW III, Nabeel I, Papanek P, Sokas R. ACOEM position statement: workplace health and safety necessitates an update to Occupational Lead standard provisions for medical removal protection, medical surveillance triggers, and the action level and permissible exposure level for lead in workplace air: ACOEM response to OSHA. J Occup Environ Med. 2023;65(3):e170–6.

Krugh M, Maani CV. Misoprostol. In: StatPearls [Internet]. Treasure Island, FL: StatPearls; 2023. https://www.ncbi.nlm.nih.gov/books/NBK539873/. Accessed 1 Dec 2023.

Lust EB, Barthold C, Malesker MA, Wichman TO. Human health hazards of veterinary medications: information for emergency departments. J Emerg Med. 2011;40(2):198–207.

McBride J, Altman D, Klein M, White W. Green tobacco sickness. Tob Control. 1998;7(3):294–8.

McReynolds T. 8 Veterinary drugs with human health hazards. 2023. https://www.aaha.org/publications/newstat/articles/2023-4/8-veterinary-drugs-with-human-health-hazards/. Accessed 24 Nov 2023.

Meadowcroft D, Robertson MN, Denny M, Rayner M, Stone A, Johnson J, Buys D. Perceptions of opioid misuse in Mississippi agricultural communities: focus group findings. J Agric Saf Health. 2023;29(1):47–56.

Meggs WJ. Chemical hazards faced by animal handlers. Occup Med. 1999;14(2):213–24.

Meyer RE. Anesthesia hazards to animal workers. Occup Med. 1999;14:225–34.

Moline JM, Landrigan PJ. Lead. In: Rosenstock L, Cullen M, Brodkin C, Redlich C, editors. Textbook of clinical occupational and environmental medicine. 2nd ed. Philadelphia, PA: Elsevier Saunders; 2005. p. 967–78.

Morning Consult. Polling presentation. Washington, DC: U. S. American Farm Bureau Federation; 2017.

MSD (Merck Sharp & Dohme Corp.). ESTRUMATE-cloprostenol sodium injection. 2023. https://dailymed.nlm.nih.gov/dailymed/fda/fdaDrugXsl.cfm?setid=634a706f-4a00-4a04-86ae-a4d8c22b8271&type=display#:~:text=Women%20of%20childbearing%20age%2C%20asthmatics,skin%20should%20therefore%20be%20avoided. Accessed 23 Nov 2023.

Murphy DJ. Safety and health hazards. In: Safety and health for production agriculture. St. Joseph, MO: American Society of Agricultural Engineers; 1992. p. 15–42.

Myers ML. Review of occupational hazards associated with aquaculture. J Agromedicine. 2010;15(4):412–26.

N.C. DHHS (North Carolina Department of Health and Human Services). How to select a well water treatment system for your home. 2018. https://epi.dph.ncdhhs.gov/oee/docs/HowtoSelect a WellWaterTreatmentSystemforYourHome.pdf. Accessed 21 Oct 2023.

N.C. DHHS. Total hardness calcium magnesium and private wells. 2019a. https://epi.dph.ncdhhs.gov/oee/docs/TotalHardnessCalciumMagnesiumAndPrivateWells.pdf; https://epi.dph.ncdhhs.gov/oee/docs/pdf. Accessed 19 Oct 2023.

N.C. DHHS. Indoor environmental quality. 2019b. https://epi.dph.ncdhhs.gov/oee/programs/iaq.html. Accessed 20 Nov 2023.

N.C. DHHS. Arsenic. 2019c. https://epi.dph.ncdhhs.gov/oee/a_z/as.html. Accessed 5 Oct 2023.

N.C. DHHS. PFAS water testing and filtration resources. 2022a. https://epi.dph.ncdhhs.gov/oee/pfas/PFAS_TestingFiltration.pdf. Accessed 22 Nov 2023.

N.C. DHHS. Mercury and private wells. 2022b. https://epi.dph.ncdhhs.gov/oee/docs/Mercury_WellWaterFactSt.pdf. Accessed 15 Oct 2023.

N.C. DHHS. Radionuclides & private wells. 2022c. https://epi.dph.ncdhhs.gov/oee/docs/Radionuclides_WellWaterFactSt.pdf. Accessed 1 Nov 2023.

N.C. DHHS. Private wells. 2023a. https://epi.dph.ncdhhs.gov/oee/programs/wellwater.html. Accessed 15 Oct 2023.

N.C. DHHS. Mold. 2023b. https://epi.dph.ncdhhs.gov/oee/a_z/mold.html. Accessed 20 Nov 2023.

NAS (National Academies of Sciences, Engineering, and Medicine). Guidance on PFAS exposure, testing, and clinical follow-up. Washington, DC: The National Academies Press; 2022.

NIOSH (National Institute for Occupational Safety and Health). Preventing worker deaths and injuries when handling Micotil 300®. DHHS (NIOSH) Publication No. 2007-124. 2007.

NIOSH. Waste anesthetic gases: occupational hazards in hospitals. DHHS (NIOSH) Publication No. 2007-151. 2007.

NIOSH. Safe handling of hazardous drugs for veterinary healthcare workers. 2010. https://www.cdc.gov/niosh/docs/wp-solutions/2010-150/pdfs/2010-150.pdf. Accessed 21 Nov 2023.

Norbert C, Joseph A, Rossi SS, Bhalla S, Gutierrez FR. Asbestos-related lung disease: a pictorial review. Curr Probl Diagn Radiol. 2015;44(4):371–82.

O'Donnell J, Gladden RM, Mattson CL, Kariisa M. Notes from the field: overdose deaths with Carfentanil and other fentanyl analogs detected—10 states, July 2016–June 2017. MMWR Morb Mortal Wkly Rep. 2018;67(27):767–8.

Olson KR. Carbon monoxide. In: Olson KR, editor. Poisoning & drug overdose. 7th ed. New York: McGraw Hill; 2018. p. 182–4.

OSHA (Occupational Safety and Health Administration). Anesthetic gases: guidelines for workplace exposures. 2000. https://www.osha.gov/waste-anesthetic-gases/workplace-exposures-guidelines. Accessed 22 Nov 2023.

PESHU (Pediatric Environmental Health specialty Units). Recommendations on management of childhood lead exposure: a resource for clinicians. 2021. https://www.pehsu.net/_Library/facts/PEHSU_Fact_Sheet_Lead_Management_Health_Professionals_9_2021.pdf. Accessed 21 Nov 2023.

Peters J. Silicosis. In: Occupational respiratory disease. USDHHS NIOSH Publication No 86–102; 1986. p. 243–84.

Popendorf WA, Reynolds AI. Industrial hygiene evaluations in agriculture. In: Langley RL, McLymore RL, Meggs WJ, Roberson GT, editors. Safety and health in agriculture, forestry, and fisheries. Rockville, MD: Government Institutes; 1997. p. 439–68.

Reddy MNT, Ashok N. Green tobacco sickness—a brief review. WNOFNS. 2019;24:209–14.

Redlich C, Balmes J. Occupational and environmental lung disease. In: Chest medicine essentials of pulmonary and critical care medicine. 3rd ed; 1995. p. 371–3.

Rees D, Murray J. Silica, silicosis, and tuberculosis. Int J Tuberc Lung Dis. 2007;11(5):474–84.

Scheftel JM, Elchos BL, Rubin CS, Decker JA. Review of hazards to female reproductive health in veterinary practice. J Am Vet Med Assoc. 2017;250(8):862–72.

Schenker M. Exposures and health effects from inorganic agricultural dusts. Environ Health Perspect. 2000;108(Suppl 4):661–4.

Shaver CS, Tong T. Chemical hazards to agricultural workers. Occup Med. 1991;6(3):391–413.

Smalling K, Romanok KM, Bradley PM, Morriss MC, Gray JL, Kanagy LK, Gordon S, Williams B, Breitmeyer S, Jones D, DeCicco LA, Eagles-Smith C, Wagner T. Per- and polyfluoroalkyl substances (PFAS) in United States tapwater: comparison of underserved private-well and public-supply exposures and associated health implications. Environ Int. 2023;178:108033.

Smith AN, Klahn S, Phillips B, Parshley L, Bennett P, Flory A, Calderon R. ACVIM small animal consensus statement on safe use of cytotoxic chemotherapeutics in veterinary practice. J Vet Intern Med. 2018;32(3):904–13.

Stone S, Anderko L, Berger M, Butler C, Cascio W, et al. Wildfire smoke: a guide for public health officials revised 2019. EPA/452/R-19/901. Washington, DC: U.S. EPA Office of Research and Development; 2019.

Suran M. Raging wildfires are exposing more people to smoky air—here's what that means for health. JAMA. 2023;330(14):1311–4.

U.S. CPSC (United States Consumer Products Safety Commission). Asbestos in the home. 2019. https://www.cpsc.gov/safety-education/safety-guides/home/asbestos-home. Accessed 21 Oct 2023.

U.S. DHHS (United States Department of Health and Human Services). Surgeon General Releases National Health Advisory on Radon. 2005. https://www.adph.org/radon/assets/surgeon_general_radon.pdf. Accessed 23 Oct 2023.

U.S. DOL (United States Department of Labor Occupational Safety and Health Administration). Occupational safety and health hazards. In: Agriculture: a review of the literature; 1994.

U.S. EPA (United States Environmental Protection Agency). Lead in your home: a parent's reference guide. EPA-747-B-99-003. 1999.

U.S. EPA. Home Buyer's and Seller's Guide to Radon. 402-K-00-008. 2000.

U.S. EPA. Drinking water from household Wells. September 2002. EPA 816-K-02-003 2002.

U.S. EPA. Protect your family from lead in your home. EPA747-K-99-001. 2003a.

U.S. EPA. Air Quality Index A Guide to air quality and your health. EPA-454/K-03-002. 2003b.

U.S. EPA. A citizen's guide to radon: the guide to protecting yourself and your family from radon. EP 402/K-12/002. 2012. https://www.epa.gov/sites/default/files/2016-12/documents/2016_a_citizens_guide_to_radon.pdf. Accessed 1 Nov 2023.

U.S. EPA. Consumer's guide to radon reduction how to fix your home. 2016. https://www.epa.gov/sites/default/files/2016-12/documents/2016_consumers_guide_to_radon_reduction.pdf. Accessed 1 Nov 2023.

U.S. EPA. Reducing PFAS in drinking water with treatment technologies. 2018a. Accessed 22 Nov 2023.

U.S. EPA. Technical assistance document for the reporting of daily air quality—the Air Quality Index (AQI). EPA 454/B-18-007. 2018b. https://www.airnow.gov/sites/default/files/2020-05/aqi-technical-assistance-document-sept2018.pdf. Accessed 11 Oct 23.

U.S. EPA. Blood lead level. 2022. https://cfpub.epa.gov/roe/indicator.cfm?i=63. Accessed 2 Nov 2023.

U.S. EPA. National primary drinking water regulations. 2023a. https://www.epa.gov/ground-water-and-drinking-water/national-primary-drinking-water-regulations#Inorganic. Accessed 15 Oct 2023.

U.S. EPA. Mercury. What to do if you have mercury spill? 2023b. https://www.epa.gov/mercury. Accessed 1 Oct 2023.

U.S. EPA. Protect your home's water. 2023c. https://www.epa.gov/privatewells/protect-your-homes-water. Accessed 21 Nov 2023.

U.S. EPA. What is vermiculite? 2023d. https://www.epa.gov/asbestos/what-vermiculite. Accessed 12 Nov 2023.

U.S. EPA. Our current understanding of the human health and environmental risks of PFAS. 2023e. https://www.epa.gov/pfas/our-current-understanding-human-health-and-environmental-risks-pfas. Accessed 21 Nov 2023.

U.S. EPA. The inside story: a guide to indoor air quality. 2023f. https://www.epa.gov/indoor-air-quality-iaq/inside-story-guide-indoor-air-quality. Accessed 19 Oct 2023.

U.S. EPA. Wildfires and indoor air quality (IAQ). 2023g. https://www.epa.gov/indoor-air-quality-iaq/wildfires-and-indoor-air-quality-iaq. Accessed 15 Nov 2023.

U.S. EPA. How does radon get into your home? 2023h. https://www.epa.gov/radon/how-does-radon-get-your-home. Accessed 12 Nov 2023.

U.S. EPA. Biomonitoring-lead. 2023i. https://www.epa.gov/americaschildrenenvironment/biomonitoring-lead. Accessed 12 Nov 2023.

U.S. EPA. Why wildfire smoke is a health concern. 2023j. https://www.epa.gov/wildfire-smoke-course/why-wildfire-smoke-health-concern. Accessed 12 Nov 2023.

U.S. EPA. Private drinking water wells. 2023k. https://www.epa.gov/privatewells. Accessed 1 Nov 2023.

U.S. EPA. Chemical contaminant rules. 2023l. https://www.epa.gov/dwreginfo/chemical-contaminant-rules. Accessed 12 Nov 2023.

U.S. FDA (United States Food and Drug Administration). FDA Animal Drug Safety Communication: Micotil 300 User Safety Alert. 2017. https://wayback.archive-it.org/7993/20190424114815/https:/www.fda.gov/AnimalVeterinary/NewsEvents/CVMUpdates/ucm575194.htm. Accessed 27 Nov 2023.

U.S. FDA Per- and Polyfluoroalkyl Substances (PFAS). 2023. https://www.fda.gov/food/environmental--contaminants-food/and-polyfluoroalkyl-substances-pfas. Accessed 21 Nov 2023.

UGAE (University of Georgia Extension). Nitrate and nitrite in water. 2022. https://extension.uga.edu/publications/deatil.html?number=C858-5&title=nitrate-and-nitrite-in-water. Accessed 22 Oct 2023.

UNEP (United Nation Environment Programme). Spreading like wildfire the rising threat of extraordinary landscape fires. 2022. https://www.unep.org/resources/report/spreading-wildfire-rising-threat-extraordinary-landscape-fires. Accessed 21 Oct 2023.

USGS (United States Geological Survey). Hardness of water. 2018. https://www.usgs.gov/special-topics/water-science-school/science/hardness-water. Accessed 15 Oct 2023.

Vagi SJ, Sheikh S, Brackney M, Smolinske S, Warrick B, Reuter N, Schier JG. Passive multistate surveillance for neutropenia after use of cocaine or heroin possibly contaminated with levamisole. Ann Emerg Med. 2013;61(4):468–74.

Vargo J, Lappe B, Mirabelli MC, Conlon KC. Social vulnerability in US communities affected by wildfire smoke, 2011 to 2021. Am J Public Health. 2023;113(7):759–67.

Wahl M, Finke B. Mercury. In: Toxicology secrets. Philadelphia: Hanley & Belfus; 2001. p. 162–3.

Wahl M, Friede R. Lead. In: Toxicology secrets. Philadelphia: Hanley & Belfus; 2001. p. 156–60.

Weimer MB. Evidence-based guidance on responsible prescribing, effective management, and harm reduction. In: North Carolina Medical Licensure Program. Jacksonville, FL: InforMed Continuing Medical Education; 2019. p. 1–33.

Whitmer M. Farmers and asbestos. 2023. https://www.asbestos.com/occupations/farmers/. Accessed 15 Oct 23.

WHO (World Health Organization). Guideline for clinical management of exposure to lead. 2021. https://www.who.int/publications/i/item/9789240037045. Accessed 20 Oct 2023.

WHO. Arsenic. 2022. https://www.who.int/news-room/fact-sheets/detail/arsenic. Accessed 20 Oct 2023.

Wikipedia. Agricultural lime. 2023. https://en.wikipedia.org/wiki/Agricultural_lime. Accessed 28 Sept 2023.

Wingert WE, Mundy LA, Nelson L, Wong SC, Curtis J. Detection of clenbuterol in heroin users in twelve postmortem cases at the Philadelphia medical examiner's office. J Anal Toxicol. 2008;32(7):522–8.

Young S, Chen L, Palatnick W, Wong P, Wong J. Led Astray. N Engl J Med. 2020;383(6):578–83.

Zoetis. Lutalyse sterile solution, safety data sheet. 2017. https://www.zoetisus.com/content/_assets/docs/vmips/safety-data-sheets/lutalyse.pdf. Accessed 23 Nov 2023.

21 Cancer and Neurodegenerative Disorders Associated with Chemical Exposures Among Farm Workers

Avian White, Stephanie L. Richards, and Jo Anne G. Balanay

Introduction

Agricultural farm workers consist of seasonal and migrant workers, self-employed farmers, contract laborers, and hired workers. Worldwide, an estimated 880 million to one billion people are employed by the agricultural sector (Togawa et al. 2021). Farm workers may perform a multitude of jobs such as rancher, nursery worker, laborer, and manager. These workers may have an increased risk of exposure to pesticides due to type of farm work performed (Das et al. 2001). Tasks involved in these positions may involve exposure to various classes of pesticides (e.g., herbicides, insecticides, fungicides, and rodenticides) used to preserve quality and quantity of harvests and prevent damage to farm structures and equipment (rodenticides). Use of chemicals, such as pesticides, is deemed necessary as production loss due to pests (i.e., fungus, insects, and rodents) and disease may be 78%, 54%, and 32% for crops such as fruits, vegetables, and cereals, respectively (Tudi et al. 2021). Workers may experience repeated exposure to pesticides, and this could lead to serious health concerns. Pesticide exposure has been linked to acute and long-term health effects, including but not limited to neurologic diseases and multiple types of cancers (Hoang et al. 2021; Mostafalou and Abdollahi 2017). Pesticide exposure has also been linked to hormone disruption, developmental issues, and respiratory diseases (Kim et al. 2017; Van Maele-Fabry et al. 2010; Ye et al. 2013). This chapter aims to provide an overview of cancers and chronic diseases that may disproportionality affect farm workers.

Pesticide Exposure

As the global population continues to grow, farmers are tasked with producing an increased level of food supplies while having finite land-based resources. Studies indicate that agricultural yields would need to increase 70–100% by 2050 (Reid and Greene 2012) to feed a projected nine billion people. Compounding this issue are factors such as agricultural pests (i.e., weeds, insects, and rodents). Thus, farmers often use pesticides to mitigate harvest loss and improve yield quality and quantity. In this effort, farm workers may experience pesticide exposure in multiple ways, typically greater than workers in non-agricultural occupations. However, the frequency and level of pesticide exposure among farm workers may vary depending on job description and use and availability of proper protective equipment.

A. White (✉) · S. L. Richards · J. A. G. Balanay
Environmental Health Sciences Program, Department of Health Education and Promotion, College of Health and Human Performance, East Carolina University, Greenville, NC, USA
e-mail: whiteav15@ecu.edu; richardss@ecu.edu; balanayj@ecu.edu

W. J. Meggs, R. L. Langley (eds.), *Farm Toxicology*, https://doi.org/10.1007/978-3-031-80441-0_21

Workers who are certified pesticide applicators may have more exposure than others due to more frequent use and or exposure to higher concentrations of pesticides. However, regardless of job description, all farm workers may experience indirect pesticide exposure.

Levels of pesticide exposure may vary by exposure route (e.g., ingestion, dermal contact, and inhalation) and can be classified as acute, sub-chronic, or chronic (Damala and Koutroubas 2016). Acute toxicity generally refers to a single exposure or multiple exposures in a time frame producing deleterious effects immediately or within 24 h post-exposure (Chimedu et al. 2013; Damala and Koutroubas 2016). Effects seen within 1–3 months following repeated pesticide exposure and those observed after 3 months are classified as sub-chronic and chronic, respectively (Mohammadpour et al. 2019). People may also experience chronic effects after acute pesticide exposure (United States Environmental Protective Agency (EPA) 2013). Regardless of exposure type, acute, sub-chronic, and chronic pesticide exposure may result in adverse health issues.

Agricultural workers experience high rates of skin disorders and chemical injuries compared to other occupations (NC Farmworker Health Program 2023) with exposures linked to neurologic disorders, certain cancers, respiratory, metabolic, and thyroid effects (Curl et al. 2020).

Pesticides and Cancer

Many pesticides to which farm workers are exposed are classified as mutagenic and/or tumor promotors. Additionally, carcinogenic solvents may be used in pesticide-formulated products (Petrelli et al. 1993; Alavanja et al. 2004). Hence, the International Agency for Research on Cancer (IARC) has labeled some pesticides as "probable human carcinogens" (IARC 1991; Alavanja et al. 2013). Research and knowledge of incidence and prevalence of cancer in farm workers is important in public health practice for this occupational group. A study that investigated the incidence of cancer in California farm workers noted that, while the population experienced decreased risk in certain causes of death, there were also higher risks of some cancers (Mills and Shah 2014; Curl et al. 2020). Lerro et al. found farm workers to have a lower overall cancer rate of 9% (Standardized Incidence Ratio [SIR] = 0.91, 95% CI, 0.89–0.93). The behavior and lifestyle of some farm workers, such as decreased smoking rates and increased rates of physical activity, may contribute to lower risk of certain cancers (i.e., lung, bladder, and kidney). This may suggest an environmental or occupational association with the elevated risk of other cancers (i.e., prostate, ovarian, lymphatic, and hematopoietic) in farm workers (Blair and Zahm 1995; Blair et al. 1992; Koutros et al. 2010; Curl et al. 2020). Exposure to endotoxins (i.e., working around stored grains and farm animal proximity) may have a protective effect against lung cancer (Lenters et al. 2010; Mastrangelo et al. 1996; Lerro et al. 2019). Indeed, some research has indicated endotoxin exposure has been found to suppress tumor growth in some mammalian models (Pance et al. 2002; Lenters et al. 2010). This may be due to the immune response initiated in response to endotoxin exposure (Lundin and Checkoway 2009; Liebers et al. 2006). However, the direct mechanism is not known and may vary based on dose and exposure.

Prostate Cancer

Globally, prostate cancer is the second most diagnosed cancer among males and is expected to increase in incidence due to growth of an aging population (Culp et al. 2020; Nguyen-Nielsen and Borre 2016; Mink et al. 2008). Recent studies have implicated farm work as an occupational risk factor for prostate cancer (Alavanja et al. 2003; Parent and Siemiatycki 2001; Krstev et al. 1998) and rates of prostate cancer among farm workers exceed the general population. Excess prostate cancer rates, compared to the general population, have been seen in farmers and commercial pesticide applicators: SIR = 1.19 (95% CI, 1.14–1.25), SIR = 1.28 (95% CI, 1.00–1.61) (Koutros et al. 2013). Increased prostate cancer incidence rates have been observed after adjustment for risk factors such as diet and age (Alavanja et al. 2003). Meyer et al. (2007) found a correlation between years of farming and incidence of prostate cancer in South Carolina (SC), with those farming less than 4 years having higher rates. This has been attributed to the possibility that short-term farmers are most often manual laborers and exposed to higher levels of contaminants (Meyer et al. 2007; Zahm and Blair 1993). One farm worker task highly associated with prostate cancer was the application of and/or mixing of pesticides. The aforementioned SC study found the prostate cancer risk of those who applied or mixed pesticides had an adjusted odds ratio (aOR) of 1.6; 95% CI, 1.2 to 2.2 (Meyer et al. 2007). The same study indicated those who had applied or mixed pesticides had 60% greater odds of developing prostate cancer. These results were similar to those of a study that examined a cohort of licensed pesticide applicators in Florida (FL). Here, researchers compared pesticide applicators to the general (FL) population and found a significant elevation of prostate cancer cases among pesticide applicators, SIR = 1.91; 95% CI, 1.72–2.13 (Fleming et al. 1999).

The direct mechanism in which pesticides interact with body systems to induce prostate cancer is unclear, although initiation of DNA damage or hormone signaling pathway alteration has been suggested (Koutros et al. 2013). Few studies have examined links between pesticide exposure and tumor characteristics, including a study showing no association (Boers et al. 2005) and another suggesting an association with tumors and significant pesticide exposure (>2400 h) (Potti et al. 2003). A preliminary study of prostate cancer in males (aged 40–49) and part of predominantly rural farming communities, sought to study incidence of aggressive cancer in this population. More than half of the participants were asymptomatic, with hematuria as the most common presentation. Additionally, patients typically presented to healthcare clinicians with Stage III cancer and a mean Gleason score of 7.5 (Potti et al. 2003) (Gleason scores, ranging from 2 to 10, are used to assign a severity grade for prostate cancer and are determined based on microscopic examination of tissue samples (Epstein et al. 2016)). Further study found the mean survival rate of prostate cancer patients with pesticide exposure was 11.3 months compared to 20.1 months for patients without pesticide exposure, thus, implying an association between pesticide exposure and aggressive prostate adenocarcinoma (Potti et al. 2003). Data analyzed from the Agricultural Health Study (AHS), consisting of licensed pesticide applicators from North Carolina and Iowa, showed possible correlations between specific pesticides and aggressive prostate cancer (Koutros et al. 2013). Researchers in this study classified aggressive prostate cancer as having either or a combination of a Gleason score ≥7, tumor characterized as poorly differentiated, distant stage, or fatal prostate cancer (Koutros et al. 2013). Analysis of these characteristics combined with pesticide exposure data indicated a significant association with aggressive prostate cancer among those exposed (compared to nonexposed) to organophosphates: fonofos, malathion, and terbufos, and the organochlorine aldrin. Of note, exposure to both fonofos and aldrin had an indicated increased risk of prostate cancer that interacted with family history (Koutros et al. 2013). Thus, there is evidence of a relationship between pesticide exposure and prostate cancer and this type of cancer should be considered as a disease among farm workers.

Thyroid Cancer

Thyroid cancer, an endocrine malignancy, is more common in women than men and has a global incidence rate of 10.2 per 100,000 and 3.1 per 100,000, respectively. Thyroid cancer incidence has tripled over the past four decades (Norouzi et al. 2023; Han et al. 2019). This indicates that environmental exposures may play a role, potentially putting workers in some occupations at increased risk of thyroid cancer. One potential environmental exposure of concern is pesticides. Multiple studies show some pesticides (i.e., fungicides, hexachlorobenzene, and dichlorodiphenyltrichloroethane [DDT]) having thyroid-disrupting effects (Boas et al. 2006; Rakitsky et al. 2000; Goldner et al. 2010). Additionally, some studies have shown associations between thyroid cancer and agricultural workers exposed to pesticides, although others have not shown this association. A case-control study on thyroid cancer patients found most were diagnosed with papillary thyroid cancer, and those working in building cleaning and pest control had significantly increased risk of thyroid cancer, OR = 2.36, 95% CI, 1.02–5.50 (Ba et al. 2017). A study focusing on atrazine, a chlorinated herbicide, suggested exposure to this chemical may lead to an increased risk of thyroid cancer (Beane-Freeman et al. 2011); however, the study was limited by small sample size.

In the general public, thyroid cancer incidence rates are 2.9 times higher in women than men (Rahbari et al. 2010). This incidence disparity is also seen in aggressive cases of thyroid cancer. The number of women involved in farming has continued to climb, reaching 28.1% in 2021 (United States Department of Agriculture (USDA) 2023). Hence, it may be important to consider the possibility of the risk of thyroid cancer from pesticide exposure in women. In a Connecticut population-based case-control study, Zeng et al. (2017) found that women exposed to pesticides experienced an increased risk of thyroid cancer, albeit not statistically significant. This has also been seen in European population studies (Lope et al. 2005; Pukkala et al. 2009; Zeng et al. 2017). Thus, with the increasing female population of farm workers, thyroid cancer may be considered a disease that health care providers should be aware of in both female and male farm workers.

Hematopoietic Cancers

Hematologic or blood cancers refer to cancers originating in the immune system or blood-forming tissue. There are three main types: leukemia (cancer of bone marrow and blood), myeloma (cancer of plasma cells), and lymphoma (cancer of immune cells) (Centers for Disease Control and Prevention (CDC) 2022; Alavanja et al. 2013; Merhi et al. 2007; Matasar and Zelenetz 2008). There may be an association between pesticide exposure and leukemia (IARC 2012; Alavanja et al. 2013). One study examining pesticide exposure and hematopoietic cancers stratified by long-term exposure (> 10 years) found an increased risk of developing non-Hodgkin's Lymphoma and myelodysplastic syndromes (may progress to leukemia) by a factor of 1.65, 95% CI, 1.08–2.51 and 2.97, 95% CI, 1.67–5.31, respectively (Merhi et al. 2007). A significantly positive association was shown for all hematopoietic cancers for those in pesticide-related occupations, OR = 1.3, 95% CI, 1.2–1.5 (Merhi et al. 2007). Data from the AHS analyzing the association between organophosphates and cancer found an increased leukemia risk for pesticide applicators RR = 2.24; 95% CI, 0.94–5.34, $P_{\text{trend}} = 0.07$ for those in the highest lifetime exposure category (>20 lifetime exposure days) (Mahajan et al. 2006). Additionally, using a cumulative exposure index (intensity-weighted exposure days) researchers found an elevated risk for leukemia, RR = 2.67; 95% CI, 1.06–6.70, $P_{\text{trend}} = 0.04$ (Mahajan et al. 2006). Further analysis of this study population also found that in the intensity-weighted highest exposure days category, there was an elevated risk for non-Hodgkin lymphoma (Purdue et al. 2007). An association between pyrethroids and cancer has been implicated following a Rusiecki et al. 2009 study on a small subset of the aforementioned AHS population. Here, a statistically significant risk was observed for multiple myeloma and permethrin, a pyrethroid, in the highest levels of both intensity-weighted lifetime exposure days and lifetime exposure, RR = 5.01; 95% CI, 2.41–10.42 and RR = 5.72; 95% CI, 2.76–11.87, respectively (Rusiecki et al. 2009). A follow-up study on the AHS cohort indicated an increased risk of acute myeloid leukemia among those exposed to glyphosate in the highest exposure group (Andreotti et al. 2018). Evidence on glyphosate exposure and cancer has been mixed with most showing a weak association (Mink et al. 2011). However, some studies have found correlations between glyphosate-based herbicides and cancer risk (i.e., non-Hodgkin lymphoma (Zhang et al. 2019)).

Further investigation of AHS data on leukemia found elevated risk in age-adjusted high and low exposure categories for multiple leukemia subtypes, including chronic lymphocytic, chronic myelogenous, acute myelogenous, and others (Mahajan et al. 2006). Other studies have linked monoclonal gammopathy of undetermined significance (MGUS) to pesticide exposure (Mills and Shah 2014). Multiple studies have indicated MGUS as a precursor to the development of multiple myeloma (Landgren et al. 2009; Van de Donk et al. 2021).

Studies are now focusing on disease characteristics that may aid practitioners as an early warning system for potential health issues. Specific morphological changes in body systems, and chromosomal aberrations on chromosome 5 and 7 (Cuneo et al. 1992) have been observed in a study comparing pesticide-exposed patients to those nonexposed. Here, differences in chromosomal aberrations, cytologic characteristics, and peripheral blood and bone marrow indices were found. There was also treatment resistance to cancer therapies observed in pesticide-exposed compared to non-pesticide–exposed patients (Cuneo et al. 1992; Mahajan et al. 2006).

Other Cancers

Research has shown that farm workers may also be at increased risk of other cancers such as melanoma, skin, and lip cancer (Curl et al. 2020). Environmental hazards, such as sun exposure (length of time working outside), may have an impact on the incidence of these cancers. Szewczyk et al. (2016) found that farmers have increased incidence and risk of recurrence of basal cell carcinoma. A study that investigated skin cancer prevalence among farm workers in Spain found that actinic keratosis was detected in 41.4%, squamous cell carcinoma in 1.4%, and basal cell carcinoma in 9.8% of 215 farm workers (Navarro-Bielsa et al. 2022). Exposure factors, such as lack of photoprotection, combined with chemical exposures may influence metabolic and cell signaling pathways, increasing the risk of certain cancers (e.g., skin and lip).

Neurodegenerative Diseases

The progressive loss of neurons in structure or function is the hallmark of neurodegenerative disease. Clinical features of this type of disease may include parkinsonism, dementia, and/or motor neuron disease (Duggar and Dickson 2017). Within this realm, there are three major neurodegenerative diseases that are considered most common: Alzheimer's disease, Parkinson's disease, and Amyotrophic Lateral Sclerosis (ALS) (Migliore and Coppedè 2009; Lamptey et al. 2022). These conditions may be influenced by environmental stressors. Evidence shows that farm workers may have an increased risk of developing neurodegenerative disease (Shresthra et al. 2020; Kamel et al. 2007). Much of this evidence has been linked to environmental exposure to pesticides (Parrón et al. 2011). Additionally, a few studies have indicated chronic exposure to pesticides may be associated with neurochemical alteration in the brain (Kori et al. 2020; Menegon et al. 1998).

Parkinson's Disease

Parkinson's disease, a progressive disorder, may affect 1%—2% of the public aged 50 and older (Migliore and Coppedè 2009; Shresthra et al. 2020). This condition is characterized by unsteady gait and balance, tremors, muscle stiffness, and difficulty coordinating movement (Lamptey et al. 2022; Migliore and Coppedè 2009). The presence of Lewy bodies may be used to microscopically characterize Parkinson's disease (Lamptey et al. 2022). Data from the aforementioned AHS indicated the incidence of Parkinson's disease was associated with cumulative pesticide use days when comparing those of high use to low use, OR = 2.3, 95% CI, 1.2–4.5; $P_{\text{trend}} = 0.009$. During follow-up from this study, newly diagnosed patients with Parkinson's disease reported experiencing changes in smell or taste and increases in hand tremors (Kamel et al. 2007). Kamel et al. (2007) found an association between Parkinson's disease and pesticide exposure with increasing lifetime use. Others examined motor neuron disease and found increased Parkinson's disease in farmers located in France (Kab et al. 2017).

Some farm workers may experience nonmotor symptoms before Parkinson's disease diagnosis. Indeed, results from the AHS showed a reduced sense of smell and dream-enacting behaviors were nonmotor symptoms experienced by this cohort (Shresthra et al. 2017). A number of nonmotor symptoms (i.e., impaired olfaction, constipation, and daytime sleepiness) were examined in relation to Parkinson's disease and indicated an increase in Parkinson's disease incidence to 215 per 10,000 person-years for persons experiencing at least three nonmotor symptoms from 16 per 10,000 person-years for those not experiencing nonmotor symptoms (Ross et al. 2012; Shresthra et al. 2017). Thus, it may be beneficial for practitioners to evaluate these nonmotor symptoms as part of a pre-screening tool for Parkinson's disease among farm workers.

Studies have indicated chemicals such as trichloroethylene (TCE) and paraquat exposure may contribute to neurodegenerative diseases (Dorsey et al. 2023; Berry et al. 2010). Trichloroethylene is a solvent that may be used in both commercial and private settings. It has been especially useful in degreasing equipment, which is helpful in keeping farm equipment working properly. Animal model studies have linked TCE exposure with dopamine neuron loss and striatonigral fiber degeneration (Gash et al. 2008). These data supported an earlier study on worker's long-term exposure to TCE, showing some of those working adjacent to TCE and having chronic dermal and inhalation exposure developing Parkinson's along with workers operating distant from TCE, but having inhalation exposure, displaying parkinsonism features (Gash et al. 2008). Rodent studies have also implicated paraquat (herbicide) exposure as a risk factor for Parkinson's disease including leading to lesions and degeneration of neurons in *Substantia nigra, Pars compacta* (Berry et al. 2010; See et al. 2023). However, the few studies showing increased risk of Parkinson's due to paraquat exposure are limited.

Amyotrophic Lateral Sclerosis

Amyotrophic lateral sclerosis (ALS) is a rapidly progressive disease of the spinal cord and affects upper and lower motor neurons (Wang et al. 2020; Morris 2015; Kang et al. 2014). The disease, also known as Lou Gehrig's disease, typically progresses to paralysis due to its effects on motor neurons and affected patients have a life expectancy of 2 to 5 years (Wang et al. 2020; Morris 2015). Researchers have sought to determine an association between ALS and farm workers. A systematic review by Kang et al. (2014) found that farm workers had a significantly increased risk of ALS, OR = 1.42; 95% CI, 1.17–1.73. Investigators also performed a geospatial analysis of crop-applied pesticides and their potential as a risk factor for ALS. Results of that analysis supported pesticides as a potential risk factor for ALS (Andrew et al. 2021). The AHS also found risk of ALS with use of some pesticides such as pyrethroids, herbicides, fumigants, and organochlorines, though this was not significant (Kamel et al. 2012).

Alzheimer's Disease and Dementia

Dementia is characterized as progressive loss of memories and cognitive abilities, while Alzheimer's disease is a form of dementia (Lane et al. 2017). Alzheimer's disease dementia is characterized by the onset of a progression of functional and cognitive decline (Lopez et al. 2019). Data from the Health and Retirement Study found an association between persons employed in agriculture, fishing, and forestry occupations and dementia, with 46% increase in the odds of being diagnosed with dementia (Arora et al. 2021). This study also found lower cognitive functioning among agricultural workers at earlier stages of aging when compared to those in other occupations (Arora et al. 2021). A study of residents aged 65 and older in Cache County, Utah, an agricultural community, found associations between occupational pesticide exposure and dementia and Alzheimer's disease, Hazard ratio [HR] = 1.38, 95% CI, 1.09–1.76 and HR 1.42, 95% CI 1.06–1.91, respectively (Hayden et al. 2009).

The type of farm work may influence the risk of cognitive decline. Many farm workers experience hearing loss due to exposure to excessive noise during their workday (e.g., power equipment, tractors). This population has a higher likelihood of experiencing noise-induced hearing loss (Humann et al. 2012). Hearing loss has been associated as a risk factor for dementia (Arora et al. 2021). In addition to hearing loss, studies have found that olfactory impairment may also be a risk factor for Alzheimer's disease. Analysis of a longitudinal clinical pathologic study of subjects, with a mean age of 79.3 years, found Alzheimer's disease pathology in the brains of patients who did not present with clinical manifestations of the disease at the time of study enrollment, but showed olfactory dysfunction (Wilson et al. 2009).

Recent research has indicated farm workers may be at increased risk of mental health issues and suicidal ideations (Zanchi et al. 2023). Pesticides, while of public health concern, may be associated with neurobehavioral effects on occupationally exposed populations (Srivastava et al. 2023). These effects may impact the aforementioned mental health issues, but it is important to note that this is a multifaceted issue (Miller and Rudolphi 2022). However, neurological disorders may impact farm worker health in a multitude of ways and should be treated as a chronic medical issue with implications in various aspects of workers' lives.

Conclusion

Farm workers may face a myriad of health issues due to multiple exposures. This combination of exposures may lead to difficulty in determining causation for a particular health outcome. Additionally, these exposures may exacerbate other health issues and/or enhance genetic predispositions for adverse health outcomes. It is important for health practitioners to have an awareness of chronic conditions to which farm workers may have an increased risk. Here, an overview is provided of neurological conditions and cancers that have been studied in the literature. However, aside from the most notable long-term AHS, many published studies are based on small sample sizes, hence many adverse health outcomes require further research. This underscores the importance of farm worker surveillance systems that may be imperative in helping practitioners in their awareness of diseases that may be common among this population.

References

Alavanja MCR, Semanic C, Dosemeci M, Lubin J, Tarone R, Lynch CF, Knott C, Thomas K, Hoppin JA, Barker J, Coble J, Sandler DP, Blair A. Use of agricultural pesticides and prostate cancer risk in the agricultural health study cohort. Am J Epidemiol. 2003;157(9):800–14.

Alavanja MCR, Hoppin JA, Kamel F. Health effects of chronic pesticide exposure: cancer and neurotoxicity. Ann Rev Pub Health. 2004;25:155–97.

Alavanja MCR, Ross MK, Bonner MR. Increased cancer burden among pesticide applicators and others due to pesticide exposure. CA Cancer J Clin. 2013;63(2):120–42.

Andreotti G, Koutros S, Hofmann JN, Sandler DP, Lubin JH, Lynch CF, Lerro CC, De Roos AJ, Parks CG, Alavanja MCR, Silverman DT, Beane Freeman LE. Glyphosate use and cancer incidence in the Agricultural Health Study. J Natl Cancer Inst. 2018;110(5):509–16.

Andrew A, Zhou J, Gui J, Harrison A, Shi X, Li M, Guetti B, Nathan R, Tischbein M, Pioro EP, Stammel E, Bradley W. Pesticides applied to crops and amyotrophic lateral sclerosis risk in the U.S. Neurtoxicology. 2021;87:128–35.

Arora K, Xu L, Bhagianadh D. Dementia and cognitive decline in older adulthood: are agricultural workers at greater risk? J Gerontol B Psychol Sci Soc Sci. 2021;76(6):1629–43.

Ba Y, Huang H, Lerro C, Li S, Zhao N, Li A, Ma S, Udelsman R, Zhang Y. Occupation and thyroid cancer: a population-based case-control study in Connecticut. J Occup Environ Med. 2017;58(3):299–305.

Beane-Freeman LE, Rusiecki JA, Hoppin JA, Lubin JH, Koutros S, Andreotti G, Zahm SH, Hines CJ, Coble JB, Barone-Adesi F, Sloan J, Sandler DP, Blair A, Alavanja MCR. Atrazine and cancer incidence among pesticide applicators in the agricultural health study (1994–2007). Environ Health Perspect. 2011;119(9):1253–9.

Berry C, La Vecchia C, Nicotera P. Paraquat and Parkinson's disease. Cell Death Differ. 2010;17:1115–25.

Blair A, Zahm SH. Agricultural exposures and cancer. Environ Health Perspect. 1995;103(Suppl 8):205–8.

Blair A, Zahm SH, Pearce NE, Heineman EF, Fraumeni JF Jr. Clues to cancer etiology from studies of farmers. Scand J Work Environ Health. 1992;18(4):209–15.

Boas M, Feldt-Rasmussen U, Skakkebæk NE, Main KM. Environmental chemicals and thyroid function. Eur J Endocrinol. 2006;154(5):599–611.

Boers D, Zeegers MP, Swaen G, Kant I, van den Brandt PA. The influence of occupational exposure to pesticides, polycyclic aromatic hydrocarbons, diesel exhaust, metal dust, metal fumes, and mineral oil on prostate cancer: a prospective cohort study. Occup Environ Med. 2005;62(8):531–7.

Centers for Disease Control and Prevention (CDC). Hematologic cancer incidence, survival, and prevalence. USCS Data Brief, no. 30. Atlanta, GA: Centers for Disease Control and Prevention, US Department of Health and Human Services; 2022.

Chimedu E, Arome D, Ameh FS. A new method for determining acute toxicity in animal models. Toxicol Int. 2013;20(3):224–6.

Culp MB, Soerjomataram I, Efstathiou E, Bray F, Jemal A. Recent global patterns in prostate cancer incidence and mortality rates. Eur Urol. 2020;77(1):38–52.

Cuneo A, Fagioli F, Tallarico A, Previati R, Piva N, Garli MG, Balboni M, Castoldi G. Morphologic, immunologic and cytogenetic studies in acute myeloid leukemia following occupational exposure to pesticides and organic solvents. Leuk Res. 1992;16(8):789–96.

Curl CL, Spivak M, Phinney R, Montrose L. Synthetic pesticides and health in vulnerable populations: agricultural workers. Curr Environ Health Rep. 2020;7(1):13–29.

Damala CA, Koutroubas SD. Farmers' exposure to pesticides: toxicity types and ways of prevention. Toxics. 2016;4(1):1. https://doi.org/10.3390/toxics4010001.

Das R, Steege A, Baron S, Beckman J, Harrison R. Pesticide-related illness among migrant farmworkers in the United States. Int J Occup Environ Health. 2001;7(4):303–12.

Dorsey ER, Zafar M, Lettenberger SE, Pawlik ME, Kinel D, Frissen M, Schneider RB, Kieburtz K, Tanner CM, De Miranda BR, Goldman SM, Bloem BR. Trichloroethylene: an invisible cause of Parkinson's disease? J Parkinsons Dis. 2023;13(2):203–18.

Duggar BN, Dickson DW. Pathology of neurodegenerative diseases. Cold Spring Harb Perspect Biol. 2017;9(7):a028035. https://doi.org/10.1101/cshperspect.a028035.

Epstein JL, Zelefsky MJ, Sjoberg DD, Nelson JB, Egevad L, Magi-Galluzzi C, Vickers AJ, Parwani AV, Reuter VE, Fine SW, Eastham JA, Wiklund P, Han M, Reddy CA, Ciezki JP, Nyberg T, Klein EA. A contemporary prostate cancer grading system: a validated alternative to the Gleason score. Eur Urol. 2016;69(3):428–35.

Fleming LE, Bean JA, Rudolph M, Hamilton K. Cancer incidence in a cohort of licensed pesticide applicators in Florida. J Occup Environ Med. 1999;41(4):279–88.

Gash DM, Rutland K, Hudson NL, Sullivan PG, Bing G, Cass WA, Pandya JD, Liu M, Choi D-Y, Hunter RL, Gerhardt GA. Trichloroethylene: parkinsonism and complex 1 mitochondrial neurotoxicity. Ann Neurol. 2008;63(2):184–92.

Goldner WS, Sandler DP, Fang Y, Hoppin JA, Kamel F, Levan. Pesticide use and thyroid disease among women in the agricultural health study. Am J Epidemiol. 2010;171(4):455–64.

Han X, Meng L, Li Y, Li A, Tury ME, Yang R, Wang P, Xiao K, Li W, Zhao J, Zhang Q, Jiang G. Associations between exposure to persistent organic pollutants and thyroid function in a case-control study of East China. Environ Sci Technol. 2019;53(16):9866–75.

Hayden KM, Norton MC, Darcy D, Østbye T, Zandi PP, Breitner JCS, Welsh-Bohmer KA. Occupational exposure to pesticides increases the risk of incident AD. Neurology. 2009;74(19):1524–30.

Hoang TT, Cancan Q, Paul KC, Lee M, White JD, Richards M, Auerbach SS, Long S, Shrestha S, Wang T, Freeman LEB, Hoffmann JN, Parks C, Xu CJ, Ritz B, Koppelman GH, London SJ. Epigenome-wide DNA methylation and pesticide use in the Agricultural Lung Health Study. Environ Health Perspect. 2021;129(9):097008.

Humann MJ, Sanderson WT, Gerr F, Kelly KM, Merchant JA. Effects of common agricultural tasks on measures of hearing loss. Am J Ind Med. 2012;55(10):904–16.

International Agency for Research on Cancer (IARC). Occupational exposures in insecticide applications, and some pesticides. In: IARC monograph on the evaluation of carcinogenic risk to humans, vol. 53. Lyon: IARC; 1991.

International Agency For Research on Cancer (IARC). A review of human carcinogens, chemical agents and related occupations. In: IARC monograph on the evaluation of carcinogenic risk to humans. Lyon: IARC; 2012.

Kab S, Moisan F, Elbaz A. Farming and incidence of motor neuron disease: French Nationwide Study. Eur J Neurol. 2017;24(9):1191–5.

Kamel F, Tanner CM, Umbach DM, Hoppin JA, Alavanja MCR, Blair A, Comyns K, Goldman SM, Korell M, Langston JW, Ross GW, Sandler DP. Pesticide exposure and self-reported Parkinson's disease in the Agricultural Health Study. Am J Epidemiol. 2007;165(4):364–74.

Kamel F, Umbach DM, Bedlack RS, Richards M, Watson M, Alavanja MCR, Blair A, Hoppin JA, Schmidt S, Sandler DP. Pesticide exposure and amyotrophic lateral sclerosis. Neurotoxicology. 2012;33(3):457–62.

Kang H, Cha ES, Choi GJ, Lee WJ. Amyotrophic lateral sclerosis and agricultural environments: a systematic review. J Korean Med Sci. 2014;29(12):1610–7.

Kim KH, Kabir E, Jahan SA. Exposure to pesticides and the associated human Health effects. Sci Tot Environ. 2017;575:525–35.

Kori RK, Mandrah K, Hasan W, Patel DK, Roy SK, Yadav RS. Identification of markers of depression and neurotoxicity in pesticide exposed agriculture workers. Biochem Mol Toxicol. 2020;34(6):e22477. https://doi.org/10.1002/jbt.22477.

Koutros S, Alavanja MC, Lubin JH, Sandler DP, Hoppin JA, Lynch CF, Knott C, Blair B, Beane-Freeman LE. An update of cancer incidence in the Agricultural Health Study. J Occup Environ Med. 2010;52(11):1098–105.

Koutros S, Beane-Freeman LE, Lubin JH, Heltshe SL, Androetti G, Barry KH, DellaValle CT, Hoppin JA, Sandler DP, Lynch CF, Blair A, Alavanja MCR. Risk of total and aggressive prostate cancer and pesticide use in Agricultural Health Study. Am J Epidemiol. 2013;177(1):59–74.

Krstev S, Barsi D, Stewart P, Dosemeci M, Swanson GM, Greenberg RS, Schoenberg JB, Schwartz AG, Liff JM, Hayes RB. Occupational risk factors and prostate cancer in U.S. blacks and whites. Am J Ind Med. 1998;34(5):421–30.

Lamptey RNL, Chaulagain B, Trivedi R, Gothwal A, Layek B, Singh J. A review of the common neurodegenerative disorders: current therapeutic approaches and the potential role of nanotherapeutics. Int J Mol Sci. 2022;23(3):1851.

Landgren O, Kyle RA, Pfeiffer RM, Hoppin JA, Beane-Freeman LE, Cerhan JR, Katzmann JA, Rajkmar SV, Alavanja MC. Monoclonal gammopathy of undetermined significance (MGUS) consistently precedes multiple myeloma: a prospective study. Blood. 2009;113:5412–7.

Lane CA, Hardy J, Schott JM. Alzheimer's disease. Eur J Neurol. 2017;25(1):59–70.

Lenters V, Basinas I, Beane-Freeman LE, Bofetta P, Checkoway H, Coggon D, Portengen L, Sim M, Wouters IM, Heederik D, Vermeulen. Endotoxin exposure and lung cancer risk: a systematic review and meta-analysis of the published literature on agriculture and cotton textile workers. Cancer Causes Control. 2010;21:523–55.

Lerro CC, Koutros S, Andreotti G, Sandler DP, Lynch CF, Louis LM, Blair A, Parks CG, Shrestha S, Lubin JH, Albert PS, Hoffmann JN, Beane-Freeman LE. Cancer incidence in the Agricultural Health Study after 20 years of follow-up. Cancer Causes Control. 2019;30(4):311–22.

Liebers V, Bruning T, Raulf-Heimsoth M. Occupational endotoxin-exposure and possible health effects on humans. Am J Ind Med. 2006;49(6):474–91.

Lope V, Pollán M, Gustansson P, Plato N, Pérez-Goméz B, Aragonés N, Suárez B, Carrasco JM, Rodríguez S, Ramis R, Boldo E, López-Abente G. Occupation and thyroid cancer risk in Sweden. J Occup Environ Med. 2005;47(9):948–57.

Lopez JAS, González HM, Léger GC. Chapter 13. Alzheimer's disease. Handb Clin Neurol. 2019;167:231–55.

Lundin JI, Checkoway H. Endotoxin and cancer. Environ Health Perspect. 2009;117(9):1344–50.

Mahajan R, Blair A, Lynch CF, Schroeder P, Hoppin JA, Sandler DP. Fonofos exposure and cancer incidence in the agricultural health study. Environ Health Perspect. 2006;114(2):1838–42.

Mastrangelo G, Marzia V, Marcer G. Reduced lung cancer mortality in dairy farmers: is endotoxin exposure the key factor? Am J Ind Med. 1996;30:601–9.

Matasar MJ, Zelenetz AD. Overview of lymphoma diagnosis and management. Radiol Clin North Am. 2008;46(2):175–98.

Menegon A, Board PG, Blackburn A, Mellick GD, Le Couteur DG. Parkinson's disease, pesticides, and glutathione transferase polymorphisms. Lancet. 1998;352(9137):1344–6.

Merhi M, Raynal H, Cahuzac E, Vinson F, Cravedi JP, Gamet-Payrastre L. Occupational exposure to pesticides and risk of hematopoietic cancers: meta-analysis of case-control studies. Cancer Causes Control. 2007;18(10):1209–26.

Meyer TE, Coker A, Sanderson M, Symanski E. A case-control study of farming and prostate cancer in African American and Caucasian men. Occup Environ Med. 2007;64(3):155–60.

Migliore L, Coppedè F. Genetics, environmenta factors and the emerging role of epigenetics in neurodegenerative diseases. Mutat Res. 2009;667(1–2):82–97.

Miller CDM, Rudolphi JM. Characteristics of suicide among farmers and ranchers: using the CDC NVDRS 2003–2018. Am J Ind Med. 2022;65(8):675–89.

Mills PK, Shah P. Cancer incidence in California farm workers, 1988–2010. Am J Ind Med. 2014;57(7):737–47.

Mink P, Adami HO, Trichopoulos D, Britton N, Mandel JS. Pesticides and prostate cancer: a review of epidemiologic studies with specific agricultural exposure information. Eur J Cancer Prev. 2008;17(2):97–110.

Mink PJ, Mandel JS, Lundin JI, Sceurman BK. Epidemiologic studies of glyphosate and non-cancer health outcomes: a review. Regul Toxicol Pharmacol. 2011;61(2):172–84.

Mohammadpour A, Dobrovolskaia MA, Cheney DL, Greish KF, Ghandehari H. Subchronic and chronic toxicity evaluation of inorganic nanoparticles for delivery applications. Adv Drug Deliv Rev. 2019;144:112–32.

Morris J. Amyotrophic lateral sclerosis (ALS) and related motor neuron diseases: an overview. Neurodiagn J. 2015;55:180–94.

Mostafalou S, Abdollahi M. Pesticides: an update of human exposure and toxicity. Arch Toxicol. 2017;91(2):549–99.

Navarro-Bielsa A, Gracia-Cazaña T, García Malinis AJ, Quintana C, Gavin N, Martinez R, Puertolas P, Zazo

E, Gilaberte Y. Skin cancer prevalence in farm workers in Spain. Eur J Dermatol. 2022;32:724–30. https://doi.org/10.1684/ejd.2022.4374.

NC Farmworker Health Program. Farmworker health facts. 2023. https://ncfhp.ncdhhs.gov/farmworker-health-facts/.

Nguyen-Nielsen M, Borre M. Diagnostic and therapeutic strategies for prostate cancer. Semin Nucl Med. 2016;46(6):484–90.

Norouzi F, Alizadeh I, Faraji M. Human exposures to pesticides and thyroid cancer: a worldwide systematic review of the literatures. Thyroid Res. 2023;16(13):13. https://doi.org/10.1186/s13044-023-00153-9.

Pance A, Reisser D, Jeannin JF. Antitumoral effects of lipid A: preclinical and clinical studies. J Investig Med. 2002;50:173–8.

Parent ME, Siemiatycki J. Occupation and prostate cancer. Epidemiol Rev. 2001;23(1):138–43.

Parrón T, Requena M, Hernández AF, Alarcón R. Association between environmental exposure to pesticides and neurodegenerative diseases. Toxicol Appl Pharmacol. 2011;256(3):379–85.

Petrelli G, Siepi G, Miligi L, Vineis P. Solvents in pesticides. Scand J Work Environ Health. 1993;19:63–5.

Potti A, Panwalker AW, Langness E. Prevalence of pesticide exposure in young males (</ = 50 years) with adenocarcinoma of the prostate. J Carcinog. 2003;2:4. https://doi.org/10.1186/1477-3163-2-4.

Pukkala E, Martinsen JI, Lynge E, Gunnasdottir HK, Sparén P, Tryggvadottir L, Weiderpass E, Kjaerheim K. Occupation and cancer-follow-up of 15 million people in five Nordic coutries. Acta Oncol. 2009;48(5):646–790.

Purdue MP, Hoppin JA, Blair A, Dosemeci M, Alavanja MCR. Occupational exposure to organochlorine insecticides and cancer incidence in the Agricultural Health Study. Int J Cancer. 2007;120(3):642–9.

Rahbari R, Zhang L, Kebebew E. Thyroid cancer gender disparity. Future Oncol. 2010;6(11):1771–9.

Rakitsky VN, Koblyakov VA, Turusov VS. Nongenotoxic (epigenetic) carcinogens: pesticides as an example. A critical review. Teratog Carcinog Mutagen. 2000;20(4):229–40.

Reid A, Greene SE. How microbes can help feed the world: report on an American Academy of Microbiology colloquium Washington, DC, December 2012. Washington, DC: American Society for Microbiology; 2012. https://doi.org/10.1128/AAMCol.

Ross GW, Abbott RD, Petrovitch H, Tanner CM, White LR. Pre-motor features of Parkinson's disease: the Honolulu-Asia aging study experience. Parkinsonism Relat Disord. 2012;18(Suppl 1):S199–202.

Rusiecki JA, Patel R, Koutros S, Beane-Freeman L, Landgren O, Bonner MR, Coble J, Lubin J, Blair A, Hoppin JA, Alavanja MCR. Cancer incidence among pesticide applicators exposed to permethrin in the Agricultural Health Study. Environ Health Perspect. 2009;117(4):581–6.

See WZC, Naidu R, Tang KS. Paraquat and Parkinson's disease: the molecular crosstalk of upstream signal transduction pathways leading to apoptosis. Curr Neuropharmacol. 2023;22(1):140–51.

Shresthra S, Kamel F, Umbach DM, Beane Freeman LE, Koutros S, Alavanja MCR, Sandler DP, Chen H. Nonmotor symptoms and Parkinson disease in the United States farmers and spouses. PLoS One. 2017;12(9):e0185510.

Shresthra S, Parks CG, Umbach DM, Richards-Baber M, Hofmann JN, Chen H, Blair A, Beane-Freeman LE, Sandler DP. Pesticide use and incident Parkinson's disease in a cohort of farmers and their spouses. Environ Res. 2020;191:110186. https://doi.org/10.1016/j.envres.2020.110186.

Srivastava A, Srivastava AK, Pandeya A, Pant AB. Pesticide mediated silent neurotoxicity and its unmasking: an update on recent progress. Toxicology. 2023;500:153665. https://doi.org/10.1016/j.tox.2023.153665.

Szewczyk M, Pazdrowski J, Golusinski P, Danczak-Pazdrowska A, Łuczewski Ł, Marszałek S, Majchrzak E, Golusinski W. Basal cell carcinoma in farmers: an occupational group at high risk. Int Arch Occup Environ Health. 2016;89(3):497–501.

Togawa K, Leon ME, Freeman LEB, Nordby KC, Baldi I, MacFarlane E, Shin A, Park S, Greenlee RT, Sigsgaard T, Basinas I, Hofmann JN, Kjaerheim K, Douwes J, Denholm R, Ferro G, Sim MR, Kromhout H, Schüz. Cancer incidence in agricultural workers: findings from an international consortium of agricultural cohort studies (AGRICOH). Environ Int. 2021;157:106825. https://doi.org/10.1016/j.envint.2021.106825.

Tudi M, Ruan HD, Wang L, Lyu J, Connell D, Chu C, Phung DT. Agriculture development, pesticide application and its impact on the environment. Int J Environ Res Public Health. 2021;18(3):1112. https://doi.org/10.3390/iherph18031112.

United States department of agriculture (USDA). Farm labor. Economic Research Service. 2023. https://www.ers.usda.gov/topics/farm-economy/farm-labor/#:~:text=Women%20Are%20an%20Increasing%20Share,28.1%20percent%20(in%20 2021.

United States Environmental Protective Agency (EPA). Chronic effects. In: Recognition and management of pesticide poisonings. 6th ed; 2013. https://www.epa.gov/sites/default/files/documents/rmpp_6thed_ch21_chroniceffects.pdf.

Van de Donk NWCJ, Pawlyn C, Yong KL. Multiple myeloma. Lancet. 2021;397(0272):410–27.

Van Maele-Fabry G, Lantin AC, Hoet P, Lison D. Childhood leukemia and parental occupational exposure to pesticides: a systematic review and meta-analysis. Cancer Causes Control. 2010;21:787–809.

Wang G, Rayner S, Chung R, Shi B, Liang X. Advances in nanotechnology-based strategies for the treatments of amyotrophic lateral sclerosis. Mater Today Bio. 2020;6:100055. https://doi.org/10.1016/j.mtbio.2020.100055.

Wilson RS, Arnold SE, Schneider JA, Boyle PA, Buchman AS, Bennett DA. Olfactory impairment in Presymptomatic Alzheimer's disease. Ann N Y Acad Sci. 2009;1170:730–5.

Ye M, Beach J, Martin JW, Senthilselvan A. Occupational pesticide exposures and respiratory health. Int J Environ Res Public Health. 2013;10:6442–71.

Zahm SH, Blair A. Cancer among migrant and seasonal farmworkers: an epidemiologic review and research agenda. Am J Ind Med. 1993;24(6):753–66.

Zanchi MM, Marins K, Zamoner A. Could pesticide exposure be implicated in the high incidence rates of depression, anxiety and suicide in farmers? A systematic review. Environ Pollut. 2023;331:121888. https://doi.org/10.1016/j.envpol.2023.121888.

Zeng F, Lerro C, Lavoué HH, Siemiatycki J, Zhao N, Shuangge M, Deziel NC, Friesen MC, Udelsman R, Zhang Y. Occupational exposure to pesticides and other biocides and risk of thyroid cancer. Occup Environ Med. 2017;74(7):502–10.

Zhang L, Rana I, Shaffer RM, Taioli E, Sheppard. Exposure to glyphosate-based herbicides and risk for non-Hodgkin lymphoma: a meta-analysis and supporting evidence. Mutat Res. 2019;781:186–206.

Basics of Toxicology and Risk Assessment

22

Ricky L. Langley

Introduction

Toxicology can be defined as the study of the mechanisms of action and adverse effects of xenobiotics in living organisms. Xenobiotics refer mostly to an exogenous organic or inorganic compound foreign to a living organism, in this chapter humans. The objective of toxicology is to identify the nature of adverse effects that may be produced by a xenobiotic and the range of doses over which that adverse effect occurs (Logan 1988). Pharmacology has been referred to as applied toxicology. The principles and equations used in pharmacology and toxicology are the same; the main difference is that pharmacology primarily deals with low doses and therapeutic outcomes while toxicology often studies the effects of larger doses or low doses of highly toxic agents.

One of the main mantras in toxicology is that the dose makes the poison. Any substance can be a poison if the dose is high enough. It may be more accurate to say the dose rate makes the poison. For example, a person undergoing cancer treatment will often receive massive doses of radiation that would kill the person if given all at once. Instead, the dose of radiation is given in smaller quantities over an extended period of time (fractionated), although the total radiation dose the person receives is the same. Another factor that the practitioner should consider from exposure to a chemical is not only the intrinsic toxicity of the agent, but also the degree of risk the chemical poses. Risk is the likelihood of injury, disease, or death occurrence. For example, if a highly toxic agent is carefully handled, and the worker is wearing appropriate protective equipment, the risk of adverse effects to the worker may be lower than improperly handling or using a less toxic agent.

In the United States numerous federal and state rules and regulations have been enacted over the last few decades to lessen the risk of adverse effects from environmental and occupational exposure to workplace hazards and environmental pollution. Some of the more notable Federal regulations are noted in Table 22.1.

The OSHA Act created the National Institute for Occupational Safety and Health within the U.S. Public Health Service which has a research and technical advisory role for OSHA. From CERCLA legislation (often referred to as the Superfund Act), the Agency for Toxic Substances and Disease Registry (ATSDR) was created to prevent or mitigate adverse human health effects from environmental hazards.

Terminology commonly used when describing toxicological and pharmacological testing of chemicals and when describing acceptable or

R. L. Langley (✉)
Department of Biological Sciences,
North Carolina State University, Raleigh, NC, USA
e-mail: rllangley@ncsu.edu

W. J. Meggs, R. L. Langley (eds.), *Farm Toxicology*, https://doi.org/10.1007/978-3-031-80441-0_22

Table 22.1 Major occupational and environmental US federal regulations

Regulation	Year adopted
Coal Mine Health and Safety Act	1969
Environmental Protection Agency (EPA) established	1970
Clean Air Act	1970
National Environmental Policy Act	1970
Occupational Health and Safety Administration (OSHA) established	1971
Federal Insecticide, Fungicide, and Rodenticide Act (FIFRA)	1972
Toxic Substances Control Act (TSCA)	1976, 2016 update
Resource Conservation and Reclamation Act (RCRA)	1976
Comprehensive Environmental Response, Compensation, and Liability Act (CERCLA)	1980
Superfund Amendment and Reauthorization Act (SARA)	1986
EPA Worker Protection Standard	1992, 2015 update

harmful levels of exposure and health effects often varies by agency and is sometimes confusing. Here is a list of some of the more commonly used terms:

Permissible Exposure Limit (PEL)—Established by OSHA and indicates a TWA (time-weighted average) concentration that must not be exceeded during any 8-h work shift.

Recommended Exposure Limit (REL)—Developed by National Institute for Occupational Safety and Health (NIOSH) and indicates a TWA concentration for up to 10-h workday that is meant to protect worker health.

Short-Term Exposure Limit (STEL)—A 15-min TWA concentration that should not be exceeded at any time during the workday. A "C" preceding the value means a ceiling value that should not be exceeded at any time during the workday.

Threshold Limit Values (TLV)—Concentration limits developed by the American Conference of Governmental Industrial Hygienists (ACGIH), a private nongovernmental corporation, and represent conditions under which ACGIH believes that nearly all workers may be repeatedly exposed without adverse effects without consideration for economic or technical feasibility.

Effective Dose (ED)—Effective dose is a term often used in pharmacologic evaluation of drugs and is the minimal dose that produces a biological response. The therapeutic range of a drug is generally defined by the range between the minimum effective dose (MED) and the maximum tolerated dose (MTD).

Minimum effective dose (MED)—The lowest dose that provides a clinically significant response in efficacy and is significantly superior to a placebo response.

Maximum tolerated dose (MTD)—The highest tolerable dose with respect to clinical limiting toxicity. If there is a large difference between the MED and MTD, it is stated the drug has a large therapeutic window. If the difference is small, then the drug may have little practical value or the patient must be closely monitored to avoid toxic effects.

ED_{50}—The median effective dose that produces an effect in 50% of the population that takes it. The ED_{50} is commonly used as a measure of the reasonable expectancy of a drug effect, although it may not represent the dose a clinician may use as this depends on the need for the effect and also the toxicity.

LD_{50}—The median lethal dose required to kill half the members of a tested population after a specified test duration. LD_{50} values are often used as a general indicator of a substance's acute toxicity. The LD_{50} is usually expressed as the mass of substance administered per unit mass of test subject, typically as milligrams of substance per kilogram of body mass. A lower LD_{50} indicates a higher toxicity.

LC_{50}— The concentration of a material in air which, on the basis of laboratory tests, is expected to kill 50% of a tested population when administered as a single exposure (usually 1 or 4 h). The LC_{50} is expressed as parts of material per million parts of air, by volume (ppm) for gases and vapors, or as micrograms of material per liter of air (micro-g/L) or mil-

ligrams of material per cubic meter of air (mg/m^3) for dust and mists.

TD_{50}—The median toxic dose of a xenobiotic at which toxicity occurs in 50% of the cases. Toxicity need not be lethal (anemia, inflammation of organs, birth defects, etc.) The TD_{50} encompasses the category of toxicity greater than the ED50 concentration but less than the LD_{50} concentration. So in order of toxicity $ED_{50} < TD_{50} < LD_{50}$.

Immediately Dangerous to Life and Health (IDLH)—A value developed by NIOSH as a maximum airborne concentration that a worker could be exposed to without injury or irreversible health effects in the event of failure of respiratory protective equipment. The IDLH level is usually expressed in units of ppm or mg/m^3. To convert between ppm and mg/m^3 use the following formula:

$$\text{ppm} = \text{mg}/\text{m}^3 \times 24.45/\text{gram molecular weight of substance}$$

No Observed Effect Level (NOEL)—During toxicity testing, the NOEL is the highest dose given that does not elicit an observable (statistically significant) effect in the test subject.

No-Observed-Adverse-Effect Level (NOAEL)—During toxicity testing, the NOAEL is the highest dose given that does not elicit an observable (statistically significant) negative or harmful effect in the test subject.

Lowest Observed Effect Level (LOEL)—The lowest dose given to a test subject that results in an observable (statistically significant) effect.

Lowest Observed Adverse Effect Level (LOAEL)—The lowest dose given to a test subject that results in an observable (statistically significant) negative or harmful effect.

Exposure-Disease Pathway

There are numerous substances both in the workplace or the environment that can present a hazard to humans (or wildlife). Hazardous agents may be present in the air, water, soil, food, or in medications and supplements that are consumed. It is estimated that 15% of the U.S. population may use private wells for drinking water (often higher in other countries) and few regulations exist to ensure the safety of the drinking water from these private wells. These exposures (air, water, soil, food, medicines/supplements) can result in adverse effects to the body including but not limited to damage to DNA (strand breaks), non-DNA changes (epigenetic effects which can interfere with gene expression or activity), cell damage (membranes, mitochondria), metabolic changes, and hormonal effects or mimicry. The resulting diseases may include cancers, diabetes, heart disease, kidney disease, pulmonary disease, neurologic disease, and adverse effects on the reproductive, endocrine, and immunologic organs.

Common environmental exposures that the rural practitioner may encounter in his/her patient evaluation may include the following (Table 22.2):

The following Table 22.3 shows examples of organ systems often affected by toxic exposures that the practitioner should consider if their

Table 22.2 Environmental exposure and common sources/uses

Lead	Paints, batteries, ammunition, lead pipes
Arsenic	Old pesticides, ground water contamination (natural or anthropogenic)
Mercury	Old pesticides, thermometers, thermostats, some light bulbs
Carbon monoxide	Engine exhaust, poorly ventilated heaters
Solvents	Degreasers, metal cleaners, ground water contamination, and vapor intrusion from nearby industries (e.g., dry cleaners
Asbestos	Insulation, popcorn ceilings, tiles, brake linings on older vehicles, even natural deposits in certain regions of the country
Radon	Ground water and vapor intrusion
Algal blooms	Often due to eutrophication from fertilizer runoff into farm ponds and lakes
Fecal Coliform bacteria (*E. coli*)	From private well water contamination, contaminated food items, petting zoos
Mold/mildew	Floods, sewage overflows broken water pipes in homes
Ozone	Air pollution events
Particulates	Wildland fires, air pollution events
PCBs, PAHs, PFAS	Usually from water contamination from industrial discharges
Formaldehyde	Building material off-gassing, new furniture/carpets
Pesticides	Both agricultural applications as well as home use

Table 22.3 Organ systems and toxic exposures

Respiratory	Asbestos, radon, glues, various smoke and exhaust
Dermatologic	Dioxin, nickel, arsenic, mercury, chromium (cement), polychlorinated biphenyls, glues, rubber latex, radiation
Liver	Carbon tetrachloride, methylene chloride, vinyl chloride, thorium
Kidneys	Cadmium, lead, mercury, chlorinated hydrocarbon solvents
Cardiovascular	Carbon monoxide, carbon disulfide, nitrates, methylene chloride, tobacco smoke, and exhaust, and consider physical stress and excessive noise levels
Reproductive	Methylmercury, carbon monoxide, lead, ethylene oxide, dibromochloropropane (DBCP)
Hematologic	Arsenic, benzene, nitrates, radiation
Neuropsychologic	Tetrachloroethylene, mercury, arsenic, toluene, lead, methanol, vinyl chloride, thallium, excessive noise

patient reports symptoms or has evidence of disease but no apparent cause is readily identified.

Factors Affecting Toxicity of a Xenobiotic

Chemicals can have local (at the point of contact with the body) and/or systemic effects. Dermal contact often causes local effects while ingestion or inhalational exposures can result in local or systemic effects because chemicals are more easily absorbed from the gastrointestinal or respiratory tracts into the bloodstream and distributed throughout the body. However, some chemicals can be rapidly absorbed by dermal contact and cause systemic illness such as organophosphate pesticides. Adverse health effects seen from chemical exposure may include irritation of skin, mucus membranes, and airways, asphyxia (toxic gases), corrosive damage to skin and eyes (acids/bases), or cellular damage affecting ion channels resulting in cardiac dysrhythmia. Other effects may include narcosis and sensitization in which subsequent exposures to even minimal amounts of the agent can cause adverse effects such as allergic contact dermatitis or even anaphylaxis. Chemicals can act

Table 22.4 Factors affecting toxicity from exposure to a xenobiotic

Factors
Dose/dose rate (toxic manifestations usually occur with increased severity and frequency as the dose increases, often described as a dose-response relationship)
Frequency, duration, and timing of exposure
Physical state of the agent-solid, liquid, gas
Purity of the agent (any additives, metabolites, contaminants?)
Route of exposure (oral, dermal, inhalation, injection)
Individual susceptibility
Age—Young/elderly may be more at risk
Sex—Certain agents may act differently in males vs. females (especially medications)
Race/ethnicity—Difference in metabolism (e.g., alcohol)
Genetics-difference in concentration of metabolic enzymes (e.g., CYP enzymes, Paraoxonase)
Health status—Immunosuppressed, medication interactions, underlying diseases
Other factors—Temperature, humidity, barometric pressure, and UV radiation levels can have an effect on the amount of agent a person is exposed to such as volatility, drift, and air inversions, and also affect the breakdown of the toxin in the environment (photodegradation, hydrolysis)

as mutagens, teratogens, and carcinogens resulting in birth defects and cancers.

There are numerous factors that affect the toxicity resulting from exposure to a xenobiotic as noted in Table 22.4.

Toxicokinetics/Toxicodynamics

In simple terms, toxicokinetics is concerned with the kinetics of absorption, distribution, metabolism, and elimination of a xenobiotic agent to which a person was exposed. Toxicodynamics is the study of the toxicological response and outcome from a xenobiotic and its mechanism of action at the receptor site with emphasis on the dose-response or xenobiotic concentration-effect relationship.

Absorption

Absorption of the toxicant may occur after inhalation, ingestion, dermal contact, or even injection depending on chemical/physical characteristics of the agent (such as gas/liquid/solid) and the circumstances behind the exposure event (was exposure accidental, intentional, unusual method of exposure such as needle stick, etc.). Inhalational exposure involves the lungs and airways, ingestion involves the stomach and intestines, and injection may be directly into a blood vessel or into the subcutaneous tissue, or muscles. Dermal contact absorption may occur through the stratum corneum (outer layer of the skin) but also through skin appendages such as sweat and oil glands, and hair follicles.

Absorption usually requires passage of the chemical across a biological membrane unless the chemical was directly injected into the vessel. There are three mechanisms for the xenobiotic to cross biological membranes: passive diffusion, active diffusion, and facilitated transport. Passive diffusion depends on the permeability of the surface of the membrane and chemical properties of the agent. Lipid solubility (favors absorption), pK of the chemical, and pH of the medium are important chemical characteristics. Ionized and polar molecules are not very lipid soluble. The pK of the chemical and pH of the medium determine the ionized/unionized concentration ratio. Passive diffusion also depends on the concentration gradient and surface area of the membrane (increased surface area increases absorption).

Xenobiotic absorption can also occur by active processes utilizing cellular ATP to assist in transport across the membrane and/or facilitated transport involving carrier proteins.

There are other factors affecting absorption such as properties of the xenobiotic itself and the membrane it may be crossing. Chemical properties include the size, charge, and state (solid/liquid/gas) of the xenobiotic. Increasing polarity increases water solubility. Gases are more readily absorbed. Smaller molecules (<50 Dalton) more readily cross cell membranes. Lipid-soluble molecules more readily permeate membranes. Nonionized molecules are more lipid soluble and more likely to penetrate cell membranes. Generally unbound (not bound to proteins) xenobiotics are able to cross cell membranes. Water-soluble molecules can diffuse through aqueous channels or by active transport mechanisms. Tight junctions such as blood-brain barrier may inhibit or limit the entry of the xenobiotic.

The size of the xenobiotic is very important in determining if respiratory absorption will occur. Particles 5–10 μm tend to deposit in the nasal passages and blowing the nose may remove a significant amount. Particles 3–5 μm tend to deposit in the trachea, 2–3 μm in the bronchus, 1–2 μm in the bronchioles, and 0.1 to 1 μm in the alveoli where they are readily absorbed into the circulation, depending on their solubility in alveolar fluid. The alveoli have a large surface area ranging from 50 to 100 m^2 . Larger particles may be coughed out of the larger-sized airways or removed by the mucociliary clearance mechanism in the lung and either expectorated or may be swallowed. The rate and depth of respiration and the concentration of the xenobiotic in the air are other important factors that govern the absorption of inhaled substances.

Xenobiotics that absorb through the skin diffuse through the stratum corneum, which is the rate-limiting step for absorption (Logan 1988). The stratum corneum differs in thickness and degree of permeability in different areas of the body. For example, the soles of the feet have the thickest layer of skin while the scrotum has a very thin layer and xenobiotics can more readily cross thin layers of skin. Water contact can increase the water content of the stratum corneum and increase its permeability twofold to threefold, especially to organic solvent compounds. Intact skin is less permeable than damaged skin.

Absorption through the GI tract is influenced by the size of the particle and its solubility (large particles are not as well absorbed and water-insoluble material will not be as well absorbed due to limited contact with the GI mucosa), active transport mechanisms, GI motility rate, and presence of food as food may bind to the chemical and decrease absorption (Logan 1988). Decreased motility will increase absorption. The pH of gastric juices and intestinal fluids influences the ionization state of the molecule. Thus organic acids are more readily absorbed in the stomach whereas organic bases are more readily absorbed in the small intestines.

Distribution

Once absorbed the agent will enter the circulation and be distributed to various tissues within the body. Distribution is dependent upon blood flow to the site (increased flow will increase absorption) and the rate of diffusion out of the capillary bed into cells of a particular organ or target (Lehman-McKeeman 2010). Factors affecting rate of diffusion include size of molecule, lipid solubility and ionization (molecules <50 daltons and lipid soluble can readily cross cell membranes), plasma protein binding, and tissue binding. The xenobiotic may distribute to the interstitial fluid or intracellular fluid or remain in the plasma where it may bind with various proteins, especially albumin. The xenobiotic may be distributed to storage tissue in the body such as fat, liver, or bone, or bind to various receptor sites in target organs. The liver and kidney tend to concentrate more of the xenobiotic than other organs as they have a high chemical binding capacity.

Metabolism

Metabolism, often referred to as biotransformation, is the metabolic conversion of xenobiotics to more water-soluble compounds which favor excretion in the urine or feces. Volatile compounds may be eliminated by exhalation. In some cases, chemical modification by biotransformation may alter the xenobiotic and make it more active or toxic such as occurs with methanol, carbon tetrachloride, and parathion. Various enzymes are involved in the biotransformation process. Some of the most important enzymes include the cytochrome P450 (CYPs) monooxygenases, flavin-containing monooxygenases (FMOs), alcohol and aldehyde dehydrogenases, amine oxidase, cyclooxygenases (COX), reductases, hydrolases, and a variety of conjugating enzymes, including acetyl transferases, glucuronidase sulfotransferase (SULT), glutathione transferases, and methyltransferases (Hodgson 2018). The reactions initiated by biotransformation are generally divided into four categories: hydrolysis, reduction, oxidation, and conjugation. Hydrolysis, reduction, and oxidation (often referred to as phase I reactions) usually result in a small increase in hydrophilicity by introducing polar groups into the molecule that in most cases can be conjugated during phase II reactions. Conjugation reactions (Phase II) include glucuronidation, sulfonation, acetylation, methylation, and conjugation with glutathione and amino acids. Conjugation reactions result in a large increase in hydrophilicity and greatly increase the excretion of xenobiotics (Lehman-McKeeman 2010).

Metabolism can occur in many organs but mainly in the liver. A number of factors influence the rate of biotransformation, including age, sex, race, genetics, nutritional status, underlying disease, and other medications the person may be using which can induce enzymes. For example, certain populations may have different CYPs for metabolizing alcohol and may not tolerate the same level of exposure.

Elimination

Elimination includes exhalation and excretion. Xenobiotics are primarily eliminated not only through the kidneys but also through the liver and biliary system, the lungs, sweat, tears, and breast milk can all excrete chemicals from the body (Logan 1988). Xenobiotics and/or their metabolites are excreted by the kidneys through glomerular filtration, passive tubular diffusion, and active tubular secretion. At the glomerulus small molecules are filtered. Larger molecules (>69 kilodaltons) and molecules that are protein-bound are not generally filtered by a healthy glomerulus. Once filtered the chemical may remain in the filtrate or be passively reabsorbed in the renal tubules. Highly lipid-soluble non-ionic compounds are more likely to be passively reabsorbed than are ionic and polar compounds which are water soluble (Gossel 1999). The pH of a solution (e.g., urine) determines the degree to which the xenobiotic is ionized. Compounds that are ionized and polar are poorly reabsorbed and are excreted in the urine. Certain organic acids and organic bases can be actively secreted into the urine as are some protein-bound chemicals that are not filtered through the glomerulus.

Manipulation of the urine pH may enhance elimination of certain acidic or basic xenobiotics. For example, if an acidic compound is ingested, then raising the urine pH will increase the ionized form of the compound and thus increase urinary excretion of the acidic compound. Bases are excreted at a greater extent at lower urine pH levels. We can utilize the Henderson-Hasselbalch equation to determine the proportion of the xenobiotic that is in the ionized (A^- or BH^+) and non-ionized (HA or B) form (Howland 1998).

$$\text{For weak acids}\ \mathrm{HA} = \mathrm{H}^+ + \mathrm{A}^-\ K_\mathrm{a} = \left(\mathrm{H}^+\right)\left(\mathrm{A}^-\right)/\left(\mathrm{HA}\right)\left(\begin{array}{l}K_\mathrm{a} = \text{equilibrium dissociation}\\ \text{constant}\end{array}\right)$$

$$\text{For weak bases}\ \mathrm{BH}^+ = \mathrm{B} + \mathrm{H}^+\quad K_\mathrm{a} = \left(\mathrm{H}^+\right)\left(\mathrm{B}\right)/\left(\mathrm{BH}^+\right)$$

$$\text{For weak acids}\ \mathrm{pH} = \mathrm{p}K_\mathrm{a} + \log\left(\mathrm{A}^-\right)/\left(\mathrm{HA}\right)$$

$$\text{For weak bases}\ \mathrm{pH} = \mathrm{p}K_\mathrm{a} + \log\left(\mathrm{B}\right)/\left(\mathrm{BH}^+\right)$$

The lungs are the major organ in eliminating xenobiotics existing primarily as gases at body temperature or have a high vapor pressure. Elimination from blood is by simple diffusion into the alveolar space (Logan 1988).

The liver is also involved in elimination of many xenobiotics. If a xenobiotic is absorbed from the GI tract, the blood passes through the liver through the portal circulation before reaching the systemic circulation. The liver can remove some of these compounds (first-pass metabolism), thus limiting their distribution to other sites in the body. The compound may be excreted from liver cells into the bile and passed into the small intestine where they may be eliminated in the feces or they may be reabsorbed in the intestines (enterohepatic circulation). Many compounds are biotransformed into polar molecules before excretion into the biliary tract. As they become less lipid soluble, they are more likely to be excreted into the feces and not reabsorbed in the intestines.

Elimination through breast milk is a concern to infants that may be breast feeding. Breast milk has high lipid content and lipid-soluble xenobiotics are readily transferred by passive diffusion into the lipid portion of breast milk.

Elimination of xenobiotics through the sweat, saliva, tears, hair, and nails can occur but usually of much less importance.

Using Simple Toxicokinetics in the Evaluation of a Person Exposed to a Xenobiotic

The easiest method to obtain information on absorption, distribution, metabolism, and excretion of a xenobiotic to which a person was exposed is by sampling blood or plasma concentrations over time. If one assumes the concentration of the xenobiotic in blood or plasma is in equilibrium with the concentration in tissues, then changes in blood/plasma xenobiotic concentration should reflect changes in tissue concentrations (Shen 2010). Compartmental toxicokinetic models consist of a central compartment representing plasma and highly perfused tissues that rapidly equilibrates (mix uniformly) with the xenobiotic connected to one or more peripheral compartments (organs and tissues) that more slowly equilibrate with the xenobiotic. The xenobiotic is administered to the central compartment and distributed between central and peripheral compartments and is eliminated from the body (Shen 2010). Toxicokinetic analysis often uses a one- or two-compartment model to predict the plasma concentration at different doses (after the administration of an intravenous bolus), establish the time course of the xenobiotic in plasma and tissues, and the extent of xenobiotic accumulation with multiple doses. The one-compartment model assumes that changes in plasma concentration reflect proportional changes in tissue concentrations. Xenobiotics whose kinetics can be described using one-compartment model rapidly equilibrate between the plasma and tissues relative to the rate of their elimination from the body. Xenobiotics whose elimination is described by a two-compartment model require a longer time for tissue levels (peripheral compartment) to equilibrate with the plasma concentration. Concentration of the xenobiotic can be plotted on a graph of logarithm of blood/plasma concentration vs. time. The elimination rate constant is the amount of xenobiotic eliminated per unit of time divided by the blood or plasma concentration and can be determined from the slope of the log concentration versus time plot graph (i.e. $K_{el} = 2.303 \times \text{slope}$). K_{el} can also be determined for first-order kinetics with the following equation:

$$K_{el} = \mathrm{Cl}/V_d \quad \mathrm{Cl} = \text{clearance},$$
$$V_d = \text{volume of distribution}$$

The elimination rate constant describes the fraction of xenobiotics eliminated per unit of time or the rate at which plasma concentrations will decline during the elimination phase. For example, if 35% of a drug were eliminated per hour, then K_{el} would be 0.35/h. K_{el} is independent of the dose or starting concentration for xenobiotics that follow first-order kinetics. As long as elimination mechanisms are not saturated, in our example, 35% of the starting concentration will be eliminated per hour whether the starting concentration (dose) is 50 units or 500 units. The elimination rate constant (proportion per unit time) can be used to calculate the time necessary to eliminate a certain proportion of xenobiotic (Bardal et al. 2011).

Most drugs and toxicants are eliminated (based on a one-compartment model) through a first-order process which means the rate of elimination at any time is proportional to the amount of the toxicant in the body at that time (see Table 22.5 for comparison of first-order and zero-order elimination). However, as the dose of a

Table 22.5 First-order vs. zero-order elimination characteristics

First order (linear kinetics)
1. Constant proportion (%) removed per unit of time (e.g., 10% eliminated every hour)
2. Concentration dependent—The higher the concentration the faster the rate of clearance
3. For every half-life that passes, the xenobiotic concentration is halved
4. Elimination mechanisms are not saturable
5. The elimination rate constant, V_d, clearance, and half-life are independent of dose
Zero order (saturation kinetics)
1. Concentration independent
2. Constant amount removed per unit of time (e.g., 10 mg eliminated per hour)
3. Elimination mechanisms are saturable
4. A true half-life or elimination rate constant does not exist but depends on dose

chemical increases its volume of distribution or its rate of elimination may change due to saturation kinetics (the drug elimination process reaches a saturation point and only a fixed amount of drug can be removed from the body). The change from first order to saturation kinetics can lead to prolonged retention times of a xenobiotic in the body or increased concentration at the target site which may result in increased toxicity (Shen 2010).

Some xenobiotics appear to be eliminated by a hybrid of zero-order and first-order kinetics known as Michaelis-Menton kinetics (Eisenga 2001). Linear or first-order kinetics occurs at low xenobiotic concentrations and zero-order kinetics occurs at higher concentrations.

The Apparent Volume of Distribution (V_d) is a proportionality constant that relates the total amount of chemical in the body to the concentration in plasma. The volume of distribution is the apparent space (fluid volume) into which an amount of chemical would need to be uniformly dissolved in order to produce the observed concentration (specific for each chemical). Volume of distribution reflects total xenobiotic concentration and is therefore driven by the affinity of the drug for either blood or tissue. Many factors affect the V_d including blood flow rates, lipid solubility of the xenobiotic, tissue type, plasma protein binding, pH, and disease states. Chemicals that are highly lipid soluble have a high V_d whereas low lipid solubility xenobiotics have a low V_d. Acidic xenobiotics tend to be highly bound to plasma proteins, with low affinity for tissue due to repulsion by the negatively charged phospholipid membranes. Acids therefore tend to reside predominantly in the blood and consequently demonstrate a low volume of distribution. Basic drugs, on the other hand, bind to plasma proteins to an extent consistent with lipophilicity, but also readily partition into phospholipid membranes resulting in extensive tissue distribution. Basic drugs therefore tend to have a higher volume of distribution. V_d provides an indication of accessibility of the chemical to therapeutic procedures such as extracorporeal removal by dialysis. Chemicals with high V_d (>5–10 L/kg) have low blood concentrations while chemicals with low V_d (<1 L/kg) are primarily contained in the blood often due to protein binding. Chemicals with very high V_d may indicate that the chemical has been distributed to and accumulated at a particular storage site in the body. Chemicals with a very large V_d have a relatively low plasma concentration compared to total body stores. In contrast, chemicals with a low V_d (higher concentration in the plasma) may be accessible to extracorporeal removal procedures; however, highly protein bound chemicals are difficult to remove by dialysis (Olson and Vohra 2018).

$$V_d = \text{Dose to the body}(\text{mg/kg}) / \text{plasma concentration}(\text{mg/L}) = \text{L/kg}$$

Once the V_d of a chemical is known, it can be used to estimate the amount of chemical remaining in the body at any time if the plasma concentration at that time is known using the following relationship:

$$X = V_d \times C$$

where X is the amount of chemical in the body and C is the plasma concentration of the chemical.

Clearance (Cl) is the rate of chemical excreted from the body in terms of volume of fluid containing that chemical that is cleared per unit of time. Clearance has units of mL/min. Total clearance is the sum of all sources of clearance (renal excretion plus hepatic metabolism plus respiratory and skin excretion). High values of clearance indicate efficient and generally rapid removal of a chemical from the body. Clearance can be calculated if the volume of distribution and elimination rate constants (K_{el}) are known and can be defined as:

$$Cl = V_d \times K_{el}$$

A crude measurement of urinary clearance may be helpful for estimating the effectiveness of fluid therapy for enhancing renal elimination of xenobiotics not secreted or absorbed by renal tubules (Osweiler 1996).

Renal Cl = urine flow rate × urine drug conc./plasma drug conc. (If the plasma concentration is small the actual amount of xenobiotic removed is also small).

The half-life of elimination of a xenobiotic ($T_{1/2}$) is the time required for the blood or plasma concentration to decrease by one-half and is dependent on both clearance and volume of distribution. The half-life can be calculated as follows:

$$T_{1/2} = (0.693 \times V_d) / Cl$$

The half-life can also be determined by $T_{1/2} = 0.693 \times K_{el}$ (K_{el} can be determined from the slope of the line that designates the elimination phase on the log concentration versus time plot). For compounds eliminated by first-order kinetics, the time required for the plasma concentration to decrease by one-half is constant. After 7 half-lives, over 99% of the chemical is eliminated.

Evaluation of the Poisoned Patient

The results of acute toxicity testing in animals can be used to provide basic information about a xenobiotic's relative potential to cause an acute toxic effect in humans (CCOHS 2024). In animal studies, the LD_{50} is usually determined. In general, the smaller the LD_{50} value, the more toxic the chemical. The opposite is also true: the larger the LD_{50} value, the lower the toxicity. Differences in the LD_{50} toxicity ratings reflect the different routes of exposure. The toxicity rating can be different for different animals. The results of toxicity testing in animals are often reported in terms of toxicity ratings or classes and may have some clinical utility in human poisonings. Two scales that are frequently used are the Hodge and Sterner scale and the Gosselin, Smith, and Hodge scale

Table 22.6 Toxicity classes: Hodge and Sterner scale

		Routes of administration			
		Oral LD_{50}	Inhalation LC_{50}	Dermal LD_{50}	
Toxicity rating	Commonly used term	(Single dose to rats) mg/kg	(Exposure of rats for 4 h) ppm	(Single application to skin of rabbits) mg/kg	Probable lethal dose for man
1	Extremely toxic	1 or less	10 or less	5 or less	1 grain (a taste, a drop)
2	Highly toxic	1–50	10–100	5–43	4 mL (1 tsp)
3	Moderately toxic	50–500	100–1000	44–340	30 mL (1 fl. Oz.)
4	Slightly toxic	500–5000	1000–10,000	350–2810	600 mL (1 pint)
5	Practically nontoxic	5000–15,000	10,000–100,000	2820–22,590	1 L (or 1 quart)
6	Relatively harmless	15,000 or more	100,000	22,600 or more	>1 L (or 1 quart)

Table 22.7 Toxicity classes: Gosselin, Smith and Hodge

Toxicity rating or class	Dose	Probable oral lethal dose (Human) for 70-kg person (150 lbs)
6 Super toxic	Less than 5 mg/kg	1 grain (a taste—less than 7 drops)
5 Extremely toxic	5–50 mg/kg	4 mL (between 7 drops and 1 tsp)
4 Very toxic	50–500 mg/kg	30 mL (between 1 tsp. and 1 fl ounce)
3 Moderately toxic	0.5–5 g/kg	30–600 mL (between 1 fl oz. and 1 pint)
2 Slightly toxic	5–15 g/kg	600–1200 mL (between 1 pint to 1 quart)
1 Practically non-toxic	Above 15 g/kg	More than 1200 mL (more than 1 quart)

as noted below (Tables 22.6 and 22.7). These tables differ in both the numerical rating given to each class and the terms used to describe each class. For example, a chemical with an oral LD_{50} value of 2 mg/kg, would be rated as "1" and "highly toxic" according to the Hodge and Sterner scale but rated as "6" and "super toxic" according to the Gosselin, Smith, and Hodge scale. It is important to reference the scale being used when classifying the toxicity of a compound (CCOHS 2024). This rating classification can be helpful to the practitioner to recognize the potential of serious injury to an individual based on the amount of exposure to the xenobiotic and may help guide the need for rapid assessment, decontamination, and therapeutic intervention.

The World Health Organization uses the acute toxicity hazard categories as the starting point for classification of pesticide hazards (WHO 2019).

Class	LD_{50} for the rat (mg/kg body weight)	
	Oral	Dermal
Ia Extremely hazardous	<5	<50
Ib Highly hazardous	5–50	50–200
II Moderately hazardous	50–2000	200–2000
III Slightly hazardous	Over 2000	Over 2000
U	Unlikely to present acute hazard 5000 or higher	

According to the WHO: "It is highly desirable that, whenever practicable, toxicological data for each formulation to be classified should be available from the manufacturer. However, if such data are not obtainable, then the classification may be based on proportionate calculations from the LD_{50} values of the technical ingredient or ingredients, according to the following formula:

$$LD_{50}\,\text{active ingredient} \times 100 / \text{Percentage of active ingredient in formulation}$$

If the formulation contains more than one ingredient (including solvents and wetting agents) of significant toxicity-enhancing proper-

A person (weight 154 pounds) consumed 4 ounces of a pesticide product accidentally and presents to the emergency room.

Convert person's body weight to kilograms

154 pounds × 1 kg/ 2.2 pounds = 70 kg

Calculate amount of product ingested (this will often rely on estimate of amount ingested by history from the exposed person and many factors to consider such as age, reliability, and level of consciousness).

1 ounce is approximately 30 mL; 4 ounces = 120 mL (Look at density of the product formulation which may be on the label. Density = g/mL and varies by element, water had a density of 1)

This pesticide product has a density of ~1 so 1 ounce = 30 g and 4 ounces = 120 g

Calculate amount of xenobiotic (active ingredient) in each gram of pesticide product ingested (The label on the container may list the amount of active ingredient (AI) in percentages such as 0.005%).

0.005% AI in the product = 0.005 g AI/100 g product = 0.00005 g AI/1 g of pesticide product × 1000 mg/g (AI) = 0.05 mg AI/g product

Thus 0.005% xenobiotic (AI) in grams in the product = 0.05 mg xenobiotic (AI)/g product

Calculate amount of xenobiotic (AI) ingested (dosage)

0.05 mg AI/g product × 120 g product ingested = 6 mg AI ingested

Calculate dosage in mg AI/kg body weight

6 mg AI ingested/70 kg = 0.086 mg/kg

Compare to toxic values for that AI (preferably use human data and the NOAEL, LOAEL levels if known. May have to rely on animal data such as ranges of LD_{50} values reported)

(Note that pesticide formulations not only contain the AI (the chemical that targets the pest of concern) but other chemicals in the formulation (diluents, carriers, wetting agents, solvents, etc) that can have their own toxicity.

Here is another example using a pure substance. Your patient attempted suicide by eating 4 cups of sugar (sugar weighs 200 g/cup). Is his life in danger from this ingestion?

Weight of person 70 kg

Dosage 800 g (4 cups of sugar)

LD_{50} sugar = 29,700 mg/kg

Max dosage = Weight × LD_{50} = 70 kg × 29,700 mg/kg = 2,079,000 mg

Convert answer from mg to grams = 2,079,000/1000 = 2079 g

Compare ingested dosage to Max dosage = 800 g < 2079 g, so it is unlikely your patient will succumb to the sugar ingestion.

ties, then the classification should correspond to the toxicity of the mixed ingredients." The WHO has an extensive list of LD_{50} values for pesticides (WHO 2019).

Here is a quick method to estimate the risk to a person from ingestion of a known xenobiotic agent by calculating the dose of xenobiotic ingested.

When evaluating the poisoned or suspected poisoned patient, the history is of paramount importance. Additional information can be obtained from the physical examination. See Approach to Patient Chap. 1 for further details.

Many toxicants may have characteristic odors, which may be detected in the patient (Table 22.8) but the absence of odor does not necessarily mean the absence of the toxicant (Chaing 1998; Olson and Vohra 2018). For example, carbon monoxide is odorless but the detection of engine exhaust may provide a clue the person was exposed to carbon monoxide.

Some patients may have a constellation of signs and symptoms associated with exposure to certain classes of xenobiotics and these are referred to as Toxidromes. The most commonly encountered toxidromes are the: (a) anticholinergic, (b) cholinergic, (c) opioid, (d) sedative-hypnotic, and (e) sympathomimetic (also known as the adrenergic or stimulant) toxidromes. See Drugs of Abuse section in Miscellaneous Farm Toxicological and Environmental Hazards Chapter for characteristic findings on physical examination.

Readily available laboratory tests which may be useful in screening the suspected poisoned patient with uncertain diagnosis include (Olson and Vohra 2018):

Serum glucose	EKG
Serum acetaminophen level	Electrolytes
Blood alcohol level	Serum osmolality
Complete blood count	Liver function panel (AST, ALT, bilirubin)
Coagulation test (PT, PTT)	Renal panel-BUN and creatinine
Pregnancy test in females of childbearing potential	

Table 22.8 Odors associated with various xenobiotics used on farms

Odor	Xenobiotic
Acetone	Acetone, isopropyl alcohol, trichloroethane, methyl bromide
Alcohol	Ethanol, isopropyl alcohol
Disinfectants	Phenol, pine oil-based cleaners, turpentine, creosote
Fishy	Zinc phosphide, aluminum phosphide
Garlic	Phosphorous, arsenic, parathion, malathion, selenium, thallium, DMSO
Mothballs	Camphor, naphthalene, paradichlorobenzene
Mowed hay (recently)	Phosgene
Peanuts	N-3-pyridyl-methyl-N-p-nitrophenyl urea (Vacor)
Rotten eggs	Hydrogen sulfide, mercaptans, carbon disulfide
Vinegar	Acetic acid
Wintergreen	Methyl salicylate

Table 22.9 Urine color and toxicants

Urine color	Toxicant or other cause
Red-pink or orange	Pyridium, rifampin, deferoxamine, hydroxycobalamin, beets, blood, porphyrins, urates, fava beans, phenolphthalein
Violet or blue or green	Methylene blue, mthocarbamol, anthraquinone, bile pigments, resorcinol, tetrahydronapthalene, thymol
Brown or black	Phenol, myoglobin, cascara, cadmium, chlorobenzenes, napthol, nitrobenzene, aniline dyes, quinine, rhubarb
Fluorescence under UV light	Suggest antifreeze product due to added fluorescein
Crystals of calcium oxalate	Ethylene glycol

Creatine kinase check for rhabdomyolysis
Urinalysis-check for crystalluria, hemoglobinuria, or myoglobinuria. Note the urine color as it may provide clues to a toxicant (Table 22.9)

The osmol gap should be calculated. The normal measured osmolality value ranges from 275 to 295 mOsm/kg. The osmol gap can be calculated using the following formula: calculated osmolality = 2× (Na) + (glucose)/18 + (BUN)/2.8. The osmol gap is the difference between the measured serum osmolality and the calculated osmolality. The normal osmol gap is <10. The osmol gap may be elevated when low molecular weight substances such as ethanol, other alcohols, and glycols are present. Patients with diabetic ketoacidosis or alcoholic ketoacidosis or with chronic renal failure may have an elevated osmol gap.

The anion gap should also be calculated. The normal anion gap of 8–12 mEq/L accounts for unmeasured anions (phosphate, sulfates, and anionic proteins) in the plasma. The anion gap can be calculated by the following formula: Anion Gap = (Na)−(Cl)−(HCO_3).

An elevated anion gap is usually associated with metabolic acidosis. It is usually due to lactic acid accumulation but may be due to other unmeasured anions such as formate (methanol poisoning), glycolate, or oxalate (ethylene glycol poisoning), beta-hydroxybuturate (ketoacidosis patients) and 5-oxyproline. Patients with elevated anion and osmol gaps suggest methanol or ethylene glycol ingestion but also can be seen with severe alcoholic or diabetic ketoacidosis. Several mnemonics are used to help recall the differential diagnosis of high anion gap acidosis (Thomas 2022). Four are as follows:

- MUDPILES: Methanol; uremia; diabetic ketoacidosis (DKA); paraldehyde, phenformin; iron, isoniazid; lactic (i.e., carbon monoxide [CO] and cyanide); ethylene glycol; salicylates.
- DR. MAPLES: DKA; renal; methanol; alcoholic ketoacidosis; paraldehyde, phenformin; lactic (i.e., CO and HCN); ethylene glycol; salicylates.
- SLUMPED: Salicylate, lactate, uremia, methanol, paraldehyde, ethylene glycol, diabetes.
- GOLD MARK: Glycols (ethylene and propylene), oxoproline, lactate, D-lactate, methanol, aspirin, renal failure, ketoacidosis (GOLD

MARK includes newly recognized forms of metabolic acidosis and eliminates P for paraldehyde as that is now rarely seen).

A narrow anion gap may occur from an overdose with bromide, nitrates, lithium, calcium, or magnesium or be seen with severe hypoalbuminemia.

Various imaging studies can be done to look for radiopaque foreign bodies, including broken needles at injection sites, ingested tablets, drug-filled packets or condoms, and some ingested liquids (e.g., arsenic). Ultrasound can be used to assess depth and spread of tissue injury after high-pressure hydrocarbon injections (e.g., hydraulic fluid) or snakebites. CT scans of chest and abdomen can be used to assess extent of injury from corrosive chemicals along with endoscopy. CT or MRI can identify neurologic complications of poisonings such as basal ganglia infarcts from carbon monoxide or cyanide exposure, cerebral hemorrhage (methanol), anoxic/ischemic injury, leukoencephalopathy (toluene and vaporized heroin), or even gas emboli (concentrated hydrogen peroxide).

Toxicology panels are available for many xenobiotic agents. However, many have long turnaround times (days) or may not be available or have reliability issues, therefore the focus should be on supportive clinical management of the patient (Olson and Vohra 2018). Before ordering toxicology screens, it is recommended that two questions be asked: (ATSDR 2023) How will the results of the test alter the approach to the treatment of the patient? and (Bardal et al. 2011) Can the result of the test be returned in time to have a positive impact on the treatment of the patient? (Olson and Vohra 2018).

Blood and urine should be obtained and stored temporarily by the laboratory in cases of suspected poisoning of unknown cause. Selective screens with rapid turnaround times (e.g., drugs of abuse) can be useful to confirm clinical impressions and may aid in further management decisions (Olson and Vohra 2018). There are various methods to hasten the removal of a xenobiotic after an exposure occurs. Consultation with a toxicologist or call the Poison Control Center (1-800-222-1222) for assistance in managing cases of poisoning is recommended.

Risk Assessment

If a person or community is concerned that they may be exposed to an environmental pollutant (e.g. pesticide contamination of ground water), then a risk assessment can be performed and the risk to the person/community can be characterized, and remediation/treatments offered if there is an indication of toxic levels of exposure or adverse health effects may occur or are occurring.

Risk assessment is the systematic scientific characterization of potential adverse health effects resulting from exposure to a hazardous agent, situation, or event (Faustman and Omenn 2010). Hazard is the intrinsic toxic properties of a hazardous agent. Risk is the probability of an adverse outcome from exposure to a hazardous agent (usually a chemical). The four steps in the risk assessment process include hazard identification, dose-response assessment, exposure assessment, and risk characterization (Fig. 22.1). The first step is identifying the hazards (chemical or chemicals) that are of concern and determin-

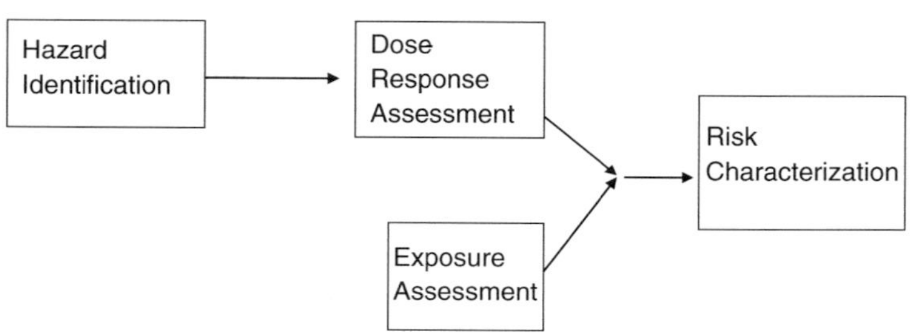

Fig. 22.1 The four-step risk assessment process

ing what health problems can be caused by the chemical, both acute and chronic. This will often require a review of the medical literature. One of the weaknesses in case reports or human epidemiology studies is the dose a person was exposed to may not be known or exposures may be to a mixture of chemicals (often in occupational studies). In many if not most cases, the hazard properties of the xenobiotic will rely on animal toxicity studies. In addition, if OSHA permissible exposure levels (PELs) are being used then remember these values are often outdated and may not have the latest health effect information to protect the worker (Ziem and Castleman 1988).

The second step, referred to as a dose-response assessment, is to determine what adverse effects or health problems may occur at different exposure levels. In these cases, animal studies are often utilized to determine what exposure levels are associated with no observed adverse effects (NOAEL), lowest observed adverse effect observed (LOAEL), and often lethal dose levels from exposures (LD). Sometimes occupational studies in humans can be used to estimate the NOAEL and LOAEL levels. A dose-response curve is plotted (Fig. 22.2) and used to find these levels. For most non-carcinogens, a threshold level usually exists below which no adverse effects occur. Carcinogenic chemicals are often considered to have no safe threshold level (especially from regulatory agency point of view). Depending on the chemical and the body's detoxification mechanisms, different shapes of the dose-response curve can occur. For example, the dose-response curve for vitamins may be U-shaped as both too low and too high exposure levels may lead to toxicity. The dose-response curve may also indicate a low margin of safety and this is especially relevant when xenobiotics are used for therapeutic purposes. If animal studies are relied upon to determine what level of exposure may result in minimal or no risk to humans, then safety factors are incorporated to account for differences between animals and humans. Additional safety factors may also be applied to account for differences in variability among humans, chronic exposures, etc.

As an alternative to the no-observed-adverse-effect level (NOAEL) approach for assessing noncancer risks associated with hazardous compounds the benchmark dose method has been proposed. The benchmark dose method is a more powerful statistical tool than the traditional NOAEL approach. The benchmark dose method involves fitting a mathematical model to all the dose-response data within a study, and thus more biological information is incorporated in the resulting estimates of guidance values such as acceptable daily intakes (ADIs) (Fillipson et al. 2003).

The third step is exposure assessment. How much of the pollutant (xenobiotic) are people exposed to during a specific time period? How many people are exposed? What are the sources

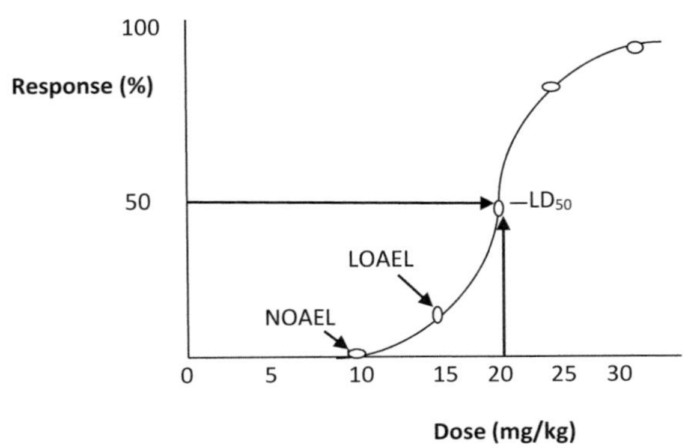

Fig. 22.2 Dose-response curve for Agent X. 6 different doses (5, 10, 15, 20 25, 30 mg/kg) of Agent X were given to 100 rats. No observed adverse effects noted at 5 and 10 mg/kg dose (NOAEL). 10% of rats developed liver inflammation at the 15 mg/kg dose (LOAEL). 50% of rats died at 20 mg/kg dose (LD_{50}). All rats died at 30 mg/kg dose

of the pollutant and how might people be exposed (air, water, food)? Major routes of exposure include inhalation, ingestion, dermal contact, and more rarely injection. Are certain populations more sensitive than others? Sensitivity can be affected by age, genetics, health status, race, and ethnicity.

There are properties of the chemical and the environment that can affect exposure, including volatility (e.g. pesticide drift), polarity (water solubility), lipophilicity (lipid soluble, may accumulate in animal fat, and skin absorption), octanol to water partition coefficient (an indicator of bioaccumulation), and degradation (soil bacteria, hydrolysis, and photolysis). Volatility (how readily it vaporizes) and depth of penetration if inhaled are influenced by particle size. Smaller particles tend to be more volatile and have lower melting points. Low-volatile compounds are more likely to exist as solids.

By using questionnaires and taking detailed patient histories we can assess the length and frequency of exposure. Biological samples of blood, urine, feces, hair, and breath may give an indication of degree of exposure. Additionally, environmental sampling of soil, water, fish, air, and dust can provide information on the amount of pollutant that may be present in the environment where a person may live or play.

After an exposure occurs, the dose or amount of xenobiotic the patient was exposed to can be generally calculated using the following formula (ATSDR 2023):

$$D = C \times IR \times AF \times EF / BW$$

where

D = exposure dose.

C = contaminant concentration.

IR = intake rate of contaminant medium.

AF = bioavailability factor (assume to be 1).

EF = Exposure factor (time exposed to pollutant).

BW = body weight (kg).

The final step is risk characterization where we compare the person/community exposure to levels that are shown to cause health effects. The risk is usually expressed as a probability and the information is put into context. For example, for cancer, we usually compare to a risk of 1 in one million. We look at the excess individual lifetime cases of cancer (beyond what would be expected to occur on average) that will occur in response to a specific exposure. Be aware that in risk assessment major assumptions, scientific judgment, and estimates of uncertainties are identified. For noncancer endpoints, the estimated or known exposure is compared to information from the dose-response assessment to determine if the exposure levels are high enough to be concerned about adverse health effects.

Once the risk assessment has been completed then decisions must be made on managing (including treatment) the risk from pollutant exposure. This is known as risk management. A risk management model based on the probability of exposure and the health impact from the exposure is noted in Table 22.10.

If a source of pollutant has been identified, then involvement of several local or state agencies may need to be initiated (if not already involved). Effective interventions to control further risk focus on the source, pathway of exposure, and the person or community affected. Can the source of the pollutant be modified, rede-

Table 22.10 Risk management model

	Probability of exposure		
Impact	Low	Medium	High
Severe/critical	Substantial preparation and monitoring required	Monitor and manage risks	Extensive monitoring and management required
Moderate	May accept risks but monitor risks	Management efforts useful	Management of risks required
Limited/minor	Accept risks	Accept risks but monitor risks	Monitor and manage risks

signed, relocated, or enclosed, or can another substitute product be used? Is it possible to control the pathway of exposure by absorbing, blocking, and diluting the pollutant so the person or community is not exposed or levels of pollutant exposure decreased? Are there actions that community members can take themselves to lessen exposure such as better home air filtration and ventilation, use of filters on water supply, avoiding consumption of wildlife/fish that may be contaminated, or as a last resort relocation.

After an individual has been exposed, the practitioner can counsel the person on activities that may modify the risk from pollutant exposure such as his/her diet, alcohol, and tobacco use (both of which can worsen or act synergistically with certain chemical exposures such as solvents and alcohol, smoking and air pollutants). Periodic health examinations and monitoring for subclinical disease should be offered depending on the pollutant and duration and magnitude of exposure. Therapeutic interventions should be offered as necessary such as the use of inhalers in individuals with reactive airways that exercise outdoors where air pollutants may be present.

References

ATSDR. Public Health Assessment Guiance Manual. 2023. https://www.atsdr.cdc.gov/pha-guidance/index.html. Accessed 25 Jan 2024.

Bardal SK, Waechter JE, Martin DS. Applied pharmacology. St. Louis, MO: Elsevier/Saunders; 2011.

CCOHS (Canadian Center for Occupational Health and Safety). Chemicals and materials. 2024. https://www.ccohs.ca/oshanswers/chemicals/ld50.html. Accessed 12 Jan 2024.

Chaing WK. Otolaryngologic principles. In: Goldfrank LR, Flomenbaum NE, Lewin NA, Weisman RS, Kowland MA, Hoffman RS, editors. Goldfrank's toxicologic emergencies. 6th ed. Stanford, CT: Appleton & Lange; 1998. p. 457–72.

Eisenga BH. Pharmacokinetic principles. In: Ling LJ, Clark RF, Erickson TB, Trestral JH, editors. Toxicology secrets. Philadelphia, PA: Hanley & Belfus; 2001. p. 19–22.

Faustman EM, Omenn GS. Risk assessment. In: Klassen CD, Watkins JB, editors. Cassarett & Doull's essentials of toxicology. 2nd ed. New York, NY: McGraw-Hill; 2010. p. 47–56.

Fillipson AF, Sand S, Nilsson J, Victorin K. The benchmark dose method—review of available models, and recommendations for application in health risk assessment. Crit Rev Toxicol. 2003;33(5):505–42.

Gossel TA. Pharmacology. A profile on pharmacokinetics. Pharmacist. 1999;71–73.

Hodgson E. Phase I and phase II metabolism and metabolic interactions: a summary. In: Smart RC, Hodgson E, editors. Molecular and biochemical toxicology. 5th ed. Hoboken NJ: Wiley; 2018. p. 189–204.

Howland MA. Pharmacokinetics and toxicokinetics. In: Goldfrank LR, Flomenbaum NE, Lewin NA, Weisman RS, Kowland MA, Hoffman RS, editors. Goldfrank's toxicologic emergencies. 6th ed. Stanford, CT: Appleton & Lange; 1998. p. 173–94.

Lehman-McKeeman LD. Absorption, distribution, and excretion of toxicants. In: Klassen CD, Watkins JB, editors. Cassarett & Doull's essentials of toxicology. 2nd ed. New York, NY: McGraw-Hill; 2010. p. 57–70.

Logan DC. Toxicology. In: McCunnney RJ, editor. Handbook of occupational medicine. Boston/Toronto: Little, Brown; 1988. p. 265–81.

Olson KR, Vohra R. Emergency evaluation and treatment. In: Poisoning and drug overdose. New York, NY: McGraw-Hill; 2018. p. 29–61.

Osweiler GD. Toxicology. Philadelphia, PA: William & Wilkins; 1996.

Shen DD. In: Klassen CD, Watkins JB, editors. Cassarett & Doull's essentials of toxicology. 2nd ed. New York, NY: McGraw-Hill; 2010. p. 99–108.

Thomas CP. What are the mnemonics used to recall the differential diagnoses of high anion gap acidosis? 2022. https://www.medscape.com/answers/242975-154572/what-are-the-mnemonics-used-to-recall-the-differential-diagnoses-of-high-anion-gap-acidosis;?form=fpf. Accessed 10 Jan 2024.

WHO (World Health Organization). The WHO Recommended classification of pesticides by hazard and guidelines to Classification. 2019. Accessed 12 Jan 2024.

Ziem GE, Castleman BI. Threshold limit values: historical perspectives and current practice. J Occup Med. 1988;31(11):910–8.

23 Occupational Hazards of Farming: An Overview

Gregory D. Kearney

Introduction

The occupational hazards and workplace exposures associated with farming have long been recognized. Among the first documented was Magnus's cautionary statement in 1555, noting respiratory concerns of farmers inhaling grain dust while threshing wheat (Magnus 1555). In 1755, Ramazzini laid the foundation of occupational medicine through his pivotal contributions to the health effects of worker's exposure to toxic materials and factors contributing to musculoskeletal problems (Ramazzini 1940). His research brought attention to the health risks associated with certain occupations and called for protective measures for workers. Even today, many of these occupational and safety concerns still exist in modern agricultural practices, given the inherent dangers present in farm environments.

Many of the topics listed in this chapter could take an entire book to describe. However, this chapter aims to provide a basic overview of the occupational hazards and health risks associated with those individuals who work in the farming environment. Some of the primary highlights in the chapter include the alarming rates of both fatal and nonfatal injuries within agriculture and the daily activities that inherently expose workers to various risks, such as working with heavy machinery, livestock, and harmful chemicals, and describes proactive preventive measures aimed at mitigating risks and protecting the health and well-being of those engaged in farming activities. Also included is an overview of the approaches and data sources used in occupational surveillance to monitor the health of the agricultural workforce, important for clinicians, public health practitioners, researchers, and policymakers. Additionally, it describes vulnerabilities of specific worker demographics, including children, women, immigrants, and older workers, underscoring susceptibility within the agricultural labor force.

Agricultural Workforce in the United States

Farming has long formed the backbone of the American workforce, playing essential roles in powering the economy and producing food for domestic consumption and commodities for the world. In the United States, agriculture represents a broad sector encompassing the largest employment sectors in the United States and many related industries accounting for an estimated 22.1 million jobs or 10.4% of the total US workforce (Economic Research Service, USDA 2022). As shown in Fig. 23.1, direct on-farm

G. D. Kearney (✉)
Department of Public Health, Brody School of Medicine, East Carolina University, Greenville, NC, USA
e-mail: kearneyg@ecu.edu

W. J. Meggs, R. L. Langley (eds.), *Farm Toxicology*, https://doi.org/10.1007/978-3-031-80441-0_23

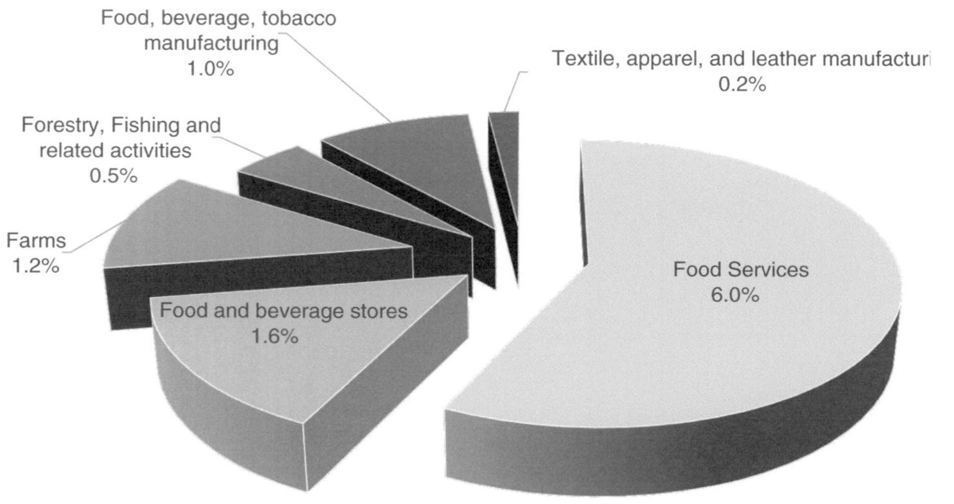

Fig. 23.1 US employment in agriculture, food, and related industries, 2022. *Agricultural and food service sectors represent 22.1 million jobs or 10.4% of total US employment. (Source: USDA, Economic Research Service using data from the US Department of Commerce, Bureau of Economic Analysis (September 29, 2023). https://www.ers.usda.gov/data-products/ag-and-food-statistics-charting-the-essentials/ag-and-food-sectors-and-the-economy)

employment accounted for 1.2% or approximately 2.6 million jobs in 2022 of the total US employment (Economic Research Service, USDA 2022).

Farm employment in the United States is defined as the number of farm owners and farm labor workers directly producing agricultural commodities, either livestock or crops (Economic Research Service, USDA 2023). The US Department of Agriculture (USDA) distinguishes the US agricultural workforce by two groups of workers: (1) self-employed farm operators and their families, and (2) hired workers (Economic Research Service, USDA 2023). The first group usually comprises agricultural establishment owners or managers who oversee the farm's operations, decision-making processes, and management. They are often responsible for various tasks such as planting, cultivating, harvesting, and managing livestock. They typically work beyond regular hours and have a personal and financial investment in the farm's success and sustainability.

The second group comprises hired workers who are employed by farm operators or larger agricultural establishments to perform specific tasks or provide labor-related services. Hired workers make up less than 1% of all US wage and salary workers, but play a vital role in agriculture (Economic Research Service, USDA 2023). Hired workers are often involved in various agricultural activities, such as planting, harvesting, tending to crops or livestock, operating machinery, and maintaining farm infrastructure. The duration of their employment varies from seasonal to temporary, depending on the demands of agricultural cycles and specific farm operations. Hired workers often possess specialized skills and labor, which are utilized to support the overall functioning of the farm, especially during peak seasons or for specific tasks that require additional workforce.

Farming and Demographic Characteristics

For over 175 years, the Census of Agriculture has been a crucial source for gathering agricultural data in the United States. To capture a complete count of farms, ranches, and the people who operate them, the US Department of Agriculture administers the Census of Agriculture survey every 5 years (NASS 2017). The survey is designed to capture many characteristics associated with farming, including land ownership, production practices, income, and demographics. The results of the census are beneficial for monitoring farming practices and informing policy.

Farming in the United States has long been dominated by family owned farms and operated businesses (MacDonald et al. 2018; NASS 2017). According to the latest agricultural census, in 2017, there were 2.2 million farms in the United States with approximately 96% reported as being family owned and operated (NASS 2017; NIFA 2017). "Family farms" are classified as "any farm in which the majority of the business is owned by an operator and any individuals related to them by blood, marriage, or adoption, including relatives who do not live in the operator's household" (Economic Research Service, USDA 2023). Note that dynamic challenges, such as evolving regulatory standards and the diversity of enterprises in the agricultural industry, have contributed to the difficulty in comparing trends accurately (Donham and Thelin 2016). For example, the definition of "farm" has been updated nine times since it was first established in 1850.

In 2017, the Census of Agriculture questionnaire was updated to better reflect the demographic data collected to better capture the contributions of persons involved in farm operations and agricultural production. The revised questions identified persons involved in making decisions for the farm as producers. This led to a 6.9% increase in the number of people identifying themselves as producers compared to the 2012 survey (NASS 2017).

As shown in Table 23.1, in 2017, the Ag Census reported that 96% of all farms in the United States were family owned. Small family

Table 23.1 Demographic characteristics among family farms in the United States (2017)

Characteristic	Small farms	Mid-size farms	Large scale farms
Number of family farms	1,798,439	108,304	52,592
Sex			
Male	62.0	74.0	78.0
Female	38.0	26.0	22.0
Age			
<35	8.0	11.0	10.0
35–64	57.0	65.0	68.0
65 and older	35.0	24.0	22.0
Race			
White	95.1	98.2	98.3
American Ind/Alaska	1.9	0.4	0.2
Black/African American	1.5	0.2	0.1
Asian	0.6	0.9	1.0
Nat Hawaiian/Pacific islander	0.1	0.0	0.0
More than one race	0.8	0.3	0.3
Hispanic	3.0	2.0	2.0
Number of years farming			
10 or less	28.0	15.0	13.0
11 or more	72.0	85.0	87.0
Lived on their farm	76.0	77.0	68.0
Primary occupation			
Farming	37.0	79.0	85.0
Other	63.0	21.0	15.0
With military service	12.0	5.0	5.0

Notes: The total number of family farm producers is 3,235,214. Totals may not add up to 100% due to rounding or exclusion of certain categories. Also, the revised definition of producer allowed data collection for up to four producers per farm

Source: USDA, Economic Research Service using data from the US Department of Commerce, Bureau of Economic Analysis (September 29, 2023). https://www.ers.usda.gov/data-products/ag-and-food-statistics-charting-the-essentials/ag-and-food-sectors-and-the-economy

farms accounted for the majority, or 88%, mid-size farms accounted for 5%, and large-scale family farms made up less than 3% of all US farms. Small family farm producers in the United States have a higher percentage of female farmers aged 65 or older, and a percentage of new or beginning farmers (farming for 10 years or less), more likely to have worked off the farm and served in the military. In contrast, mid-size and large-scale family farm producers share similar demographics, with farming as their primary occupation and fewer individuals having served in the military or being new farmers. Large-scale farms tend to have multiple individuals involved in farming operations, with 11% of mid-size farms and 26% of large and very large farms reporting three or more producers. This suggests a higher level of complexity in their farming practices (NASS 2017).

Hired Farmworkers

According to the USDA's Economic Research Service (ERS), in 2017, farmers reported hiring approximately 2.4 million farm workers. However, that number is an underestimate as it does not include nonfarm employers such as labor contractors (Costa 2023). As shown in Table 23.2, data from the US Census Bureau (2021) comparing hired farm laborers to all US private wage and salary workers were considerably less educated, slightly younger, more than four times likely to be of Mexican origin, and approximately half as likely to be a US citizen than the entire US wage and salary workforce.

Although not shown in Table 23.2, a higher percentage of female laborers in crops and related support industries and a greater diversity of ethnic backgrounds among crop workers than among livestock workers. Crop laborers also tended to

Table 23.2 Demographic characteristics of hired farm workers in the United States

Characteristic	Farm laborers	Farm managers	All other occupations in agriculture	Agriculture: all occupations	All US private wage and salary workers
Gender					
Female	28.0	17.0	33.0	28.0	44.0
Age (average in years)	39.7	43.7	42.0	40.9	40.6
Under 25 years of age	21.0	10.0	15.0	18.0	18.0
Over 44 years of age	39.0	48.0	44.0	41.0	41.0
Marital status					
Married	47.0	62.0	54.0	51.0	48.0
Race/ethnicity/ancestry					
White, not Hispanic	31.0	65.0	63.0	45.0	59.0
Black, not Hispanic	3.0	2.0	3.0	3.0	11.0
Other, not Hispanic	4.0	6.0	6.0	5.0	11.0
Hispanic: Mexican origin	54.0	22.0	23.0	40.0	12.0
Hispanic: Other	9.0	4.0	5.0	7.0	8.0
Born in US (incl. Puerto Rico)	48.0	80.0	77.0	61.0	81.0
US citizens	56.0	88.0	85.0	69.0	91.0
Education					
No high school diploma	45.0	16.0	16.0	32.0	8.0
High school diploma (includes equivalency)	34.0	33.0	31.0	33.0	29.0
Some college	22.0	51.0	53.0	35.0	63.0

Notes: Farm Laborers include farm graders and sorters; Farm managers include supervisors and inspectors
Source: USDA, Economic Research Service analysis of data from US Department of Commerce, Bureau of the Census, American Community Survey, 2021

have lower education, with 50% lacking a high school degree compared to 32% found in livestock workers (USDA 2022; Census Bureau 2021). These findings highlight the need for targeted support and resources to address the unique challenges facing farmworkers in the United States.

H-2A Workers

The H-2A visa program also referred to as the H-2A temporary agricultural workers program, was initially created to assist farmers fill employment gaps by recruiting workers from other countries. The H-2A program allows farm employers to hire temporary migrant workers when there is a shortage of American workers to fill seasonal or temporary positions. According to the Department of Labor (DOL) data, more than 90% of H-2A workers are employed on crop farms (DOL 2022). Over the years, the program has seen a significant expansion, quadrupling in size in the past decade. As of 2022, an estimated 300,000 temporary or H-2A visas were issued to workers to enable them to travel to the United States for farm employment. However, this is likely an underestimate given reporting difficulties and the exclusion of part-time workers involved in ancillary farming activities (Costa 2023; DOL 2022).

Vulnerable Workgroups

Although this chapter provides a detailed overview of the occupational hazards and health risks linked to farming, it is important to understand that the term "risk" can be intricate and differ depending on many factors. While all workers are exposed to workplace hazards, certain groups within the farming community are more susceptible to harm due to inherent risk factors, including worker demographic and socioeconomic characteristics. In this section, selected farm labor workgroups that have been highlighted as being vulnerable, include immigrant and foreign-born workers, women, children, and older workers.

Immigrant and Foreign-Born Workers

Farmworkers in the United States are a marginalized population due to their socioeconomic status and the nature of their work. Typically, many farmworkers are low-income, immigrants and/or foreign-born from Mexico and Central America, and often lack authorization to work in the United States. Farmworkers frequently engage in physically demanding labor, and their exposure to pesticides in the agricultural sector poses potential health risks (Arcury and Quandt 2009). Numerous studies have shown that immigrant and foreign-born farmworkers experience considerable workplace hazards, resulting in physical accidents, injuries, various mental health issues, and death (Arcury and Quandt 2009; Smith-Appelson et al. 2021; Riester et al. 2019; Keeney et al. 2022).

In the United States, farmworkers are typically classified as either migrant or seasonal. Migrant farmworkers travel from place to place, staying in temporary housing, while seasonal workers live in one community year-round and work on the same farm the following year. The seasonal and temporary nature of their work creates many challenges such as limited access to healthcare, inadequate housing, and language barriers. Overall, the intersection of economic, social, and occupational factors makes farmworkers particularly susceptible to exploitation and hardship, emphasizing the need for comprehensive support systems and policy measures to address their unique challenges (Arcury and Quandt 2009).

Hispanic and Latino workers represent a significant percentage of the agricultural labor force in the United States. Unfortunately, this demographic workgroup continues to disproportionately experience high fatal and nonfatal work-related injuries across many occupations (Riester et al. 2019). According to Bureau of Labor Statistics (BLS), from 2012 to 2021, a total of 1542 fatal injuries were reported among agricultural workers, with Hispanic and Latino workers accounting for almost half of those deaths.

Occupational injuries and deaths among Hispanic and Latino farmworkers in the United States involve exposure to a range of occupational hazards. Transportation-related incidents, which include tractor overturns, roadway crashes, and motor vehicle incidents occurring off public roadways are among the leading causes of death (BLS 2023). In research studies, Latino farmworkers have the highest heat-related illness mortality rate compared with non-Latinos (Mizelle et al. 2022a, b).

For nonfatal injuries among Hispanic and Latino farmworkers, musculoskeletal disorders are among the most common (Mora et al. 2014), while occupational stress, mental health issues, and impacts from the COVID-19 pandemic have also been cited (Arcury et al. 2018, 2021; Keeney et al. 2022). Traumatic eye injuries among Latino farmworkers occur at rates exceeding those for all US crop production workforce. (Quandt et al. 2013).

Youth

Children who work on farms are exposed to a variety of hazards that can result in injuries and even fatalities (Summers et al. 2018). These dangers include heavy machinery, large livestock, bodies of water, quad bikes, motorbikes, utility vehicles/cars, tractors, and horses (Adams et al. 2021; Pickett et al. 2017, 2018). Unfortunately, these hazards put young people who live and work on farms at high risk for injury, disability, and death (Larson-Bright et al. 2007). What's more, children on farms often engage in risky activities, which only increases their chances of getting hurt (Pickett et al. 2017). Furthermore, farm machinery and vehicles often lack adequate safety features, as well as passive safety devices, which only serve to heighten the risk of injury (Pickett et al. 2012).

In the United States, the Fair Labor Standards Act (FLSA), allows children who are at least 12 years old to work outside of school hours in any non-dangerous job, with parental consent, for 7 days a week, unless there are state-specific regulations (DOL 2016). Usually, 12 is the minimum age for farm work; however, youth under 12 years of age can work on small farms outside of school hours with parental consent, as long as the work is considered safe (DOL 2016). To ensure the safety of young farm workers, it is essential to have tailored interventions, education on their rights, and stringent safety standards.

Women

Women who work in agriculture face unique challenges that can have negative impacts on their health, safety, and overall well-being. Studies have shown that they are at a higher risk of heat-related illnesses, particularly when performing physically demanding tasks in hot weather. This can have adverse effects on pregnancy health and birth outcomes (Flocks et al. 2013). Exposure to pesticides, herbicides, and other agrochemicals is another significant health issue among women in agricultural settings. Research suggests that prolonged exposure to these chemicals can lead to various adverse health outcomes, including respiratory problems, dermatological issues, and reproductive health concerns (Flocks et al. 2011). While study limitations exist, the available evidence highlights the need for continued research on the specific risks faced by women in agriculture due to pesticide exposure. Improving study designs, considering multiple factors influencing exposure and health outcomes, and incorporating longitudinal approaches can improve the reliability of findings.

In addition to chemical exposure, women in agriculture also face hazards related to musculoskeletal health due to the physically demanding nature of farm work. Ergonomic hazards such as manual handling, awkward postures, and repetitive movements can lead to musculoskeletal disorders, repetitive strain injuries, and back pain among female agricultural workers (Hathorn et al. 2009). Furthermore, sociocultural factors can make them more vulnerable, especially for migrant and seasonal female workers who may face language barriers, limited access to healthcare, and difficult living conditions (Habib and Fathallah 2012). Addressing these concerns requires targeted interventions, including adequate training, access to protective equipment, health education, and policies that prioritize the unique needs and risks faced by women in the agricultural workforce.

Older Workers

Older workers working in agriculture are often considered a vulnerable population due to a combination of age-related challenges and the demanding nature of farm work. The physical demands of farming, such as lifting, bending, and prolonged exposure to harsh environmental conditions, can pose significant health risks for older workers (Heaton et al. 2012). Age-related health issues, including joint problems and reduced stamina, may further compromise their ability to perform strenuous tasks, increasing the likelihood of injuries (Marcum et al. 2011; Heaton et al. 2012). The risk of suicide is higher among older farmers compared to the general population and other occupations, with aggregated age-specific male farmer suicide rates being the highest among farmers aged 65 years and older (Scheyett et al. 2019; Kennedy et al. 2021). Other factors including limited access to healthcare and inadequate safety measures on farms exacerbate the vulnerability of older workers. These findings emphasize the need for targeted interventions and support systems to address the unique occupational health challenges faced by older farmers.

Occupational Health Hazards in Farming

The diverse nature of farming presents a multitude of work hazards that pose significant risks to health and safety that extend beyond the obvious daily dangers posed by machinery and equipment. Although there are variations of names and definitions of these hazards, they can generally be categorized into groups as either chemical and dust hazards, physical hazards, psychosocial or work organization hazards, ergonomic hazards, safety hazards, and biological risk hazards. A diagram illustrating these types of occupational hazards and descriptions of health risks are described later (Fig. 23.2).

Chemical and dust hazards (and the main focus of this book) pose risks including respiratory issues, skin irritation, and systemic toxicity due to exposure to agricultural chemicals and dust particles. Physical hazards, including machinery-related injuries and falls, can result in fractures, cuts, lacerations, and amputations. Psychosocial hazards arise from factors such as long working hours and social isolation, leading to stress and potential mental health issues. Ergonomic hazards, characterized by poor ergonomic conditions, repetitive motions, and awkward position, can lead to musculoskeletal disorders including back and joint pain, and carpal tunnel syndrome. Safety

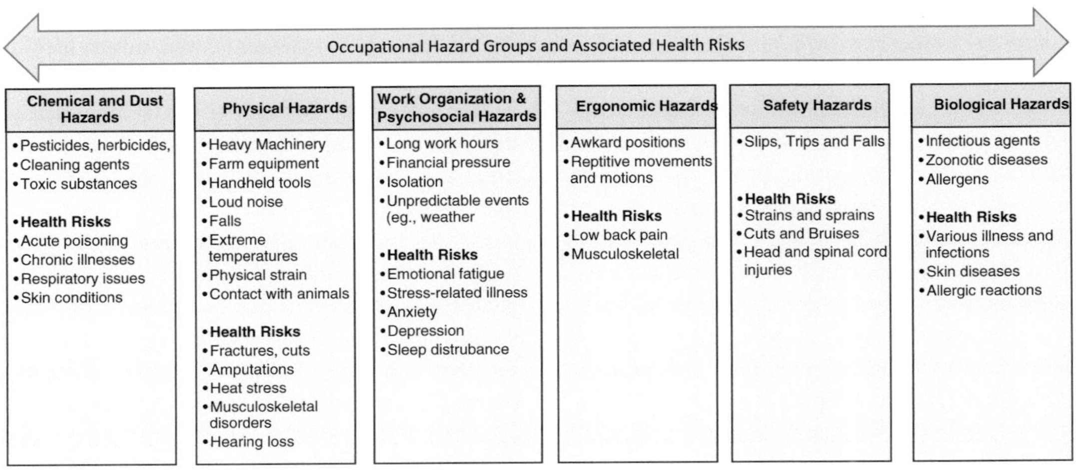

Fig. 23.2 Common occupational hazards and health risks associated with farming. (Source: USDA, Economic Research Service analysis of data from US Department of Commerce, Bureau of the Census, American Community Survey, 2021)

hazards on farms encompass a wide range, from machinery accidents to electrical shocks, leading to injuries that range from minor cuts to severe, life-threatening incidents. Biological risk hazards arise from exposure to animals and their waste, posing the risk of contracting infections and diseases such as Q fever and avian influenza.

Farming Injuries, Illnesses, and Fatalities in the United States

The agricultural sector continues to experience a disproportionately higher rate of occupational injuries and work-related fatalities compared to other industries, despite efforts in safety training and improvements (Donham and Thelin 2016; NIOSH 2023, 2024). In 2022, the Bureau of Labor Statistics (BLS) reported that agriculture (farming along with fishing and forestry) occupations had the highest fatality rate among all US occupational groups, reporting 23.5 fatalities per 100,000 full-time workers (FTEs), in contrast to 3.7 per 100,000 FTEs for all other occupations (BLS 2022).

The most commonly reported causes of fatal injuries associated with farming are primarily related to machinery and equipment, with tractor overturns being a significant contributor (Myers et al. 2008; Pickett et al. 2012). Other fatal incidents associated with work hazards on the farm include manure-handling systems, livestock handling, falls, and quad-bike operations. These also contribute to increased worker injuries on modern farms (Gorucu et al. 2022; Pate and Gorucu 2020). Heat stroke has increasingly been identified as a leading cause of nonfatal injuries among agricultural workers, underscoring the occupational risks associated with environmental conditions and physical exertion (Jackson and Rosenberg 2010). Exposure to agrochemicals during various farming activities has also been highlighted as a significant risk factor for nonfatal injuries, emphasizing the need for proper safety measures and protective equipment (Francis et al. 2014).

Nonfatal work-related incidents, including cuts, lacerations injuries, and musculoskeletal disorders, illustrate the diverse range of nonfatal injuries prevalent in the agricultural sector (Asamani 2022). A comprehensive study analyzing agricultural-related injuries between 2015 and 2019 found that over 62,000 individuals sought medical care in emergency departments. Common nonfatal injuries involved fractures, open wounds, and amputations. Vehicle incidents, particularly tractor accidents, were among common sources of injuries (Weichelt et al. 2021).

Human Health Impacts of Pesticides

Pesticides have played a prominent role in agricultural practices throughout history, dating back approximately 4500 years to ancient Mesopotamia when the Sumerians utilized sulfur compounds for pest control (Umetsu and Shirai 2020). The era of World War II witnessed a rapid evolution in pest control with the development of synthetic chemicals like DDT, BHC, and Aldrin, marking a transformative period. DDT, renowned for its efficacy against diseases such as malaria and typhus, initially demonstrated broad-spectrum pest control but raised concerns about housefly resistance and adverse ecological impacts (Unsworth 2010). By the year 2000, global pesticide production had surged, exceeding five million tons annually, yet only a fraction effectively targeted intended pests, resulting in widespread contamination of non-target environments (Tudi et al. 2021). The persistence of pesticide residues in ecosystems continues to pose substantial threats to both environmental and human health.

The harmfulness of pesticides to farmers and workers can vary depending on factors such as the specific chemical composition, concentration, application methods, and personal protective measures. However, some classes of pesticides are generally associated with higher risks to human health. In general, organophosphates and carbamates, which are types of insecticides, are often considered more hazardous to farmers and workers due to their neurotoxic effects. These pesticides can affect the nervous system and may lead to acute poisoning in cases of exposure. Additionally, fumigants, which are pesticides designed to gas or vaporize to control pests, can pose significant risks if not handled properly. Fumigants are known for their high toxicity, and inhalation or skin contact can result in severe health effects.

It is important to understand that the risks associated with pesticide exposure depend on various factors. The proper use of personal protective equipment and adherence to safety guidelines are crucial in minimizing potential harm. Farmers and workers should receive adequate training on the safe handling and application of pesticides to reduce these risks. Furthermore, mounting evidence suggests that pesticide exposure can have detrimental effects on the immune system. Although the impact of altered cytokine levels on chronic diseases remains uncertain, studies indicate that pesticide exposure can influence immune function. The severity of immune disorders is contingent upon the dose and duration of exposure (Gangemi et al. 2016).

Limitations in Research

Research involving pesticide exposure and related health impacts remains of critical importance. However, there are various epidemiological limitations and challenges including study design, methodology, and documenting exposure effects. Many studies grapple with limitations, including insufficient data on exposure levels, variations in pesticide administration methods, challenges in assigning significance to subtle observed changes, and difficulties in interpreting results. The primary challenge lies not only in understanding the effects of individual pesticides and their combinations but also in discerning the manner and duration of exposure. Untangling the toxic effects on the immune system necessitates consideration of these factors in tandem (Nesheim et al. 2020).

Monitoring Agricultural Workers for Pesticide Exposure

The Worker Protection Standard (WPS) was established by the US EPA in 1992 to protect agricultural workers from potential pesticide exposure in farms, forests, nurseries, and greenhouses. The WPS sets guidelines for how pesticides should be handled, applied, and disposed of in agricultural settings, aiming to safeguard the health of workers and their families. The standard has been updated over time to enhance protections and align with new scientific findings and safety practices. In 2015, the WPS update emphasized actively reducing pesticide exposure cases among farmworkers and their families. The update aimed to ensure a healthier workforce and fewer economic setbacks from lost wages, medical expenses, and work or school absences (EPA 2024).

Prevention Strategies

The hierarchy of hazard control is a methodical approach to managing workplace risks and minimizing workers' exposure to hazards. This system is widely accepted by the industry and is considered a standard for workplace safety. The hazard controls prioritize measures that consist of five levels: elimination, substitution, engineering controls, administrative controls, and personal protective equipment. In the context of agricultural farming, this hierarchy can be effectively employed to manage various risks to enhance overall safety and productivity for workers (Fig. 23.3).

The hierarchy of hazard control measures prioritizes eliminating hazards at the top of the list, followed by substitution, engineering controls, administrative controls, and personal protective equipment as a last resort. Eliminating hazards could mean removing toxic chemicals and using organic farming methods. Substitution involves replacing hazardous materials with safer alternatives. Engineering controls isolate people from hazards, while administrative controls change the way people work. Personal protective equipment is the final line of defense.

Implementing these measures involves assessing risks and adopting appropriate measures at each level. This could mean safer machinery, proper training on chemical handling, ventilation systems, and protective gear. By following this

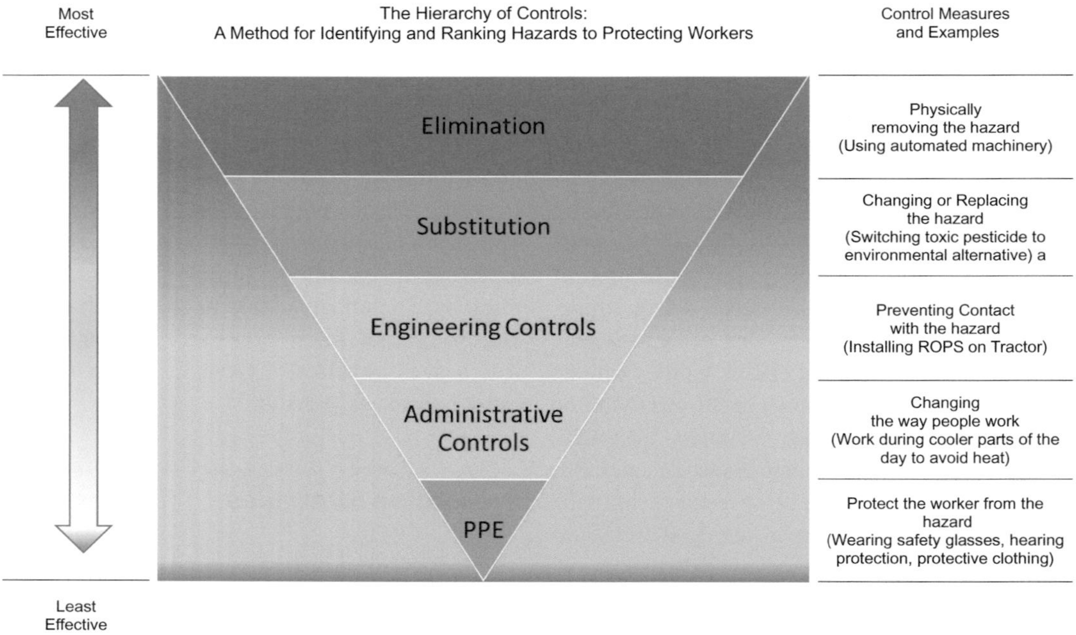

Fig. 23.3 The hierarchy of hazard controls and ranking of effectiveness for protecting workers on the farm. (Source: Adapted from the National Institute of Occupational Safety and Health (NIOSH))

hierarchy, farmers can reduce risks and create a safer environment for themselves and others. This approach aligns with the growing demand for sustainable and environmentally friendly agricultural practices while ensuring the well-being of all involved.

Occupational Health Surveillance and Data Sources

Each year, thousands of workers are killed, and millions are injured or become ill on the job because of health hazards in their workplace (NASS 2017). Identifying how these problems occurred and preventing them from happening again is the primary aim of health surveillance.

Public health surveillance is defined as the "ongoing, systematic collection, analysis, and interpretation of health-related data essential to planning, implementation, and evaluation of public health practice" (Thacker and Birkhead 2008). The information derived from surveillance data plays a vital role in occupational health by identifying trends, risk factors, and emerging health concerns related to farming-related injuries, accidents, and fatalities. As illustrated below, there the three general approaches used to monitor population health issues, including (1) active surveillance, (2) passive surveillance, and (3) sentinel surveillance.

Active Surveillance Systems

As the name implies, "active" surveillance involves the proactive approach of collecting health data to monitor a health outcome or issue. Active surveillance is resource-intensive and involves healthcare workers reporting. One of the primary characteristics of active surveillance is the collection of data through systematic outreach. Examples include interviews, or health assessments among specific groups of workers. This method ensures more comprehensive and detailed information on health events, offering a clearer picture of trends and risks.

- *Agricultural Health Study (AHS)*: The AHS was launched in 1993 as a research project to gain insights into how genetic, and lifestyle factors affect the health of farming populations (National Cancer Institute 2024). With nearly 90,000 participants, the prospective study includes licensed pesticide applicators and their spouses in Iowa and North Carolina. The AHS is led by the National Cancer Institute, the National Institute of Environmental Health Sciences, and the US Environmental Protection Agency.
- *Occupational Safety and Health Administration (OSHA) Inspections*: Proactive inspections identifying and mitigating safety hazards in agricultural settings. (Some state Departments of Labor sections also do proactive surveillance such as the migrant housing program in North Carolina)
- *Farm Injury Surveillance Systems*: Established in specific regions or states, collecting data from healthcare facilities regarding farm-related injuries.

Passive Surveillance Systems

Passive surveillance relies on the voluntary reporting of health events by healthcare providers or workers themselves. While it offers a less resource-intensive approach, it might lead to underreporting and incomplete data. Examples of passive surveillance systems include:

- *NIOSH (National Institute for Occupational Safety and Health) FACE Program and Bureau of Labor Statistics (BLS), Census of Fatal Occupational Injuries (CFOI)*: Passive collection of data on fatal occupational injuries in agriculture from various sources.
- *State-Based Health Departments and State Departments of Agriculture*: Passive systems gathering information on agricultural injuries and fatalities and pesticide poisonings from on-site investigations, hospital records, death certificates, etc.
- *National Ag Safety Database (NASD) and National Agricultural Workers Survey (NAWS)*: Repositories and surveys offering insights into agricultural safety and worker health.

Sentinel Surveillance

Sentinel systems focus on selected sites or specific groups, aiming to monitor particular conditions or diseases. This targeted approach provides in-depth insights into specific health issues prevalent within a defined population or location. Examples include the following.

- *Occupational Health Clinics for Agriculture (OHCA)*: Monitoring injuries and illnesses specific to agricultural workers.
- *NIOSH and the Sentinel Event Notification System for Occupational Risks (SENSOR) Pesticide Surveillance Program*: State-based occupational reporting of acute pesticide exposures to monitor outbreaks and emerging pesticide-related issues.
- *Other Collaborative Efforts*: Regional or national collaborations pooling data from multiple sources to comprehensively monitor agricultural injuries and fatalities (Fig. 23.4).

Each surveillance method has its strengths and limitations, making a combination of these approaches beneficial for comprehensive occupational health monitoring and timely intervention.

Data Sources

The data generated by surveillance systems often serve as the basis for generating information crucial for developing focused interventions, policies, and safety measures aimed at mitigating risks and enhancing the well-being of farmers and agricultural workers (Patel et al. 2017; Weichelt et al. 2021). While there is not an official comprehensive dataset covering all agricultural injuries and fatalities, leveraging a variety of data sources can help address specific information gaps. Listed below are a few highly recognized data sources that either collect, analyze, or monitor data for

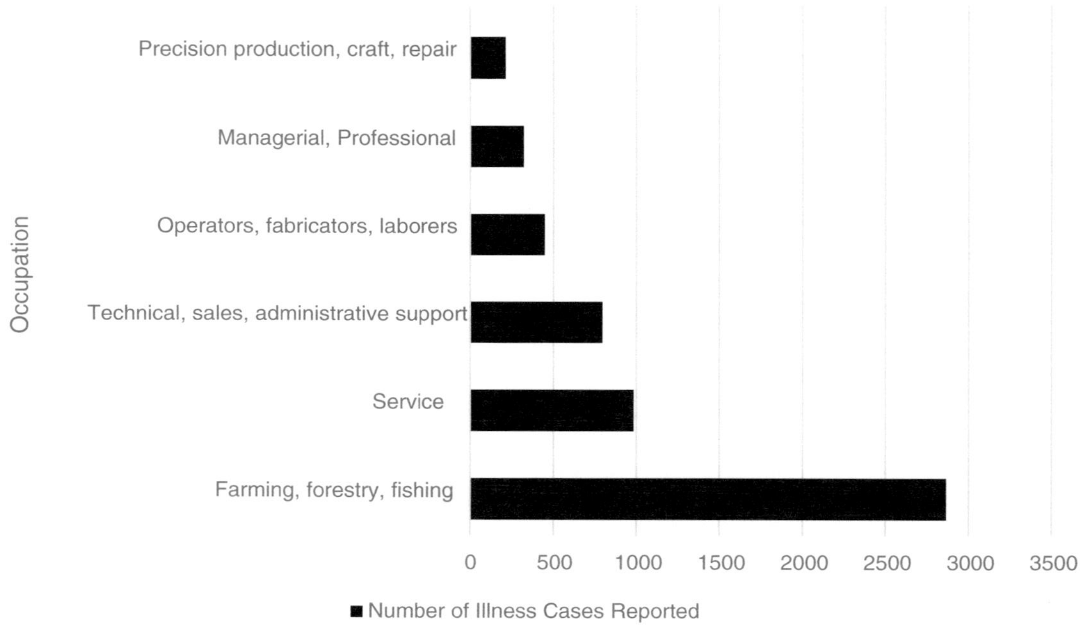

Fig. 23.4 Number of acute pesticide-related illnesses by occupation among states participating in the Sentinel Event Notification System for Occupational Risk (SENSOR) Program (1998–2011). (Source: NIOSH, SENSOR Pesticide Database (Nov 2020). Available at https://www.cdc.gov/niosh/topics/pesticides/overview.html)

accidents, injuries, and fatalities in agricultural workplaces in the United States.

Governmental Data Sources

- **Bureau of Labor Statistics (BLS)**:
  Provides reports and data via programs like the Census of Fatal Occupational Injuries (CFOI) and the Survey of Occupational Injuries and Illnesses (SOII), offering comprehensive insights into work-related incidents among agricultural workers.
- **National Institute for Occupational Safety and Health (NIOSH)**:
  Offers research and reports on agricultural safety and health, including specialized programs like the Agricultural Health and Safety Network (AgriSafe) and the Fatality Assessment and Control Evaluation (FACE) Program.
- **Occupational Safety and Health Administration (OSHA)**:
  Furnishes information on agricultural safety regulations, statistics, and resources pertinent to workplace safety, aiding in understanding and preventing farm-related injuries.
- **Agricultural Resource Management Survey (ARMS)**:
  Jointly sponsored by ERS and USDA, the National Agricultural Statistics Service (NASS), provides valuable insights into the management aspects of agriculture, which may encompass data on labor-related incidents.
- **Farm Labor Survey (USDA)**:
  Conducted by the USDA, offering specific information on labor within the agricultural sector, potentially including data on injuries and illnesses among farmworkers.
- **Census of Agriculture (USDA)**:
  Conducted every 5 years, offering a comprehensive overview of every farm in the country, providing detailed data on various aspects of agricultural operations, potentially including occupational incidents.

Nongovernmental Data Sources

- **National Farm Medicine Center**:
  Conducts research and provides reports specifically focusing on-farm injuries, fatalities, and illnesses, contributing significant insights into agricultural health and safety.
- **National Safety Council (NSC)**:
  Offers resources related to agricultural safety and may provide valuable data on injuries and fatalities in the agricultural sector through specialized reports.
- **Agricultural Safety and Health Council of America (ASHCA)**:
  Provides resources, conducts research, and generates reports dedicated to agricultural safety and health, potentially offering valuable data on incidents within the sector.

Academic Institutions and Universities

- **University Agricultural Safety & Health Centers (many partially supported by NIOSH funding)**:
  Institutions such as the Great Plains Center for Agricultural Health and the Upper Midwest Agricultural Safety and Health Center conduct extensive research and provide data on agricultural injuries, illnesses, and fatalities.
- **Scholarly Articles and Journals**:
  Academic publications in fields such as occupational health, public health, and agricultural science present studies and statistics on agricultural worker injuries and health outcomes, contributing to a comprehensive understanding of the sector's health and safety dynamics.

Surveys such as the Census of Agriculture, and Farm Labor Survey offer specific labor-related data, including incidents, aiding in comprehensive analysis. Non-governmental entities like the National Farm Medicine Center, National Safety Council, and Agricultural Safety and Health Council of America provide specialized research and reports dedicated to agricultural safety, enriching the pool of available data. Additionally, academic institutions and scholarly publications contribute significantly to occupational health knowledge through research, studies, and articles focusing on agricultural worker injuries and health outcomes, enhancing the depth of information available for surveillance and interventions.

Summary

Despite the many technological advancements, the agricultural sector continues to have the highest rates of fatal and nonfatal injuries in the United States, making it crucial to adopt a comprehensive approach to ensuring the safety of farmers and farmworkers. Understanding prevalent workplace hazards such as pesticide exposure, machinery risks, zoonotic infections, and musculoskeletal strain is pivotal. Implementing tailored interventions, including protective gear, training, and safety protocols, can significantly reduce health risks. Regulatory frameworks can enforce standards and foster a safety culture. Proactive measures, such as mental health initiatives, can also contribute to a safer work environment, safeguarding workers' health and ensuring the sustainability of the sector. Acknowledging pesticide exposures, addressing vulnerable workgroups, and implementing prevention strategies are integral components of this comprehensive approach.

References

Adams J, Kennedy A, Cotton J, Brumby S. Child farm-related injury in Australia: a review of the literature. Int J Environ Res Public Health. 2021;18(11):6063. https://doi.org/10.3390/ijerph18116063.

Arcury TA, Quandt SA. Latino farmworkers in the eastern United States: health, safety and justice; 2009. p. 1–14. https://doi.org/10.1007/978-0-387-88347-2.

Arcury T, Sandberg J, Talton J, Laurienti P, Daniel S, Quandt S. Mental health among Latina farmworkers and other employed Latinas in North Carolina. Rural Ment Health. 2018;42(2):89–101. https://doi.org/10.1037/rmh0000091.

Arcury T, Smith S, Talton J, Chen H, Laurienti P, Quandt S. Depressive symptoms of Latinx women in rural farmworker and urban non-farmworker families in North Carolina. J Racial Ethn Health Disparities. 2021;9(6):2351–60. https://doi.org/10.1007/s40615-021-01172-8.

Asamani L. Work-related health and safety challenges of rice irrigation farmworkers. Eur J Bus Manag Res. 2022;7(1):292–9. https://doi.org/10.24018/ejbmr.2022.7.1.1296.

BLS. Labor force statistics. Washington, DC: U.S. Bureau of Labor Statistics; 2022. https://www.bls.gov/cps/cpsaat15.htm. Accessed 19 Jan 2024.

BLS. Fatal Injuries to Agricultural Workers in 2021 were the second lowest in a decade. Washington, DC: U.S. Bureau of Labor Statistics; 2023. https://www.bls.gov/opub/ted/2023/fatal-injuries-to-agricultural-workers-in-2021-were-the-second-lowest-in-a-decade.htm. Accessed 21 Dec 2023.

Costa D. How many farmworkers are employed in the United States? Economic Policy Institute; 2023. https://www.epi.org/blog/how-many-farmworkers-are-employed-in-the-united-states/. Accessed 12 Jan 2024.

Department of Labor (DOL). Wage and Hour Division. 29 CFR Part 553. 2016. https://www.ecfr.gov/current/title-29/part-553. Accessed 12 Jan 2024.

Department of Labor (DOL). H-2A: temporary agricultural employment of foreign workers. 2022. https://www.dol.gov/agencies/whd/agriculture/h2a. Accessed 12 Jan 2024.

Donham KJ, Thelin A. Agricultural medicine: rural occupational and environmental health, safety, and prevention. London: Wiley; 2016.

Economic Research Service, USDA. Ag and Food Sectors and the Economy. 2022. https://www.ers.usda.gov/topics/farm-economy/farm-labor/. Accessed 20 Jan 2024.

Economic Research Service, USDA. Ag and Food Sectors and the Economy. Farm Labor. 2023. https://www.ers.usda.gov/topics/farm-economy/farm-labor/. Accessed 20 Jan 2024.

EPA Worker Protection Standard. U.S. Environmental Protection Agency. 2024. https://www.epa.gov/compliance/worker-protection-standard-compliance-monitoring-program. Accessed 12 Jan 2024.

Flocks J, Kelley M, Economos J, McCauley L. Female farmworkers' perceptions of pesticide exposure and pregnancy health. J Immigr Minor Health. 2011;14(4):626–32. https://doi.org/10.1007/s10903-011-9554-6.

Flocks J, Mac V, Runkle J, Tovar-Aguilar J, Economos J, McCauley L. Female farmworkers' perceptions of heat-related illness and pregnancy health. J Agromedicine. 2013;18(4):350–8. https://doi.org/10.1080/1059924x.2013.826607.

Francis MR, Raja L, Inbarani E, Regi H, Nicolas J, Nitin P, et al. Perceptions of farmers' and farmworkers' wives on the use and hazards of agrochemicals in rural Vellore. New Solut. 2014;23(4):625–42. https://doi.org/10.2190/ns.23.4.f.

Gangemi S, Gofita E, Costa C, Teodoro M, Briguglio G, Nikitovic D, et al. Occupational and environmental exposure to pesticides and cytokine pathways in chronic diseases (review). Int J Mol Med. 2016;38:1012–20. https://doi.org/10.3892/ijmm.2016.2728.

Gorucu S, Michael J, Chege K. Nonfatal agricultural injuries treated in emergency departments: 2015–2019. J Agromedicine. 2022;27(1):41–50. https://doi.org/10.1080/1059924X.2021.1913271.

Habib RR, Fathallah FA. Migrant women farm workers in the occupational health literature. Work. 2012;41:4356–62. https://doi.org/10.3233/wor-2012-0101-4356.

Hathorn D, Carruth A, Agosta L, Pryor S. Self-reported back pain among farm women in Southeast Louisiana. AAOHN J. 2009;57(6):232–8. https://doi.org/10.1177/216507990905700606.

Heaton K, Azuero A, Phillips JA, Pickens H, Reed D. The effects of arthritis, mobility, and farm task on injury among older farmers. Nursing (Auckl). 2012;2:9–16. https://doi.org/10.2147/nrr.s28122.

Jackson LL, Rosenberg HR. Preventing heat-related illness among agricultural workers. J Agromedicine. 2010;15(3):200–15. https://doi.org/10.1080/1059924x.2010.487021.

Keeney A, Quandt A, Villaseñor M, Flores D, Flores L. Occupational stressors and access to COVID-19 resources among commuting and residential Hispanic/Latino farmworkers in a US-Mexico border region. Int J Environ Res Public Health. 2022;19(2):763. https://doi.org/10.3390/ijerph19020763.

Kennedy A, Cerel J, Kheibari A, Leske S, Watts J. A comparison of farming- and non-farming-related suicides from the United States' national violent deaths reporting system, 2003–2016. Suicide Life Threat Behav. 2021;51(3):504–14. https://doi.org/10.1111/sltb.12725.

Larson-Bright M, Gerberich S, Alexander B, Gurney J, Masten A, Ryan A, et al. Work practices and childhood agricultural injury. Inj Prev. 2007;13(6):409–15. https://doi.org/10.1136/ip.2006.014233.

MacDonald JM, Hoppe RA, Newton D. Three Decades of Consolidation in U.S. Agriculture, EIB-189. Washington, DC: U.S. Department of Agriculture, Economic Research Service; 2018.

Magnus O. Historia om de Nordiska folken. Roma MDLV (Reprint Gidlunds Förlag, Stockholm, 1982). 1555.

Marcum JL, Browning SR, Reed DB, Charnigo RJ. Farmwork-related injury among farmers 50 years of age and older in Kentucky and South Carolina: a cohort study, 2002–2005. J Agric Saf Health. 2011;17:259–73. https://doi.org/10.13031/2013.38186.

Mizelle E, Larson K, Doherty C. Understanding farmworker fluid intake using intersectionality theory. New Solut. 2022a;32(1):19–29. https://doi.org/10.1177/10482911221078964.

Mizelle E, Larson K, Bolin L, Kearney G. Fluid intake and hydration status among North Carolina farmworkers: a mixed methods study. Workplace Health Saf. 2022b;70(12):532–41. https://doi.org/10.1177/21650799221117273.

Mora D, Miles C, Chen H, Quandt S, Summers P, Arcury T. Prevalence of musculoskeletal disorders among immigrant Latino farmworkers and non-farmworkers in North Carolina. Arch Environ Occup Health. 2014;71(3):136–43. https://doi.org/10.1080/19338244.2014.988676.

Myers J, Layne L, Marsh S. Injuries and fatalities to U.S. farmers and farm workers 55 years and older. Am J Ind Med. 2008;52(3):185–94. https://doi.org/10.1002/ajim.20661.

National Cancer Institute. Agricultural Health Study. Bethesda, MD: National Cancer Institute, Division of Cancer Epidemiology and Genetics; 2024. https://dceg.cancer.gov/research/who-we-study/cohorts/agricultural-health-study#:~:text=Since%20it%20began%20in%201993,information%20on%20non%2Dcancer%20health. Accessed 20 Jan 2024.

National Institute of Food and Agriculture, USDA. Family farms. 2017. https://www.nifa.usda.gov/grants/programs/family-small-farm-program/family-farms. Accessed 20 Dec 2023.

Nesheim ON, Fishel FM, Mossler M. Toxicity of Pesticides. PI-13. Gainesville, FL: University of Florida (UF), Institute of Food and Agricultural Sciences (IFAS) extension; 2020. https://edis.ifas.ufl.edu/publication/PI008.

NIOSH. Agricultural safety. Centers for Disease Control and Prevention, National Institute for Occupational Safety and Health. 2023. https://www.cdc.gov/niosh/topics/aginjury/default.html Accessed 11 Nov 2023.

NIOSH. National Farm Safety and Health Week. Centers for Disease Control and Prevention. 2024. https://www.cdc.gov/niosh/newsroom/feature/national-farm-safety-and-health.html#:~:text=Data%20from%20the%20U.S.%20Bureau,19.5%20deaths%20per%20100%2C000%20workers. Accessed 20 Jan 2024.

Pate M, Gorucu S. Agricultural work-related fatalities to non-working youth: implications for intervention development. J Agric Saf Health. 2020;26(1):31–43. https://doi.org/10.13031/jash.13691.

Patel K, Watanabe-Galloway S, Gofin R, Haynatzki G, Rautiainen R. Non-fatal agricultural injury surveillance in the United States: a review of national-level survey-based systems. Am J Ind Med. 2017;60(7):599–620. https://doi.org/10.1002/ajim.22720.

Pickett W, Hagel L, Dosman J. Safety features on agricultural machines and farm structures in Saskatchewan. J Agromedicine. 2012;17(4):421–4. https://doi.org/10.1080/1059924x.2012.713836.

Pickett W, Berg R, Marlenga B. Social environments, risk-taking and injury in farm adolescents. Inj Prev. 2017;23(6):388–98. https://doi.org/10.1136/injuryprev-2016-042075.

Pickett W, King N, Marlenga B, Lawson J, Hagel L, Elliot V, et al. Exposure to agricultural hazards among children who visit farms. Paediatr Child Health. 2018;23(7):e143–9. https://doi.org/10.1093/pch/pxy015.

Quandt S, Kucera K, Haynes C, Klein B, Langley R, Agnew M, et al. Occupational health outcomes for workers in the agriculture, forestry and fishing sector: implications for immigrant workers in the southeastern US. Am J Ind Med. 2013;56(8):940–59. https://doi.org/10.1002/ajim.22170.

Ramazzini B. De morbis artificum Berardini Ramazzini diatriba [diseases of workers]. In: The Latin text of 1713 revised with translation and notes by Wilmer cave Wright. Chicago, IL: The University of Chicago Press; 1940.

Riester S, Leniek K, Niece A, Montoya-Barthelemy A, Wilson W, Sellman J, et al. Occupational medicine clinical practice data reveal increased injury rates among hispanic workers. Am J Ind Med. 2019;62(4):309–16. https://doi.org/10.1002/ajim.22949.

Scheyett A, Bayakly R, Whitaker M. Characteristics and contextual stressors in farmer and agricultural worker suicides in Georgia from 2008–2015. Rural Ment Health. 2019;43(2–3):61–72. https://doi.org/10.1037/rmh0000114.

Smith-Appelson J, Reynolds J, Grzywacz J. Assessing the extreme loneliness of immigrant farmworkers. Sociol Inq. 2021;91(3):696–717. https://doi.org/10.1111/soin.12428.

Summers P, Quandt S, Johnson C, Arcury T. Child work safety on the farms of local agricultural market producers: parent and child perspectives. J Agromedicine. 2018;23(1):52–9. https://doi.org/10.1080/1059924x.2017.1387635.

Thacker SB, Birkhead GS. Surveillance. In: Gregg MB, editor. Field epidemiology. Oxford: Oxford University Press; 2008.

Tudi M, Daniel Ruan H, Wang L, Lyu J, Sadler R, Connell D, Chu C, Phung DT. Agriculture development, pesticide application and its impact on the environment. Int J Environ Res Public Health. 2021;18(3):1112.

Umetsu N, Shirai Y. Development of novel pesticides in the 21st century. J Pestic Sci. 2020;45(2):54–74. PMID: 33132734; PMCID: PMC7581488. https://doi.org/10.1584/jpestics.D20-201.

United States Census Bureau. American community survey. American community survey 1-year estimates, Table GCT0101. Using American FactFinder. 2021. Accessed 7 Jan 2012.

United States Department of Agriculture, National Agricultural Statistics Service. 2017 Census of Agriculture. 2017. https://www.nass.usda.gov/AgCensus/. Accessed 20 Dec 2023.

Unsworth J. International Union of Pure and Applied Chemistry (IUPAC). History of pesticide use. 2010. https://agrochemicals.iupac.org/index. Accessed 11 Nov 2023.

Weichelt B, Scott E, Burke R, Shutske J, Gorucu S, Sanderson W, et al. What about the rest of them? Fatal injuries related to production agriculture not captured by the Bureau of Labor Statistics (BLS) census of fatal occupational injuries (CFOI). J Agromedicine. 2021;27(1):35–40. https://doi.org/10.1080/1059924x.2021.1956663.

Index

W. J. Meggs, R. L. Langley (eds.), *Farm Toxicology*, https://doi.org/10.1007/978-3-031-80441-0

P

MIX
Papier aus verantwortungsvollen Quellen
Paper from responsible sources
FSC® C105338

If you have any concerns about our products,
you can contact us on
ProductSafety@springernature.com

In case Publisher is established outside the EU,
the EU authorized representative is:
Springer Nature Customer Service Center GmbH
Europaplatz 3, 69115 Heidelberg, Germany

Printed by Libri Plureos GmbH
in Hamburg, Germany